Pediatric Urology for the Adult Urologist

Hsi-Yang Wu • Sutchin R. Patel
Anthony A. Caldamone
Editors

Pediatric Urology for the Adult Urologist

Springer

Editors
Hsi-Yang Wu
Surgery, Division of Urology
Alpert Medical School of Brown University
Providence, RI, USA

Anthony A. Caldamone
Surgery, Division of Urology
Alpert Medical School of Brown University
Providence, RI, USA

Sutchin R. Patel
Department of Urology
University of Wisconsin
School of Medicine and Public Health
Madison, WI, USA

ISBN 978-3-032-10305-5 ISBN 978-3-032-10306-2 (eBook)
https://doi.org/10.1007/978-3-032-10306-2

This Springer imprint is published by the registered company Springer Nature Switzerland AG
The registered company address is: Gewerbestrasse 11, 6330 Cham, Switzerland

Preface

For the first part of my career, I worked in a pediatric hospital setting where all of my patients were children, and my main interactions were with other pediatric specialists. After moving to Brown, I re-entered the adult urology call schedule to cover adult and pediatric weekend call two times per year, while my adult colleagues took pediatric call on the other weekends. There is definitely a selection bias in that adults who continue to have problems related to their pediatric condition are the ones who are having surgery or presenting to the Emergency Department, but sometimes they are having kidney stones or erectile dysfunction related to their pediatric condition.

The first half of this book covers common management questions for the initial evaluation of pediatric referrals. The children with more complex conditions will most likely have had a prenatal consultation with pediatric urology to establish postnatal care, so these conditions will not be covered. The second half of the book covers the long-term outcomes and expected complications of pediatric conditions that continue to require regular follow-up with an adult urologist. While this is not purely a Transitional Urology textbook, there are principles for transitioning care from pediatric to adult providers which can help the patient and family feel comfortable with their new team.

The difference between pediatric and adult urology is mainly a cultural gap in how we approach patients. This requires us to navigate the changes in the same condition over time as well as tailoring our discussions with parents and patients differently, as the children grow up and take over their own care. When I worked in California, I would often attend the California Bladder Exstrophy Support Team campout at Lake Tahoe during the summer. This is a great opportunity for children with bladder exstrophy to meet other children with the same condition, and to share their experiences about surgery, catheterization, and how to deal with physician practices and hospitals. As the children became older, the discussion would evolve from continence procedures to kidney stones, then sexual function and pregnancy, and then the possibility of approaching chronic kidney disease or bladder cancer. Their parents would share their experiences about finding new adult physicians for their children, and the hurdles that they had to overcome. I have been fortunate to have colleagues who will see my adult men with hypospadias (reconstructive urologists) and adult spina bifida and exstrophy patients (female pelvic medicine reconstructive surgeons or reconstructive urologists), and I have worked closely with the kidney transplant team to prepare patients with posterior urethral valves or neurogenic bladder for transplantation. Having a "warm hand-off" to the adult provider is important since it allows for important information to be passed along and avoid missing key topics and provides the families with a sense of continuity of care [1].

Ideally, the process of transitioning from pediatric to adult urology should start several years before the child will age out of a pediatric hospital, but this can vary based on whether the emerging adult patient is ready to assume their care from their parents [2]. Baseline bladder and renal function are usually what concern the adult provider the most, but understanding the patient's social support and resources (how much do the parents do for them, do they schedule the visits, arrange transportation, help get authorizations from the PCP) is not something that automatically comes to mind when a young adult is seen in clinic. In some ways, a young adult patient can be similar to a geriatric patient, in the amount of assistance needed to arrange a basic clinic visit. Having a transition coordinator or navigator (a nurse or social worker) to help with this process is a consistent recommendation in both the United States and Europe [3, 4]. However, the problem is that the amount of effort required to accomplish medical transition is not sustainable for a single provider to undertake, since it is not usually reimbursed.

Insurance coverage is often a significant problem, since many pediatric urology patients will be on public insurance plans if they have an extensive surgical history. Access to adult specialists can be more difficult to arrange than for pediatric specialists on public insurance plans. Legal guardianship issues should be worked out for those patients who continue to require a parent or guardian to make medical decisions. GotTransition.org has resources designed for both patients and their parents to assist with the transition to adult providers; this is supported by the National Alliance to Advance Adolescent Health.

The perspective from adult providers on pediatric patients entering their clinic is surprising [5]. First, the adult providers were not expecting the degree to which parents expected a specialist to be a primary care physician (PCP), or expected the PCP to provide referrals for issues that are typically handled by PCP's. For the adult spina bifida population in Canada, only 24% had a PCP caring for them [6]. The role of the PCP as a "quarterback" in adult health care needs to be explained. They also felt that patients and families were initially more resistant to making changes to medications, because they had been on the medications for so long with their pediatric provider and there was a long history of trust with the pediatric provider [5].

Second, access to prior medical records can be limited, so the information obtained directly from the patient or parent can be incomplete. If the medical record is available, it is impossible to sift through 20 years' worth of notes, labs, and x-rays. As noted by Gray et al., adult providers often request a 1–2 page short summary of the patient's history, with disease-specific markers, including which medications have worked, and which medications have not [5]. Similar to when a complex patient is transferred to another pediatric provider, the brief summary is extremely important.

Third, even if the patients have insurance, the availability of multidisciplinary clinics, social work, and mental and behavioral health specialists on the adult side is often limited. Sometimes referrals to adult providers are made from the pediatric provider without realizing that the adult provider does not accept the insurance plan that the patient has. This should be worked prior to transitioning the patient [5].

While pediatric urologists would like to believe that we have all of our adult patients in a stable condition by the time they transition to an adult provider, the bladder continues to change over a lifetime. What happens to the young adults who are transitioned to adult care? In a neurogenic bladder population at a mean age of 22 years, 71% (17/24) had a change in plan, including surgery in 58% [7]. This points out the need for continuing management of high-risk patients. Perhaps even more worrisome is what happens to the patients who fail to make a successful transition to an adult provider. The spina bifida clinic at Riley Children's in Indianapolis set up a Transitional Urology clinic across the hall from the Spina Bifida clinic, and asked patients to make an appointment within 1 year. The assumption was that the convenient location and familiarity with the Spina Bifida clinic would make it more likely that patients would successfully transition their care. At 2 years, only 40% of the patients had made an appointment, and no factor (distance to clinic, age, insurance, prior non-compliance) predicted who would successfully make the transition. When they tried to contact the patients who did not make an appointment, they were unable to contact the majority of them [8].

Patients with hypospadias, non-neurogenic urinary incontinence, and kidney stones will usually return to see an adult urologist when they have ongoing symptoms. The patients who are at risk for chronic kidney disease from high grade vesicoureteral reflux, renal dysplasia, or neurogenic bladder may not see an adult urologist if they are feeling fine. Having open lines of communication between pediatric and adult urology is a prerequisite for a successful transition of care. However, young adults in their early 20s have the highest rate of not having health insurance, with a peak of 18% at age 26 years, after they come off their parents' insurance and before they purchase insurance through their work [9]. Having walked my young adult children through the process of selecting health insurance plans and picking a PCP, I can understand how the illusion of immortality in your 20s and the desire to save money from an already paltry paycheck can lead some young adults to go without insurance. As pediatric urologists, we can prepare our patients with a concise folder of relevant information, at least one visit with their adult urologist, and reassurance that while they can still call us with questions, we are fully supportive of what their adult urologist will recommend for them. While the gaps in insurance coverage will continue to be a barrier to good follow-up for adults with a congenital urological condition, hopefully this book can provide a concise plan for the day when a young adult arrives in your office with their parents in tow, accompanied by a thick chart and a long list of medications.

Providence, RI, USA — Hsi-Yang Wu
Madison, WI, USA — Sutchin R. Patel
Providence, RI, USA — Anthony A. Caldamone

References

1. Berkowitz S, Lang P. Transitioning patients with complex health care needs to adult practices: theory versus reality. Pediatrics. 2020;145(6):e20193943.
2. Wood HM, Yerkes EB. The transition process: initial assessment and development of a treatment plan. In: Wood HM, Wood D, editors. Transition and lifelong care in congenital urology. Current clinical urology. Springer; 2015. pp. 3–10.
3. Gray WN, Schaefer MR, Resmini-Rowlinson A, Wagoner ST. Barriers to transition from pediatric to adult care: a systematic review. J Pediatr Psychol. 2018;43(5):388–502.
4. Pape L, Ernst G. Health care transition from pediatric to adult care: an evidence-based guideline. Eur J Pediatr. 2022;181:1951–8.
5. Gray W, Dorriz P, Kim H, Paritain L, Benekos E, et al. Adult provider perspectives on transition and transfer to adult care: a multispecialty, multi-institutional exploration. J Pediatr Nursing. 2021;(59):173–80.
6. Young NL, Anselmo LA, Burke TA, McCormick A, Mukherjee S. Youth and young adults with spina bifida: their utilization of physician and health resources. Arch Phys Med Rehabil. 2014;95:466–71.
7. Chan R, Scovell J, Jeng Z, Rajanahally S, Boone T, et al. The fate of transitional urology patients referred to a tertiary transitional care center. Urology. 2014;84:1544–8.
8. Szymanski KM, Cain MP, Hardacker TJ, Misseri R. How successful is the transition to adult urology care in spina bifida? A single center 7-year experience. J Pediatr Urol. 2017;13:40.e1–40.e6.
9. https://www.census.gov/library/stories/2020/10/uninsured-rates-highest-for-young-adults-aged-19-to-34.html.

Contents

1 The Development of Pediatric Urology as a Subspecialty in the United States and Europe

Sutchin R. Patel and Anthony A. Caldamone

The subspecialty of pediatric urology emerged as it became recognized that children with urologic disorders needed to be treated by those with specialized training. In the past, general urologists, pediatric surgeons, and plastic surgeons took care of many of these children, and it took the persistent work of early pioneers in the field to show that subspecialization provided better care for children with urologic disorders [1]. The purpose of our chapter is to trace the roots of pediatric urology and highlight some of the individuals who played a major role in the development of the field of pediatric urology.

Edwin Beer (1876–1938) was among the first urologists to recognize that pediatric urology was a field that needed to be developed to better care for children with urologic disorders (Fig. 1.1). Beer earned his M.D. from the College of Physician and Surgeons in 1899 and served as an intern at Mt. Sinai Hospital from 1899 to 1902 and then embarked on postgraduate study in Prague, Vienna, and Berlin [2, 3]. In Europe, he was exposed to the developments in endoscopy pioneered by Nitze. In 1910, he would return to practice in New York and would serve as Chief of Urology at Mt. Sinai Hospital. Though Beer is best known for his innovative fulguration of bladder tumors, he made significant contributions to pediatric urology, including developing the first pediatric cystoscope, and, with Abraham Hyman, coauthored the first textbook of pediatric urology, *Diseases of the Urinary Tract in Children* (1930) [2, 4, 5]. Abraham Hyman recalled,

S. R. Patel (✉)
Department of Urology, University of Wisconsin School of Medicine and Public Health, Madison, WI, USA

A. A. Caldamone
Surgery, Division of Urology, Alpert Medical School of Brown University, Providence, RI, USA
e-mail: ACaldamone@brownhealth.org

H.-Y. Wu et al. (eds.), *Pediatric Urology for the Adult Urologist*, https://doi.org/10.1007/978-3-032-10306-2_1

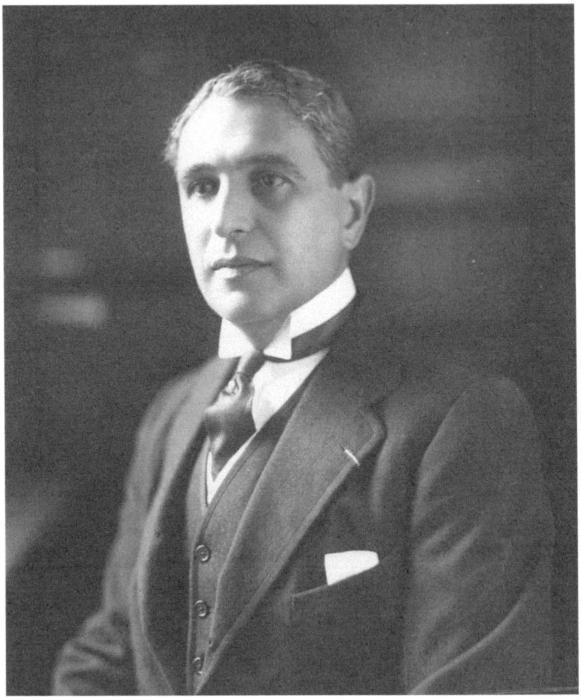

Fig. 1.1 Edwin Beer. (Courtesy of the William P. Didusch Center for Urologic History)

> We decided… to foster the investigation of urology in children… practically a neglected field. Very few children had been examined urologically the way the adults were. They didn't have children's cystoscopes until Dr. Beer, in association with the Wapplers, brought out the first baby cystoscope. So we could then cystoscope female infants practically at birth and males when they were a few months old… We met with considerable opposition… At that time… any infection with temperature and pyuria was pyelitis. Very little was known of … congenital things… [3]

Edwin Beer and Abraham Hyman's text reviewed the pediatric urology experience at Mount Sinai Hospital in New York City. In the preface they write, "the whole subject dealt with in these pages is… still in the stage of development" and that "no one has had sufficient experience to deal with the whole subject in a complete manner" [4]. The authors describe the style of their text as "each chapter is more or less a separate essay in which the material is not arranged as in the ordinary textbook." The text comprised of 14 chapters, with "illustrative cases" at the end of nine of the chapters to help the reader recognize how the pediatric patient should be approached differently from the adult patient [4].

Meredith Fairfax Campbell (1894–1968) was one of the earliest urologists to focus on pediatric urology (Fig. 1.2). Campbell earned his medical degree in 1919 from Columbia College of Physician and Surgeons and began his internship at Bellevue Hospital [6]. This was interrupted for 2 years as he underwent treatment for tuberculosis at the Trudeau Sanitarium. He returned to Bellevue and completed his training at the New York University (NYU) School of Medicine. He joined the

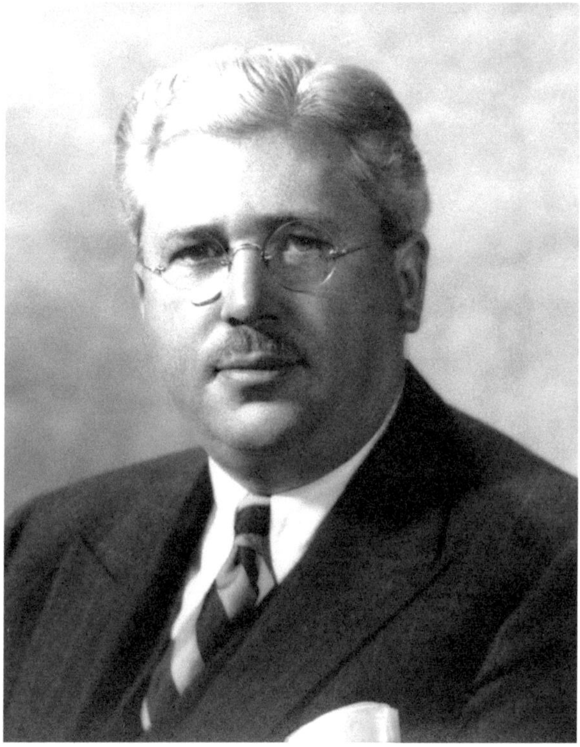

Fig. 1.2 Meredith Fairfax Campbell. (Courtesy of the William P. Didusch Center for Urologic History)

faculty of NYU and became Professor and Chair of the department in 1937 [6]. Campbell published multiple articles on pediatric urological disorders, starting as early as 1929 [6]. In 1937, he published his two-volume text, *Pediatric Urology* [7]. He solely authored 11 of the 12 chapters, and his text was based on over 24,000 necropsy studies. The text was well-referenced, as each chapter had an extensive bibliography. In the preface, Dr. Campbell wrote, "Pediatric urology is still in its diaper age and as yet comparatively few physicians are experienced in it" [7]. At the time, much of the literature published on pediatric urology consisted of small case series. Dr. Campbell aimed to correct this in his text as he presented data from relatively large case series from his practice at the time.

Frank Bartholomew Bicknell (1907–1999) attended the University of Michigan medical school from 1928 to 1932 and then trained at Detroit Receiving Hospital (1932–1936) prior to joining the faculty at Wayne State University School of Medicine [8] (Fig. 1.3). He was Chief of Urology at Harper and Hutzel Hospital and also practiced at Children's Hospital in Michigan. He developed a strong interest in pediatric urology, and it was at the 1948 AUA annual meeting in Boston, MA, that he shared a cab ride with Harry Spence of Dallas, and they talked about bringing together a small group of urologists interested in discussing urologic problems in children as part of the annual AUA meeting [8, 9].

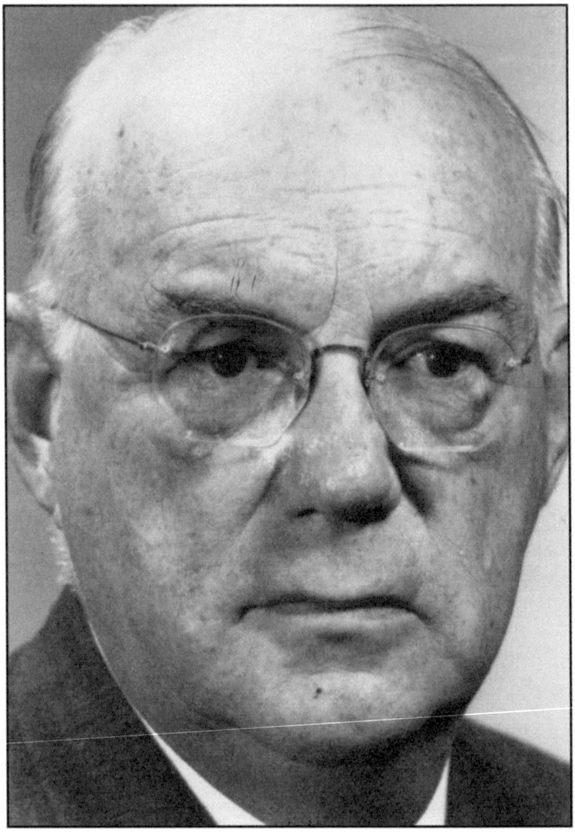

Fig. 1.3 Frank Bartholomew Bicknell. (Courtesy of the William P. Didusch Center for Urologic History)

Sir David Innes Williams (1919–2013) is known as the central founder of the modern field of pediatric urology (Fig. 1.4). He entered the Royal Army Medical Corps in 1945 and left in 1948 as a Major and surgical specialist [9]. He began training in urology at St. Peter's Hospital for Stone. The Institute of Urology offered postgraduate instruction in genitourinary surgery. The Institute came to include St. Philip's Hospital, where DI had his first pediatric ward managed by Sister Fay [9]. 1948 was an important year in the development of pediatric urology, as in addition to the taxicab conversation in Boston between Frank Bicknell and Harry Spence, DI Williams encountered a patient who would redirect his career. As DI Williams stated, "It was in 1948 when after 6 years of general surgery, in and out of the Army, I was a resident in urology at St. Peter's Hospital for Stone that I realized that the Senior staff there had no idea how to treat a boy admitted with retention from posterior urethral valves" [10]. In 1950, Williams became registrar at the Hospital for Sick Children at Great Ormond Street (GOS), London, working with Thomas Twistington Higgins, a general pediatric surgeon who also practiced urology [10]. The only other surgeon interested in pediatric urology was Denis Browne, Chief of

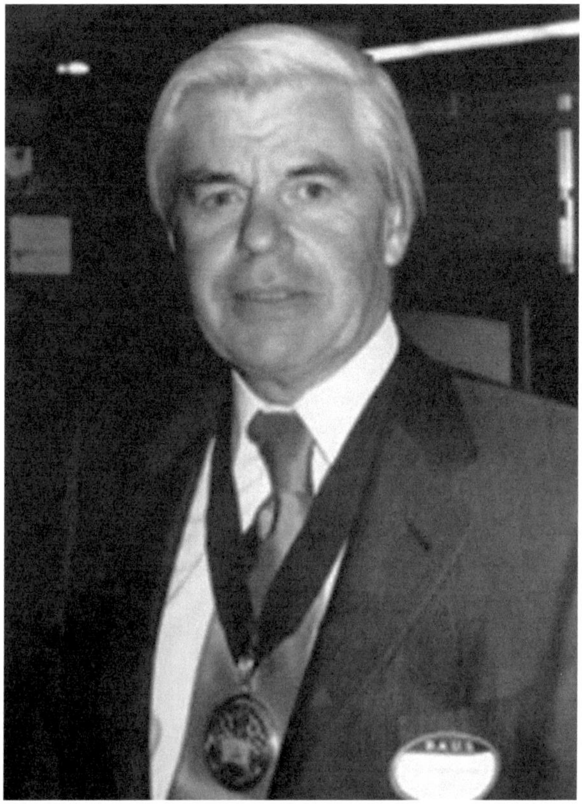

Fig. 1.4 Sir David Innes Williams. (Courtesy of the British Association of Urological Surgeons Museum)

Pediatric Surgery at GOS, and who Williams regarded as "not having an eye for cystoscopy."

Regarding the corpus of knowledge on pediatric urology at the time, DI Williams would comment, "The only major text on the subject was Meredith Campbell's two volumes published in 1931, but it was rather too heavily dependent on autopsy material from Bellevue Hospital, New York. I then obtained an attachment to the delightful (and delightfully named) Mr. Thomas Twistington Higgins, a general surgeon with an inclination towards urology and assisted him in the publication of *The Urology of Childhood* in 1951" [10]. Dr. Williams' text was also written with Ellison Nash and was the first significant work in pediatric urology since Campbell's text. In 1952, at the age of 32, Williams was appointed as a consultant surgeon at GOS.

In 1951, on the other side of the pond, nine urologists met during the AUA Meeting in Chicago in Frank Bicknell's hotel room at the Palmer House [8, 11]. The individuals included Drs. Knowlton Barber (Detroit), Frank Bicknell (Detroit), Meredith Campbell (New York City), Frank Hinman Jr. (San Francisco), Samuel Harris Johnson III (Pittsburgh), Harry Mertz (Indianapolis), Edward Shumaker (Detroit), Harry Spence (Dallas), and John Lattimer (New York City). The program consisted of three presentations: Frank Hinman Jr. described "Female

Pseudohermaphroditism," Knowlton Barber discussed "Obstructions of the UPJ in Infancy and Childhood," and Frank Bicknell spoke on "Recurrent Infections of the Genitourinary Tract in Infancy and Childhood." The concept for the creation of the Society for Pediatric Urology came from this meeting, and plans were made for a Sunday afternoon meeting at the subsequent AUA. Meredith Campbell was selected as President, and Frank Bicknell as Secretary. In the future, when Harry Spence wrote Campbell regarding the origin of the SPU, Campbell replied, "In retrospect, I feel Frank Bicknell should be given full credit as the initial instigator of the project which is truly his baby" [12].

During the early years of the subspecialty, DI Williams would comment, "Pediatric Urology was launched but still had to claim its territory, gain its corpus of in-depth knowledge, and develop its defining skills" [9, 13]. Williams would provide a steady stream of knowledge through his papers and lectures and in his collaboration with many others that were interested in the field.

In 1956, Herbert Johnston joined the Department of Paediatric Surgery, consisting of Peter Paul Rickham and Isabella Forshall, as the pediatric urologist at Alder Hey Children's Hospital in Liverpool, then an epicenter of modern pediatric anesthesia under Jackson Rees [14] (Fig. 1.5). As Alder Hey Children's Hospital had the

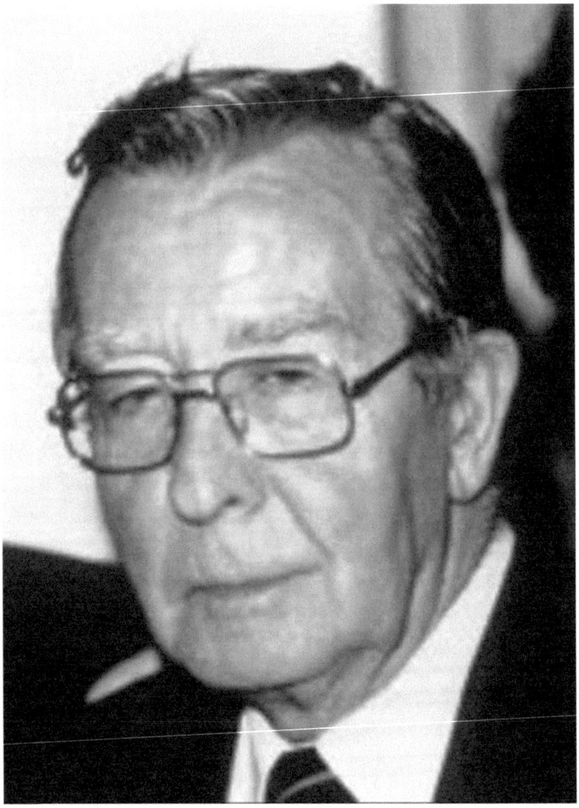

Fig. 1.5 James Herbert (Herbie) Johnston. (Courtesy of David A. Bloom)

world's first neonatal surgical unit (inaugurated in May 1953), young surgeons from around the world would come to train there [15]. In 1969, Peter Rickham and Herbert Johnston would publish the landmark textbook *Neonatal Surgery* which was to become the "bible of neonatal surgery," according to Professor Lewis Spitz [15]. Though Johnston once described himself as "the poor man's Innes Williams," his self-deprecating comment was far from the truth as both Williams and Johnston would set the standard for the practice of pediatric urology in the United Kingdon and train many future pediatric urologists from the United States and around the world [14].

Jean Cendron, a young French surgeon returning from a Fulbright scholarship in Boston with Robert Gross and Orvar Swenson, began pediatric urologic work in Paris in 1954 and frequently collaborated with DI Williams [16]. Barry O'Donnell, from Dublin, came to learn from DI Williams in 1956 and then started the first pediatric urology center in Ireland. Robert Jeffs came from Toronto in 1957 to also learn under Williams and returned to found the first pediatric urology center in North America [10].

On May 24, 1963, a group of urologists interested in pediatric urology met at the home of DI Williams in Hampstead, England. Williams would write, "In 1963 a group of us got together over the dinner table to found the Society of Paediatric Urological Surgeons, a somewhat relaxed affair which would have been called a club, but for the fact that expenses were only deductible for societies" [10]. Thus, the Society of Paediatric Urological Surgeons (SPUS) was founded, and the attendees at the dinner and first members of the society included Herbert Johnston, Richard Mogg, John Scott, John Mitchell, Herbert Eckstein, Barry O'Donnell, and Jean Cendron. SPUS grew to be an international group of the most respected leaders in the field of pediatric urology.

The American Urological Association, in conjunction with the Society for Pediatric Urology, inaugurated its Meredith Campbell Lecture in 1964 in Pittsburgh with Mr. David Innes Williams as speaker. Fittingly, the topic was posterior urethral valves [1]. Alan Retik came to study with DI in 1966, and a steady stream of international and native fellows and registrars continued until October 1978, when DI Williams retired clinically. He, however, began a new career as Director of the British Postgraduate Medical Federation, centered at the University of London [14]. Philip Ransley was appointed to be Williams' successor at the GOS and would go on to make many important contributions to the specialty, including his research with Tony Risdon, which clarified the relationship between intrarenal reflux and pyelonephritic scarring of the kidney, as well as train the next generation of future pediatric urologists [14].

Though we have discussed some of the first textbooks in pediatric urology, it is important to mention one of the first pediatric urology surgical atlases. Frank Hinman, Jr. (1915–2011) was Professor of Urology at the University of California, San Francisco [17] (Fig. 1.6). Though not a full-time pediatric urologist, he made numerous important contributions to the field of pediatric urology. His *Atlas of Urologic Surgery* (1989) and *Atlas of Pediatric Urologic Surgery* (1994), both illustrated by Paul Stempen, became some of the most widely used atlases in urology

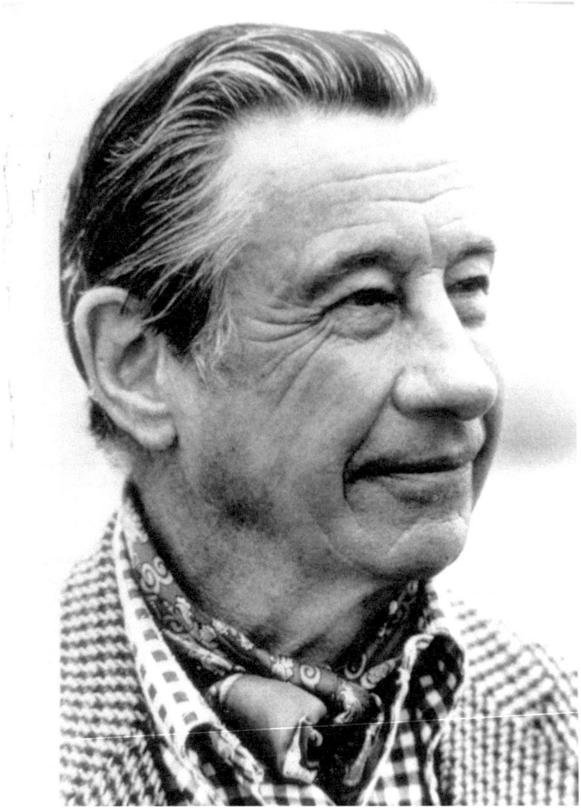

Fig. 1.6 Frank Hinman Jr. (Courtesy of the William P. Didusch Center for Urologic History)

[18, 19]. In his *Atlas of Pediatric Urologic Surgery*, Hinman Jr. dedicated chapters to the pediatric preoperative evaluation, pediatric anesthesia, operating on neonates and children, intraoperative care, and postoperative challenges. The text includes "commentaries for each operation written by prominent pediatric urologists selected from the membership of the SPU and the Section of Urology of the AAP (American Academy of Pediatrics)." Thus, Frank Hinman Jr.'s pediatric surgical text played an important role in disseminating and teaching pediatric urologic surgery for residents, general urologists, as well as pediatric urologists.

In regard to subspecialization, Frank Hinman Jr. would state, "In societal organizations, just as in embryology, ontogeny recapitulates phylogeny. Much as pediatrics split away from general medicine and urology split away from general surgery, pediatric urology's destiny was to have its own societal and elevated subunit" [20]. When trying to justify why pediatric urologists needed subcertification, one only had to look to the comments of Sir Denis Browne, the father of pediatric surgery, who stated, "Paediatric surgery exists as a specialty, not to establish a monopoly but to establish a standard" [21]. The SPU and the American Academy of Pediatrics Section on Urology (AAP–SOU) played important roles in the movement toward subcertification. The SPU became involved with the AUA annual meeting through active participation in the pediatric urology abstract selection process, making recommendations for plenary topics and speakers, and organizing the postgraduate courses in pediatric urology. The original purpose of the AAP Section on Urology was to foster close ties to pediatricians and to establish an independent identity for urologists who focused their practice on children. Furthermore, the Section on Urology was adopted by the international pediatric urology community as the major scientific meeting for pediatric urologists. The combined efforts of the SPU and AAP–SOU led to pediatric urological representation on the Residency Review Committee, which eventually led to the Accreditation Council for Graduate Medical Education (ACGME) approval of fellowships in pediatric urology in 1991 and to the ABU approval of the Pediatric Urology In-Service Examination, first administered in 1995 [22]. In 1994, the Pediatric Urology Coordinating Council (PUCC) was created, consisting of leadership from the SPU, AAP–SOU, Society for Fetal Urology (SFU), and the American Association of Pediatric Urologists (AAPU). The PUCC would negotiate a separate section of the *Journal of Urology* dedicated to pediatric urology with its own editorial board and would help organize and administer the Pediatric Urology Fellowship match. The founding of the *Journal of Pediatric Urology* in 2005, largely through the persistence of J. David Frank, its first Editor-in-Chief, allowed the field of pediatric urology to have yet another journal to publish research in the field and help establish a core content of knowledge that was required by the American Board of Medical Specialists (ABMS) to recognize a specialty [1, 22]. In 2006, the American Board of Urology (ABU) approved Subspecialty Certification in Pediatric Urology. In 2007, a subcommittee of the ABU Examination Committee constructed the first pediatric subcertification examination, which was administered to 176 applicants in 2008. There are currently 25 ACGME-accredited fellowships in Pediatric Urology [1].

The development of the field of pediatric urology is a story that began with the determination of the early pioneers in the field, nurtured by the perseverance and collaboration of many pediatric urologists, and which ultimately led to subspecialization. Frank Hinman Jr. articulated it best when he dedicated his 1991 text *American Pediatric Urology*, "To the men who taught themselves pediatric urology in order to teach the rest of us, and to the children upon whom they learned." [18].

Key Points

- Meredith Campbell played a significant role in the development of pediatric urology with the publication of his two-volume text *Pediatric Urology* in 1937.
- Sir DI Williams is considered a central founder of the field of pediatric urology and was responsible for the training of many early pediatric urologists from both Europe and the United States at The Hospital for Sick Children, Great Ormond Street.
- The development of The Society of Pediatric Urology (SPU), the Urology Section of the American Academy of Pediatrics (AAP), and the Society of Paediatric Urological Surgeons (SPUS) were important organizations that led to both the advancement and growth of pediatric urology.

- ACGME Approval of pediatric urology fellowships (1991) and American Board of Urology (ABU) approval of the Pediatric Urology In-Service Exam (1995) combined with the creation of a pediatric urology section in the Journal of Urology and the founding of the Journal of Pediatric Urology (2005) were all important final steps leading to the ABU to approve subspecialty certification in Pediatric Urology.

References

1. Caldamone AA, Cromie WJ, Patel SR, Bloom DA, Rushton HG, Rabinowitz R. The birth of pediatric urology in the United States: from pioneers to subcertification. J Pediatr Urol. 2024;20:S4–S10.
2. Herr HW. The legacy of Edwin Beer: fulguration of papillary bladder tumors. J Urol. 2005;173:1087–9.
3. Kaplan GW. Edwin Beer-a patriarch of pediatric urology. Urology. 1999;53:236–8.
4. Beer E, Hyman A. Diseases of the urinary tract in children. New York: Paul B. Hoeber Inc; 1930.
5. Beer E. Cystoscopy and ureteral catheterization in young children. Am J Surg. 1911;25:79–81.
6. Rabinowitz R. Meredith Campbell and the story behind "Campbell's urology". De Historia Urologiea Europaeae. 2017;24:42–53.
7. Campbell M. Pediatric Urology. New York: The Macmillan Company; 1937.
8. Patel SR, Bloom DA, Caldamone AA. Frank B. Bicknell: pioneer in pediatric urology and founder of the American Urological Association History Forum. Urology. 2023;173:1–4.
9. Bloom DA. A tribute to Sir David Innes Williams 12 June 1919–3 May 2013. J Pediatr Urol. 2013;9:395–7.
10. Williams DI. The history of paediatric urology: personal recollections 1948-1978. BJU Int. 2003;92(Supplement 1):1–3.
11. Bicknell F. Pediatric Urology AUA Hoffman-Roche Series; 1980. p. 1.
12. Meredith F. Campbell letter addressed to Harry M. Spence, American Urological Association archives. Linthicum: William P Didusch Center for Urologic History; 1967.
13. Gulland A. David Innes Williams: founder of the specialty of paediatric urology. BMJ. 2013;347:f5182.
14. Whitaker R. A brief history of paediatric urology in the UK. Trends in Urology & Men's Health. 2017;8:26–8.
15. Losty PD. Peter Paul Rickham: the Liverpool neonatal surgery unit 1953. Pediatr Surg Int. 2024;41:12.
16. Cendron M. Jean Cendron: the birth of pediatric urology in France. J Pediatr Urol. 2008;4:412–3.
17. Kogan BA. Frank Hinman Jr.: Clinical, Scientist and Advocate. J Urol. 1991;146:568–70.
18. Hinman Jr., F. American pediatric urology. San Francisco; Norman Publishing. 1991.
19. Hinman F Jr. Atlas of pediatric urologic surgery. Philadelphia: W.B. Saunders Company; 1989.
20. Hinman F Jr. Early pediatric urology and first steps of specialization. In: Jones LW, editor. The American Urological Association centennial history: 1902-2002. Baltimore: American Urological Association; 2002. p. 775–97.
21. Patel SR, Caldamone. Sir Denis Browne: contributions to pediatric urology. J Pediatr Urol. 2010;6:496–500.
22. Rushton HG, Kaplan GW, Mitchell ME, Caldamone AA. Road to pediatric urology subcertification: a 25-year journey. J Pediatr Urol. 2019;15:108–11.

Part I

Initial Presentation

Prenatal Hydronephrosis

2

Rebecca S. Zee and C. D. Anthony Herndon

Abbreviations

99mTc-MAG3	technetium-99m-labelled mercaptoacetyl triglycine
APRPD	anteroposterior renal pelvis diameter
BOO	bladder outlet obstruction
CAP	continuous antibiotic prophylaxis
NICU	Neonatal intensive care unit
PHN	prenatal hydronephrosis
PUV	posterior urethral valves
RUSD	renal and bladder ultrasound
SFU	societies for Fetal Urology
UPJ	ureteropelvic junction
UPJO	ureteropelvic junction obstruction
US	ultrasound
UTD	urinary tract dilation
UTI	urinary tract infection
UVJ	ureterovesical junction
VCUG	voiding cystourethrogram
VUR	vesicoureteral reflux

R. S. Zee (✉) · C. D. A. Herndon
Children's Hospital of Richmond at Virginia Commonwealth University, Department of Surgery, Division of Pediatric Urology, Richmond, VA, USA
e-mail: claude.herndon@vcuhealth.org

H.-Y. Wu et al. (eds.), *Pediatric Urology for the Adult Urologist*,
https://doi.org/10.1007/978-3-032-10306-2_2

Introduction

Prenatal hydronephrosis (PHN) is the most common congenital genitourinary anomaly affecting up to 3% of live births in the United States [24]. There are several causes of PHN, such as transient or physiologic dilation, vesicoureteral reflux (VUR), and ureteropelvic junction (UPJ) obstruction. Fortunately, most children born with PHN do not require surgical intervention. The appropriate evaluation of neonates with PHN will help identify those who are at higher risk of urologic disease. In this chapter, we review the evaluation and workup of prenatal hydronephrosis for the adult urologist.

Prenatal Imaging

The mainstay of evaluation for PHN is a renal ultrasound (RUSD) that shows images of the bladder, kidneys, and ureteral dilation (if present). PHN is commonly detected during the anatomy scan that is performed at around 20 weeks of gestation [2, 11]. Common parameters for measurement of fetal dilation are the anterior–posterior renal pelvic diameter/anterior–posterior diameter (APRPD/APD), measured at the midpoint of the renal pelvis in the transverse plane. Prenatally, some dilation may be physiologic. As urine production increases during gestation, the thresholds of normal increase for each trimester (Table 2.1) [22].

Hydronephrosis Grading Systems

Societies for Fetal Urology (SFU) Grading System

The most common system for reporting of PHN is the SFU grading system, which is a 4-point scale that describes the degree of dilation as well as the parenchymal thickness (Fig. 2.1) [32]. In this system, grade 1 dilation is the mildest, with only splitting of the renal pelvis. SFU grade 2 describes dilation of the renal pelvis and major calyces. SFU grade 3 is a dilation of both major and minor calyces. Severe dilation with thinning of the parenchyma is considered SFU grade 4 [16].

SFU grade is predictive of the potential for surgical intervention as well as renal function [15]. There is a direct correlation between the degree of dilation and

Table 2.1 Template for reporting renal ultrasound findings. Seven criteria are included, which help the clinician perform risk stratification

Definition of Antenatal Hydronephrosis by APRPD (mm)		
	Second trimester	Third trimester
Mild	4 to ≤7	4 to ≤9
Moderate	7 to ≤10	9 to ≤15
Severe	> 10	> 15

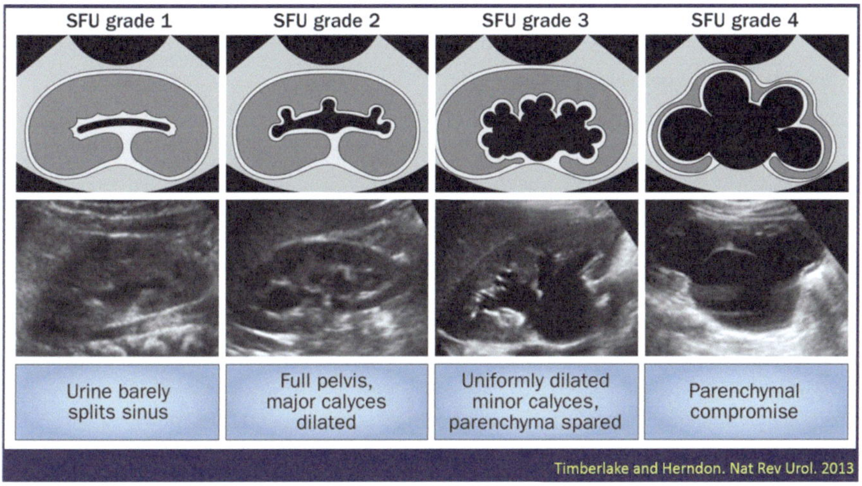

Fig. 2.1 Societies for Fetal Urology (SFU) grading system includes four categories to classify the severity of dilation. SFU grade 1 includes only the splitting of the renal pelvis. SFU grade 2 includes dilation of major calyces. SFU grade 3 describes dilation of minor and major calyces. SFU grade 4 includes dilation with thinning of the renal parenchyma. The SFU grading system does not describe any urinary structures distal to the kidney

incidence of urologic disease. In a study of 125 renal units with SFU grade 3 or 4 hydronephrosis, Ross et al. reported that 77% of patients who required surgical intervention demonstrated SFU grade 4 hydronephrosis [27]. There were significantly more renal units with SFU grade 3 hydronephrosis in the observation group [27].

The SFU system does have limitations. For instance, SFU grading does not take the appearance of bladder and ureters into account or provide any guidance for evaluation and management. Furthermore, there is little adoption of this system outside of pediatric urology.

Urinary Tract Dilation (UTD) System

The UTD system, initially published in 2014, was established by a multidisciplinary team composed of nine professional societies [24]. The purpose of the new system was to include new criteria on imaging that would provide a framework for risk stratification. An additional goal of this new system was to establish common terminology across disciplines, both prenatally and postnatally, and to avoid ambiguous terminology such as "caliectasis" or "pyelectasis."

Table 2.2 demonstrates a standardized template for reporting findings on a renal ultrasound. These criteria include: APRPD, central and peripheral calyceal dilation, parenchymal thickness, unexplained oligohydramnios, and the appearance of the renal parenchyma, ureters, and bladder [24]. The major difference between the SFU

Table 2.2 Antenatal hydronephrosis renal ultrasound criteria for risk stratification as defined by Anteroposterior Renal Pelvic Diameter (APRPD) in mm

Ultrasound findings postnatally (>48 h)				
	Normal	UTD P1	UTD P2	UTD P3
APRPD	<10 mm	10 to <15 mm	≥15 mm	≥15 mm
Calyceal dilation				
Central	Absent	Present	Present	Present
Peripheral	Absent	Absent	Present	Present
Parenchymal thickness	Normal	Normal	Normal	Abnormal[a]
Parenchymal appearance	Normal	Normal	Normal	Abnormal[a]
Ureter(s)	Normal	Normal	Abnormal	Abnormal
Bladder	Normal	Normal	Normal	Abnormal[a]
Corresponding SFU grade	0	1–2	3	4

[a]If any are present, then the patient should be stratified as high risk UTD P3

and UTD systems is that the UTD grading system takes into account APRPD and the appearance of the ureters and bladder, whereas the SFU grading system does not. Another benefit of the UTD system is the improved counseling for patient families, who are commonly uncertain of the significance of the diagnosis.

Based on these standardized parameters, three categories of risk were defined for newborns based on APD, SFU grade, and the appearance of the kidneys, ureters, and bladder on ultrasound. Risk stratification allows for straightforward work-up and management after initial postnatal US (Fig. 2.2).

Risk stratification refers to the risk of pyelonephritis, risk of needing urologic surgery, or loss of renal function. The presence of prenatal hydronephrosis predisposes patients to a higher risk of UTI than patients without PHN. There is a linear correlation between the degree of hydronephrosis and the risk of UTI. *Lee* et al. reported that the incidence of UTI was 4% for SFU grade 1, 14% for grade 2, 33% for grade 3, and 40% for SFU grade 4 [22]. We reported on a cohort of 213 PHN patients followed prospectively and found an overall incidence of 8% with a vast majority (89%) occurring in the first year of life [38].

Low-risk patients (UTD P1) comprise the largest group of patients who will present with prenatal hydronephrosis. On first postnatal US, patients will demonstrate central calyceal dilation, and APD 10 mm to <15 mm (Table 2.2). There will be no abnormalities in the appearance of the kidneys, ureters, or bladder, and a normal parenchymal thickness. Intermediate risk patients (UTD P2) will have a postnatal US that demonstrates APD ≥ 15 mm, with central and peripheral calyceal dilation and/or abnormal appearance of the ureters. High-risk patients (UTD P3) will have all features of P2, with the addition of abnormal appearance of bladder or renal parenchyma, such as renal cysts and/or thinning of the renal parenchyma. This corresponds to SFU grade 4 hydronephrosis at the kidney level. Of note, risk stratification is based on the most severe feature seen in either kidney. For example, the detection of unilateral parenchymal thinning would be considered UTD P3, or high risk (Table 2.2).

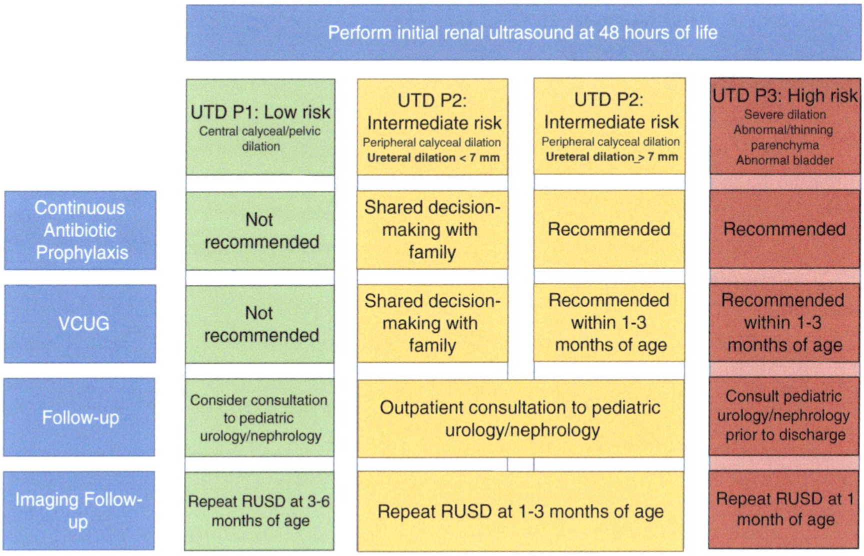

Fig. 2.2 Flow chart for workup and evaluation of UTD. For intermediate risk UTD P2, recommendations differ based on the presence of ureteral dilation. If ureteral dilation is ≥7 mm, VCUG and antibiotic prophylaxis are recommended. For ureteral dilation below 7 mm, clinicians should engage with shared decision-making with the family about whether to proceed with VCUG and/or CAP

Bilateral Dilation

For prenatal screening or neonates for whom RUSD reveals severe bilateral dilation with oligohydramnios, bladder outlet obstruction (BOO) should be suspected. BOO in the neonate may represent urethral atresia, posterior urethral valves (PUV), ureterocele, spinal dysraphism, or prune belly syndrome. Parents with prenatal findings suspicious for BOO should be counseled to deliver the baby in a facility with an available neonatal intensive care unit (NICU) where appropriate neonatal evaluation, consultant availability, and supportive care can be provided.

Patients with suspected BOO require immediate bladder decompression at birth, commencement of prophylactic antibiotics, joint nephrology and urology consultation, and prompt evaluation to elucidate the anatomy of the genitourinary tract. In neonates, we recommend urethral placement of a 6 or 8 French feeding tube attached to drainage with a Luer lock adapter. Placement of a Foley catheter in neonates can cause UVJ obstruction, or the balloon may dislodge into the dilated posterior urethra in patients with PUV. If necessary, a Foley catheter may be used without inflating the balloon. Initial imaging evaluation includes a renal US and VCUG.

Evaluation and Management of UTD

Renal US (RUSD)

All patients with PHN should have a RUSD obtained prior to discharge from the hospital to evaluate the severity of dilation. Importantly, the first postnatal US should be performed after 48 hours of age. Neonates experience significant third-spacing, which can underestimate the degree of dilation if performed prior to 48 hours of age [23]. If the initial postnatal US is normal, a repeat RUSD is recommended at 3–6 months to confirm resolution of PHN.

If the initial postnatal RUSD demonstrates dilation of the renal pelvis and central calyces, or low risk (UTD P1), consultation to pediatric urology and/or nephrology for ongoing outpatient management should be considered. The next surveillance RUSD should be performed at 3–6 months of life.

If initial postnatal RUSD demonstrates dilation of central and peripheral calyces with or without ureteral dilation, representing the intermediate risk category (UTD P2), pediatric nephrology and/or urology should be consulted prior to discharge, or an expedited referral should be obtained. Repeat RUSD should be performed at 1–3 months of life.

In cases of high risk (UTD P3) with the appearance of parenchymal thinning, abnormal appearance of the parenchyma, or bladder, pediatric urology and/or nephrology should be consulted prior to discharge from the hospital, or an expedited outpatient referral should be completed. RUSD should be repeated within 1 month of birth.

Continuous Antibiotic Prophylaxis (CAP)

The purpose of continuous antibiotic prophylaxis (CAP) is to prevent UTI and the subsequent risk of renal scarring. UTI rates in patients with PHN vary widely, from 8% to 22%, with a higher UTI rate in patients with higher degrees of dilation and patients with ureteral dilation [8, 15, 19–21, 30, 31, 37]. Other risk factors for UTI include intact foreskin, female gender, and the presence of urinary tract obstruction. [6, 15, 37, 40].

The recommendation to start continuous antibiotic prophylaxis (CAP) can also be based on UTD risk stratification. UTD P1 patients are at low risk of infection and therefore do not require CAP. In UTD P2, CAP is recommended for patients with ureteral dilation ≥7 mm. This is based on our recent data that demonstrated a higher incidence of UTI in patients with ureteral dilation ≥7 mm [20]. If there is ureteral dilation <7 mm, then the clinician should engage in shared decision-making with the family about whether or not to start CAP. All patients in the P3 category should be initiated on CAP prior to discharge from the hospital.

Amoxicillin is the most commonly used antibiotic prophylaxis in the first 3 months of life, which covers enterococcus species as well as gram-negative rods. Infants are administered 1 mL of amoxicillin suspension (125 mg/5 mL) daily until the patient is old enough to transition to trimethoprim-sulfamethoxazole liquid. Trimethoprim-sulfamethoxazole should not be given to newborns less than 2 months of age due to the risk of kernicterus. At 2 months of age, trimethoprim-sulfamethoxazole dosing should be started at 2 mg/kg daily based on trimethoprim content.

Voiding Cystourethrogram (VCUG)

A voiding cystourethrogram (VCUG) is the gold standard for detecting the presence and severity of vesicoureteral reflux (VUR). VUR is present in 15–25% of children with PHN [5, 17, 18, 26, 35]. VCUG can also identify lower urinary tract anomalies such as PUV and ureteroceles. A normal postnatal RUSD does not predict the absence of VUR, as 25% of patients with VUR will have a normal postnatal RUSD [18].

VCUG is not recommended in low-risk (UTD P1) patients due to the relatively low likelihood of infection in this group. During counseling, families should be made aware that VUR still may be present; however, testing is not recommended in the absence of infection in low-risk patients. Subsequently, any child with known UTD who develops a febrile UTI should be evaluated with a VCUG to evaluate for the presence of VUR.

VCUG should be considered in intermediate risk UTD P2. As previously stated, in UTD P2 with ureteral dilation ≥7 mm, there is a higher incidence of UTI [20]. Therefore, VCUG may be more useful in this subset of intermediate-risk patients. VCUG is recommended in the high-risk (UTD P3) group. VCUG should ideally be deferred until it can be obtained in a facility that regularly performs infant studies.

Renal Scintigraphy

Renal scintigraphy, such as a 99mTc-MAG3 (technetium-99m-labelled-mercaptoacetyl triglycine) MAG3 renal diuretic scan, is useful for detecting the differential function and presence of obstruction. Similar, less popular tests which employ the use of radiotracers include 99mTc-DMSA (technetium-99m-labelled-dimercaptosuccinic acid) and 99mTc-DTPA (technetium-99m-labelled-diethylenetriamine pentaacetic acid). MAG3 scans are unreliable in neonates and, therefore, rarely performed prior to 6–12 weeks of age [4, 10, 29, 36].

Common Causes of Urinary Tract Dilation

Transient/Physiologic Dilation

The most common cause of UTD is transient dilation, which affects up to 70% of patients with PHN. A vast majority of these patients will resolve by 4 years of age

Table 2.3 Differential diagnosis of UTD

Differential diagnosis of urinary tract dilation
Non-obstructive
Transient/Physiologic
Vesicoureteral reflux (VUR)
Multicystic Dysplastic Kidney (MCDK)
Prune Belly Syndrome
Obstructive
Ureteropelvic junction (UPJ) obstruction
Ureterocele
Ectopic ureter
Ureterovesical Junction (UVJ) obstruction
Posterior urethral valves (PUV)
Urethral Atresia
Other

and can be followed with serial RUSD in childhood [7, 39]. Causes of UTD are listed in Table 2.3.

UPJ Obstruction (UPJO)

Most UPJO-like dilation will resolve without surgical intervention and can be followed with RUSD surveillance. In a study of 104 patients with a UPJO-like pattern of dilation, only 22% required surgical intervention [33]. Several publications have demonstrated that an APD threshold of 15 mm postnatally or in the third trimester was more predictive of the need for surgery [3, 12, 28, 41].

Vesicoureteral Reflux (VUR)

VUR is the third most common cause of UTD and will be present in approximately 30% of patients with PHN [1, 18, 22, 25, 34]. Historically, screening for VUR was performed in all patients with PHN. In contemporary practice, VUR screening is now pursued based on the risk of UTI. Risk factors for UTI in PHN patients include female gender, intact foreskin, and severity of UTD [6, 8, 9, 13, 19, 21, 30, 31, 37, 38]. As previously mentioned, VCUG is recommended for UTD P2 intermediate-risk patients with ureteral dilation ≥7 mm and UTD P3 high-risk patients.

Summary

- Patients with prenatal imaging suspicious for bladder outlet obstruction (bilateral severe hydronephrosis and/or oligohydramnios) should be delivered in a facility with a high-acuity NICU, and pediatric nephrology/urology consultations should be obtained.

- Neonates with PHN should have a postnatal RUSD to assess for UTD. The timing is dictated by prenatal severity and should ideally be performed between 48 hours of age (prior to discharge) and 2 weeks postnatally (with pediatrician).
- A shared decision-making process should be used for decisions to start CAP.
  - Most neonates will have UTD P1 and will not benefit from CAP.
  - Neonates with UTD P2 with ureteral dilation ≥7 mm and UTD P3 will benefit from CAP.
- In a child with known postnatal UTD and undetermined VUR status (no prior VCUG) who develops fever (≥100.4 °F or 38 °C), the child should be evaluated for a UTI. If a UTI is present, the patient should undergo VCUG to evaluate for VUR.

References

1. Adra AMAM, Mejides AA, Dennaoui MS, et al. Fetal pyelectasis: is it always physiologic? Am J Obstet Gynecol. 1995;173:1263–6.
2. American College of Obstetricians and Gynecologists. ACOG practice bulletin 101. Obstet Gynecol. 2009;113(2 Pt 1):451–61.
3. Arora S, Yadav P, Kumar M, et al. Predictors for the need of surgery in antenatally detected hydronephrosis due to UPJ obstruction—a prospective multivariate analysis. J Pediatr Urol. 2015;11:248.e1–5. https://doi.org/10.1016/j.jpurol.2015.02.008.
4. Bayne CE, Majd M, Rushton HG. Diuresis renography in the evaluation and management of pediatric hydronephrosis: what have we learned? J Pediatr Urol. 2019;15:128–37. https://doi.org/10.1016/j.jpurol.2019.01.011.
5. Berrocal T, Pinilla I, Gutierrez J, et al. Mild hydronephrosis in newborns and infants: can ultrasound predict the presence of vesicoureteral reflux. Pediatr Nephrol. 2007;22:91–6. https://doi.org/10.1007/s00467-006-0285-1.
6. Braga LH, Farrokhyar F, D'Cruz J, et al. Risk factors for febrile urinary tract infection in children with prenatal hydronephrosis: a prospective study. J Urol. 2015;193:1766–71. https://doi.org/10.1016/j.juro.2014.10.091.
7. Braga LH, McGrath M, Farrokhyar F, et al. Society for fetal urology classification vs urinary tract dilation grading system for prognostication in prenatal hydronephrosis: a time to resolution analysis. J Urol. 2017; https://doi.org/10.1016/j.juro.2017.11.077.
8. Braga LH, Mijovic H, Farrokhyar F, et al. Antibiotic prophylaxis for urinary tract infections in antenatal hydronephrosis. Pediatrics. 2013;131:e251–61. https://doi.org/10.1542/peds.2012-1870.
9. Braga LH, Pemberton J, Heaman J, et al. Pilot randomized, placebo controlled trial to investigate the effect of antibiotic prophylaxis on the rate of urinary tract infection in infants with prenatal hydronephrosis. J Urol. 2014;191:1501–7. https://doi.org/10.1016/j.juro.2013.10.033.
10. Chung S, Majd M, Rushton HG, Belman AB. Diuretic renography in the evaluation of neonatal hydronephrosis: is it reliable? J Urol. 1993;150:765–8. https://doi.org/10.1016/S0022-5347(17)35609-4.
11. Committee on Practice Bulletins—Obstetrics and the American Institute of Ultrasound in Medicine. Practice Bulletin No. 175: Ultrasound in Pregnancy. Obstet Gynecol. 2016;128:e241–56. https://doi.org/10.1097/AOG.0000000000001815.
12. Coplen DE, Austin PF, Yan Y, et al. The magnitude of fetal renal pelvic dilatation can identify obstructive postnatal hydronephrosis, and direct postnatal evaluation and management. J Urol. 2006;176:724–7; discussion 727. https://doi.org/10.1016/j.juro.2006.03.079.

13. Easterbrook B, Capolicchio J-P, Braga LH. Antibiotic prophylaxis for prevention of urinary tract infections in prenatal hydronephrosis: an updated systematic review. Can Urol Assoc J. 2017a;11(3) https://doi.org/10.5489/cuaj.4384.
14. Easterbrook B, Capolicchio JP, Braga LH. Antibiotic prophylaxis for prevention of urinary tract infections in prenatal hydronephrosis: an updated systematic review. Can Urol Assoc J. 2017b;11:S3–S11.
15. Erickson BA, Maizels M, Shore RM, et al. Newborn society of fetal urology grade 3 hydronephrosis is equivalent to preserved percentage differential function. J Pediatr Urol. 2007;3:382–6. https://doi.org/10.1016/j.jpurol.2007.01.196.
16. Fernbach SK, Maizels M, Conway JJ. Ultrasound grading of hydronephrosis: introduction to the system used by the Society for Fetal Urology. Ped Rad. 1993;23:478–80.
17. Gloor JM, Ramsey PS, Ogburn JPL, et al. The association of isolated mild fetal hydronephrosis with postnatal vesicoureteral reflux. J Matern Fetal Neonatal Med. 2002;12:196–200. https://doi.org/10.1080/jmf.12.3.196.200.
18. Herndon CD, McKenna PH, Kolon TF, et al. A multicenter outcomes analysis of patients with neonatal reflux presenting with prenatal hydronephrosis. J Urol. 1999;162:1203–8.
19. Herz D, Merguerian P, McQuiston L. Continuous antibiotic prophylaxis reduces the risk of febrile UTI in children with asymptomatic antenatal hydronephrosis with either ureteral dilation, high-grade vesicoureteral reflux, or ureterovesical junction obstruction. J Pediatr Urol. 2014;10:650–4. https://doi.org/10.1016/j.jpurol.2014.06.009.
20. Holzman SA, Braga LH, Zee RS, et al. Risk of urinary tract infection in patients with hydroureter: an analysis from the Society of Fetal Urology Prenatal Hydronephrosis Registry. J Pediatr Urol. 2021;17:775–81.
21. Lee JH, Choi HS, Kim JK, et al. Nonrefluxing neonatal hydronephrosis and the risk of urinary tract infection. J Urol. 2008;179:1524–8. https://doi.org/10.1016/j.juro.2007.11.090.
22. Lee RS, Cendron M, Kinnamon DD, Nguyen HT. Antenatal hydronephrosis as a predictor of postnatal outcome: a meta-analysis. Pediatrics. 2006;118:586–93. https://doi.org/10.1542/peds.2006-0120.
23. Maclaurin JC. Changes in body water distribution during the first two weeks of life. Arch Dis Child. 1966;41:286–91.
24. Nguyen HT, Benson CB, Bromley B, et al. Multidisciplinary consensus on the classification of prenatal and postnatal urinary tract dilation (UTD classification system). J Pediatr Urol. 2014;10:982–98. https://doi.org/10.1016/j.jpurol.2014.10.002.
25. Nguyen HTTHT, Herndon CDADA, Cooper C, et al. The Society for Fetal Urology consensus statement on the evaluation and management of antenatal hydronephrosis. J Pediatr Urol. 2010;6:212–31. https://doi.org/10.1016/j.jpurol.2010.02.205.
26. Phan V, Traubici J, Hershenfield B, et al. Vesicoureteral reflux in infants with isolated antenatal hydronephrosis. Pediatr Nephrol. 2003;18:1224–8. https://doi.org/10.1007/s00467-003-1287-x.
27. Ross SS, Kardos S, Krill A, et al. Observation of infants with SFU grades 3-4 hydronephrosis: worsening drainage with serial diuresis renography indicates surgical intervention and helps prevent loss of renal function. J Pediatr Urol. 2011;7:266–71. https://doi.org/10.1016/j.jpurol.2011.03.001.
28. Shamshirsaz AAA, Ravangard SF, Egan JF, et al. Fetal hydronephrosis as a predictor of neonatal urologic outcomes. J Ultrasound Med. 2012;31:947–54.
29. Shulkin BL, Mandell GA, Cooper JA, et al. Procedure guideline for diuretic renography in children 3.0. J Nucl Med Technol. 2008;36:162–8. https://doi.org/10.2967/JNMT.108.056622.
30. Silay MS, Undre S, Nambiar AK, et al. Role of antibiotic prophylaxis in antenatal hydronephrosis: a systematic review from the European Association of Urology/European Society for Paediatric Urology Guidelines Panel. J Pediatr Urol. 2017; https://doi.org/10.1016/j.jpurol.2017.02.023.
31. Szymanski KM, Al-Said AN, Pippi Salle JL, Capolicchio JP. Do infants with mild prenatal hydronephrosis benefit from screening for vesicoureteral reflux? J Urol. 2012;188:576–81. https://doi.org/10.1016/j.juro.2012.04.017.

32. Timberlake MD, Herndon CDA. Mild to moderate postnatal hydronephrosis--grading systems and management. Nat Rev Urol. 2013;10:649–56. https://doi.org/10.1038/nrurol.2013.172.
33. Ulman I, Jayanthi VR, Koff SA. The long-term followup of newborns with severe unilateral hydronephrosis initially treated nonoperatively. J Urol. 2000;164:1101–5.
34. Upadhyay J, McLorie GA, Bolduc S, et al. Natural history of neonatal reflux associated with prenatal hydronephrosis: long-term results of a prospective study. J Urol. 2003;169:1837–41; discussion 1841; author reply 1841. https://doi.org/10.1097/01.ju.0000062440.92454.cf.
35. Van Eerde AM, Meutgeert MH, De Jong TPVM, Giltay JC. Vesico-ureteral reflux in children with prenatally detected hydronephrosis: a systematic review. Ultrasound Obstet Gynecol. 2007;29:463–9. https://doi.org/10.1002/uog.3975.
36. Wong JCH, Rossleigh MA, Farnsworth RH. Utility of Technetium-99m-MAG3 diuretic renography in the neonatal period. J Nucl Med. 1995;36:2214–9.
37. Zareba P, Lorenzo AJ, Braga LH. Risk factors for febrile urinary tract infection in infants with prenatal hydronephrosis: comprehensive single center analysis. J Urol. 2014;191:1614–8. https://doi.org/10.1016/j.juro.2013.10.035.
38. Zee RS, Herbst KW, Kim C, et al. Urinary tract infections in children with prenatal hydronephrosis: a risk assessment from the Society for Fetal Urology Hydronephrosis Registry. J Pediatr Urol. 2016;12 https://doi.org/10.1016/j.jpurol.2016.04.024.
39. Zee RS, Herndon CDA, Cooper CS, et al. Time to resolution: a prospective evaluation from the Society for Fetal Urology hydronephrosis registry. J Pediatr Urol Regist J Pediatr Urol. 2017a;12 https://doi.org/10.1016/j.jpurol.2016.12.012.
40. Zee RSS, Herndon CDADAA, Cooper CSS, et al. Time to resolution: a prospective evaluation from the Society for Fetal Urology hydronephrosis registry. J Pediatr Urol. 2017b;13:316.e1–5. https://doi.org/10.1016/j.jpurol.2016.12.012.
41. Zhang L, Li Y, Liu C, et al. Diagnostic value of anteroposterior diameter of renal pelvis for predicting postnatal surgery: a systematic review and meta-analysis. J Urol. 2018;200:1346–53.

Understanding Pediatric Circumcision: A Guide for Adult Urologists

3

Victor H. Figueroa and Martin A. Koyle

Key Points

1. Pediatric circumcision involves distinct anatomical, cultural, and ethical considerations that differ from those in adult cases.
2. Medical indications include phimosis, recurrent balanitis, and urinary tract infections, with the surgical intervention tailored to the child's age and condition.
3. Several techniques (Gomco, Mogen, Plastibell, sleeve excision) are available, each with unique benefits, risks, and complication profiles.
4. Safe outcomes require informed consent, effective pain management, and vigilant postoperative care to minimize adverse events.

Introduction

Circumcision, a surgical procedure involving the removal of the foreskin from the penis, represents one of the most ancient surgical interventions known to mankind [1]. Its practice spans diverse cultures and religions, carrying profound symbolic and historical significance [2]. In Judaism, for instance, circumcision, known as *Brit Milah (Bris)*, is a religious commandment symbolizing the covenant between God and Abraham and his descendants, typically performed on the eighth day of a male infant's life [3]. Within Islamic traditions, circumcision, referred to as *Khitan*, holds a significant cultural position; despite not being explicitly stipulated in the Quranic text, it is regarded as a sunnah, reflecting the practices and customs attributed to the Prophet Muhammad, and is often performed before puberty [4]. Beyond its religious contexts, circumcision is also practiced for a multitude of non-religious

V. H. Figueroa (✉) · M. A. Koyle
Department of Urology, University of Minnesota, Minneapolis, MN, USA
e-mail: figue188@umn.edu

H.-Y. Wu et al. (eds.), *Pediatric Urology for the Adult Urologist*,
https://doi.org/10.1007/978-3-032-10306-2_3

reasons, encompassing perceived hygienic benefits, cultural norms, and preventive healthcare considerations [5]. The prevalence of circumcision exhibits substantial geographical variations, with higher rates observed in regions with strong Jewish or Muslim populations, as well as in certain parts of Africa and the United States [6].

The decision to circumcise a child is multifaceted, laden with ethical, cultural, and medical considerations that evoke fervent debates across diverse perspectives [7]. Parents often grapple with the influence of cultural traditions, religious beliefs, and perceived health advantages in making this pivotal choice for their sons [8]. Medical viewpoints on circumcision are varied and nuanced, with some professional organizations acknowledging potential health benefits, such as reduced risk of urinary tract infections in infancy and decreased incidence of penile cancer and certain sexually transmitted infections later in life [9]. However, other organizations emphasize the potential risks associated with the procedure, including bleeding, infection, and pain, while highlighting the importance of respecting the child's bodily autonomy and right to make their own decisions about their body when they are old enough. Ethical debates surrounding circumcision often revolve around the principles of autonomy, beneficence, and non-maleficence [10, 11].

Historical and Cultural Perspectives on Circumcision

Historically, circumcision's roots can be traced back to ancient civilizations, where it likely originated as a tribal ritual or a marker of social identity. In ancient Egypt, archaeological evidence suggests that circumcision was practiced as early as 2300 BC, with depictions found in tombs and other artifacts, indicating its significance in their culture and society [3]. The procedure's presence in early religious texts, such as the Old Testament, underscores its enduring importance in shaping religious identity and adherence to divine commandments [12]. Anthropological studies reveal that circumcision has been practiced in various forms across different cultures worldwide, often serving as a rite of passage or a symbol of belonging to a particular group [13]. The motives behind these practices were diverse, including religious obligations, hygiene beliefs, and social customs.

The cultural significance of circumcision is deeply embedded in the traditions and beliefs of numerous societies. In many Jewish communities, circumcision is not merely a medical procedure but a sacred ritual performed by a trained mohel, symbolizing the covenant between God and the Jewish people, where it reinforces communal identity and intergenerational continuity [1, 14]. Similarly, in Islamic societies, circumcision is widely practiced as a religious tradition, often celebrated with elaborate ceremonies and festivities, signifying a boy's entry into manhood and adherence to Islamic customs [15, 16]. Even in cultures where circumcision is not explicitly tied to religious beliefs, it may still hold cultural significance as a marker of social status, hygiene practices, or conformity to societal norms [14, 15]. Understanding these historical and cultural perspectives is crucial for appreciating the diverse meanings and values associated with circumcision across different societies and communities.

Medical Indications for Circumcision

From a medical standpoint, circumcision has been suggested to offer several potential health benefits, although these are subject to ongoing debate and scrutiny. One of the frequently cited advantages is a reduced risk of urinary tract infections in infancy, particularly during the first year of life, as the foreskin can act as a reservoir for bacteria, increasing the likelihood of infection [17–19]. While the occurrence of penile cancer is notably infrequent, particularly in regions with well-developed healthcare systems and access to advanced medical interventions, certain epidemiological investigations have indicated a potential inverse association between circumcision and the risk of developing this malignancy; some researchers hypothesize that the removal of the foreskin may decrease the accumulation of carcinogenic substances and improve hygiene, thereby diminishing the probability of penile cancer development [20–22]. Furthermore, studies have explored the potential role of circumcision in reducing the transmission of certain sexually transmitted infections, including HIV and HPV, with some evidence suggesting that circumcision may offer partial protection by altering the genital microbiome and reducing the availability of target cells for infection [21].

It is essential, however, to acknowledge that the medical benefits of circumcision are not universally accepted, and professional medical organizations offer varying recommendations based on a comprehensive assessment of the available evidence. Some organizations, such as the American Academy of Pediatrics, have acknowledged the potential health benefits of circumcision but emphasize that the decision should be made by parents in consultation with their pediatrician, taking into account their individual circumstances and values [23]. Conversely, other organizations, such as the Canadian Paediatric Society, do not recommend routine circumcision for all newborn males, citing concerns about potential risks and the lack of conclusive evidence demonstrating significant health benefits [23]. These divergent perspectives highlight the complexity of medical evidence and the need for individualized decision-making based on a thorough evaluation of the potential benefits and risks.

Phimosis

Phimosis is a physiological condition characterized by the inability to retract the foreskin. In children, phimosis is commonly observed and typically resolves spontaneously without intervention, as the foreskin gradually separates from the glans penis [24, 25]. In certain instances, phimosis may persist beyond childhood, leading to discomfort, foreskin laceration, or penile pain [24, 26]. Pathologic phimosis can arise as a result of chronic inflammation, scarring, or underlying skin conditions, resulting in a constricted foreskin that is difficult or impossible to retract (Fig. 3.1) [7]. In such cases, circumcision may be considered as a therapeutic intervention to alleviate symptoms and prevent complications.

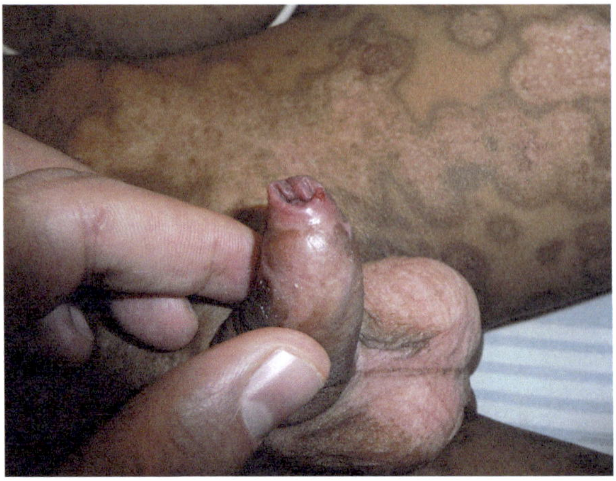

Fig. 3.1 Patient with a history of Stevens–Johnson syndrome and subsequent pathologic phimosis. Note the chronic inflammatory changes in the distal foreskin

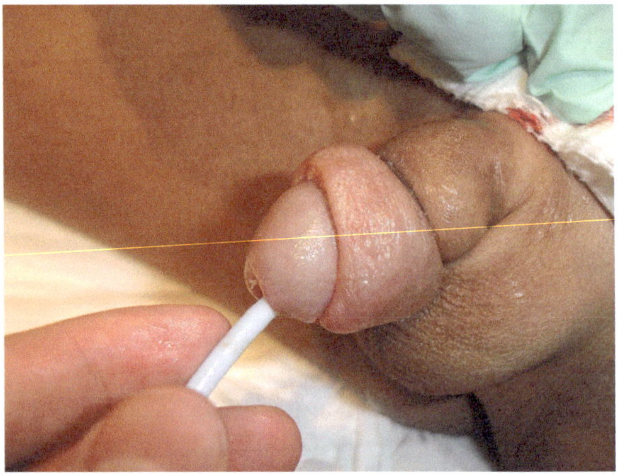

Fig. 3.2 Paraphimosis in a young boy after Foley catheter placement

The decision to perform circumcision for phimosis should be based on a thorough clinical evaluation, considering factors such as the severity of symptoms, the presence of complications, and the patient's overall health status [26]. Conservative measures, such as topical corticosteroid creams, may be attempted initially to soften the foreskin and facilitate retraction; however, if these measures prove ineffective or if complications arise, circumcision may be recommended as the definitive treatment option [25].

Paraphimosis

Paraphimosis is a condition in an uncircumcised male, in which the phimotic ring is stuck behind the glans penis, leading to pain and discomfort (Fig. 3.2). Prompt reduction of the foreskin is essential to prevent complications such as edema, ischemia, and necrosis of the glans [27]. If manual reduction is not possible, surgical intervention, such as a dorsal slit or circumcision, may be necessary to relieve the constriction and restore normal blood flow. In addition to addressing the acute episode of paraphimosis, topical steroids with manual reduction or circumcision may be considered as a prophylactic measure to prevent recurrence, particularly in individuals with underlying phimosis or a history of recurrent episodes [24].

Balanitis

Balanitis, defined as the inflammation of the glans penis, and balanoposthitis, the inflammation of the glans and foreskin, can occur in uncircumcised males due to poor hygiene, infection, or underlying skin conditions (Fig. 3.3) [24, 28]. Recurrent episodes of balanitis or balanoposthitis can result in discomfort, pain, and potential complications such as pathologic phimosis or adhesions between the foreskin and glans. While proper hygiene practices and topical treatments can effectively manage most cases of balanitis, circumcision may be considered as a preventive measure in individuals with recurrent or chronic infections [29]. By removing the foreskin, circumcision eliminates the space where bacteria and other pathogens can accumulate, reducing the risk of future infections and associated complications. However, the decision to perform circumcision for recurrent balanitis should be made on a case-by-case basis, weighing the potential benefits against the risks and considering alternative treatment options [28, 30].

Recurrent Urinary Tract Infections

Recurrent urinary tract infections in infancy can pose a significant health concern, particularly in boys younger than 12 months of age [30]. While urinary tract infections are more common in females, uncircumcised infant males, in their first 6 months of life have a higher risk of developing these infections compared to their

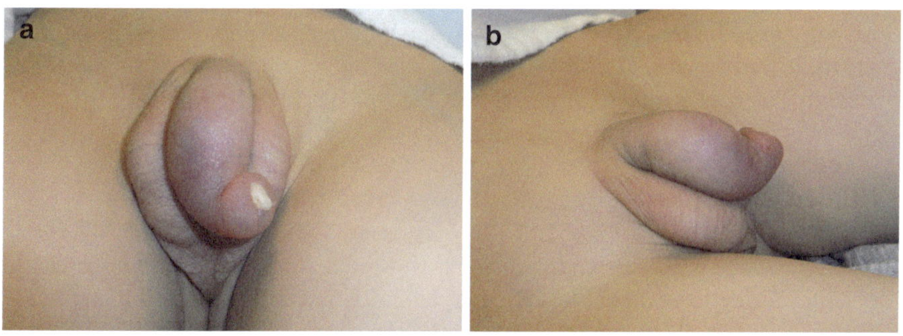

Fig. 3.3 Anterior (**a**) and lateral views (**b**) of a boy with bacterial balanitis with swelling and drainage from the foreskin

circumcised counterparts. The foreskin can serve as a reservoir for bacteria, increasing the likelihood of ascending infection into the urinary tract [19, 31, 32]. For infant males with recurrent UTIs, especially those who have a detected coincidental urology abnormality such as high-grade vesicoureteral reflux and/or posterior urethral valves, circumcision could be considered to prevent recurrent UTI and potentially offer long-term renal protection [33]. The American Academy of Pediatrics suggests that circumcision can lower the risk of UTI, but it does not advocate for routine circumcision [34]. The decision to perform circumcision for recurrent UTIs should be made with medical consultation, considering factors such as the character of the infections (upper and lower urinary tract), frequency and severity of infections, age, presence of other risk factors, and the potential benefits and risks of the procedure.

Potential Benefits of Neonatal Circumcision

While circumcision is a personal decision with cultural, religious, and medical considerations, it is crucial to understand the potential benefits associated with the procedure. Multiple studies have explored the protective effects of circumcision against various medical conditions, including urinary tract infections, penile cancer, and sexually transmitted infections.

Reduced Risk of Urinary Tract Infections

Circumcision is associated with a decreased risk of urinary tract infections in infancy, particularly in the first year of life. However, the overall incidence of UTIs in infant males is low, and the number needed to treat to prevent one UTI through circumcision is relatively high [35]. The protective effect of circumcision is thought to result from the removal of the foreskin, which can harbor bacteria, increasing the risk of infection [36].

The risk of UTI for boys is the highest in the first year of life. This risk is significantly higher in uncircumcised boys, but this trend begins normalizing after 6 months, to a similar risk after 1 year. Circumcision provides about a ten-fold decrease in the risk of UTIs [35]. The risk is even higher for boys with an additional risk factor, such as an underlying urologic abnormality [37].

Reduced Risk of Sexually Transmitted Infections

Research indicates that male circumcision can reduce the risk of certain sexually transmitted infections, including HIV, herpes simplex virus type 2, and human papillomavirus [7]. A meta-analysis of randomized controlled trials found that male circumcision reduced the risk of HIV acquisition in men by approximately 60% [23]. Circumcision should not be offered as the only strategy for HIV and other STI reduction and prevention; other methods of risk reduction, including safe sexual practices and barrier methods, should be emphasized [35].

The protective effects of circumcision against STIs may be attributed to the removal of the foreskin, which can harbor pathogens and facilitate transmission. However, other STIs, such as chlamydia, gonorrhea, genital herpes, and human papillomavirus, are not as significantly impacted by circumcision [38].

Prevention of Penile Cancer

Circumcision has been linked to a lower incidence of penile cancer, a rare malignancy that primarily affects uncircumcised men. Although circumcision can reduce the risk of penile cancer, the overall incidence of this disease is low, and other risk factors, such as HPV infection and poor hygiene, may play a more significant role [39]. Research indicates that the protective effect of circumcision performed in childhood or adolescence against invasive penile cancer is not sustained when analyses are limited to individuals without a history of phimosis [40]. In contrast, there was some evidence that circumcision in adulthood was associated with an increased risk of invasive penile cancer [23, 35]. Human papillomavirus is the causative agent for penile cancer and cervical cancer, and is more commonly carried by uncircumcised men [41].

For all indications and potential benefits, circumcision should only be performed after obtaining informed consent and confirming that a thorough history and physical examination have identified no contraindications. The patient and/or their parents must be counseled on the potential benefits, risks, and limitations of the procedure, as well as any reasonable alternatives. Preoperative planning should include a discussion of anesthetic options and pain management strategies appropriate for the child's age. The choice of surgical technique, postoperative dressing, and detailed aftercare instructions should also be clearly communicated and tailored to the individual case.

Contraindications

Circumcision should be deferred in the presence of medical conditions that increase the risk of bleeding or impair wound healing. Neonatal circumcision is contraindicated in infants with known bleeding disorders, such as hemophilia or von Willebrand disease. If circumcision is considered in these patients, it should be performed in a controlled surgical setting, with appropriate hematologic support and meticulous hemostasis [35, 42]. Adequate vitamin K administration is also essential prior to circumcision, as vitamin K deficiency in the newborn period can increase the risk of bleeding [43, 44]. In North America, intramuscular vitamin K is routinely administered at birth, and many providers will not proceed with circumcision unless it has been given. In contrast, some European countries favor oral vitamin K regimens, which may vary in efficacy and timing [45]. These differences in practice should be taken into account when planning circumcision in the neonatal period.

In premature or medically unstable infants, the procedure is typically postponed until the child's condition has stabilized, ensuring optimal tolerance to the intervention and minimizing potential complications [46, 47]. While there is no universally accepted age or weight cutoff, some practitioners recommend avoiding newborn circumcision techniques in infants older than 6 weeks or weighing more than 5 kilograms, due to an increased risk of bleeding or suboptimal outcomes [48, 49]. However, these thresholds are not absolute, and many practitioners continue to use newborn techniques beyond these limits based on clinical judgment and institutional protocols.

Anatomical contraindications to circumcision include congenital penile anomalies such as micropenis, significant penile torsion, concealed penis, penoscrotal webbing, ambiguous genitalia, epispadias, chordee, and most cases of hypospadias (Fig. 3.4). However, if hypospadias is confirmed to be truly distal and the foreskin removal will not affect potential future repair, neonatal circumcision may be safely performed [50]. In general, the foreskin is an important tissue for reconstructive penile procedures, and premature circumcision in the presence of these anomalies may compromise surgical planning, limit reconstructive options, and negatively impact both functional and cosmetic outcomes [46, 51].

Surgical Techniques for Newborn Circumcision

Gomco Clamp

The Gomco clamp technique, a widely employed surgical method for newborn circumcision, involves the use of a specialized instrument consisting of a metal clamp, a cone-shaped base, and a screw mechanism (Fig. 3.5). During the procedure, the foreskin is drawn over the cone and secured in place with the clamp, which compresses the foreskin and restricts blood flow. After a period of several minutes, the compressed foreskin is surgically excised, leaving a clean, circular incision. The Gomco clamp technique offers several advantages, including precise control over the amount of foreskin removed and a relatively low risk of bleeding [52].

However, it is crucial to select the correct size of the Gomco bell and clamp, properly position the foreskin through the hole of the Gomco base plate, and accurately assess the amount of foreskin to be removed, to avoid complications such as poor cosmetic outcomes [52].

Mogen Clamp

The Mogen clamp technique, an alternative surgical method for newborn circumcision, utilizes a compressive instrument with two opposing flat arms that are advanced along the redundant foreskin, and, after assuring that the glans lies below these

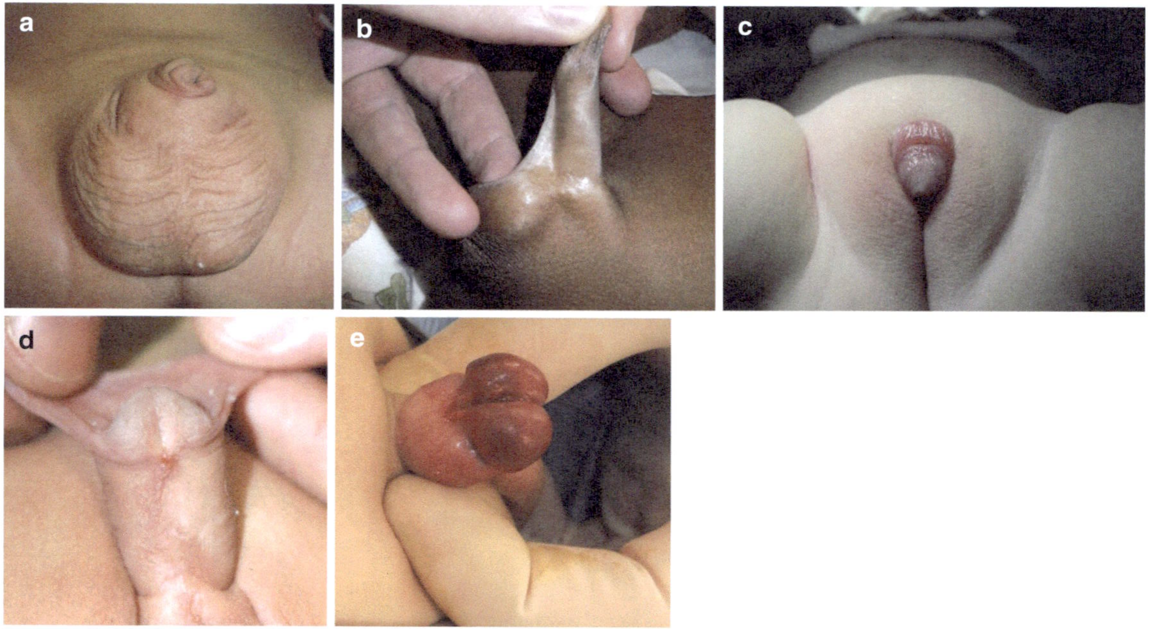

Fig. 3.4 Penile anomalies that contraindicate circumcision. (**a**) Concealed penis, (**b**) Webbed penis, (**c**) Ambiguous genitalia, (**d**) Hypospadias, (**e**) Epispadias

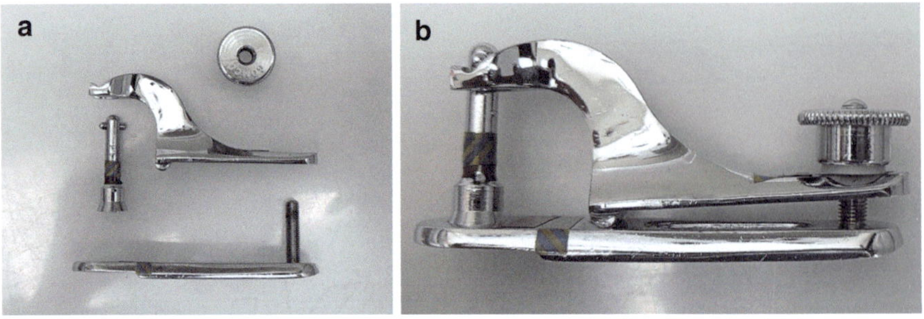

Fig. 3.5 Gomco clamp: (**a**) shows the disassembled clamp: bell, base plate, yoke, and nut; (**b**) assembled clamp

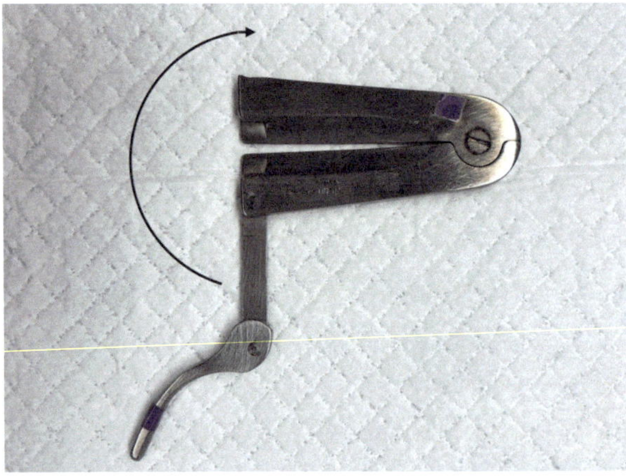

Fig. 3.6 Mogen clamp

arms, they are closed to clamp and compress the redundant distal foreskin (Fig. 3.6). The foreskin is drawn through the clamp and positioned for excision, after which the blades are closed to crush and cut the foreskin simultaneously along a line that is 1 mm wide, and the foreskin is excised distal to the clamp [53]. The Mogen clamp technique offers a short surgical time, typically lasting only seconds to a few minutes, and allows for good control over the amount of foreskin removed, making it suitable for use on small penises [54].

Similar to the Gomco, the most common complications associated with the Mogen clamp technique include bleeding and inadequate foreskin removal, both of which may necessitate revision surgery. Careful attention to surgical technique and proper patient selection are essential to minimize the risk of complications and ensure optimal outcomes with the Mogen clamp technique [53, 54]. Although generally considered safe, instances of partial glans amputation have been reported with the Mogen clamp, underscoring the importance of caution and experience when using this device [55, 56].

This technique is known for its speed and simplicity, making it a popular choice among some practitioners, in particular Jewish mohels performing Brit Milah [53, 54].

Plastibell Device

The Plastibell technique involves placing a plastic ring over the glans and tying a suture around the foreskin, constricting blood flow to the foreskin distal to the ring (Fig. 3.7). Over the next few days, the foreskin dries and falls off, typically within 5–10 days. The Plastibell technique offers the advantage of not requiring surgical excision of the foreskin, reducing the risk of bleeding and infection [57, 58].

However, complications such as ring migration, delayed separation, and discomfort have been reported. Parents should be informed of the expected timeframe for Plastibell separation and instructed to seek medical attention if complications arise [24, 59].

In summary, the choice of surgical technique for circumcision depends on factors such as surgeon preference, patient age, anatomical considerations, and the presence of underlying medical conditions.

Modified Circumcision Clamp

Inspired by the classic Mogen clamp, a modified circumcision clamp features a large hollow center with atraumatic edges, designed to keep the glans penis away from the surgical field [60]. Unlike the standard Mogen clamp, the modified version incorporates a sliding bar that adjusts to accommodate varying penis sizes, ensuring

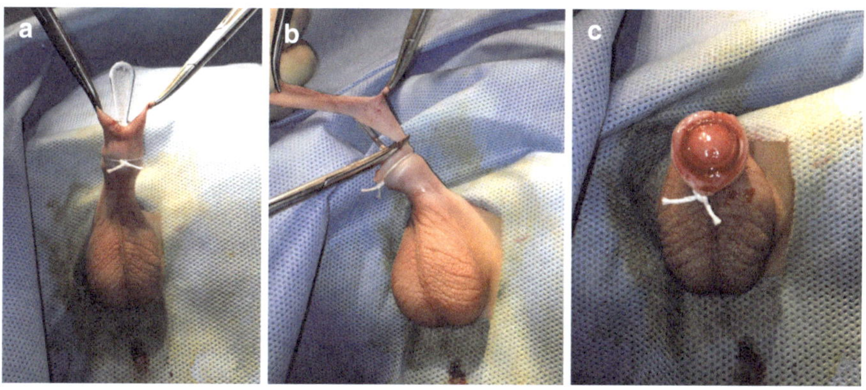

Fig. 3.7 Plastibell device: after release of glanular adhesions, the device is placed over the glans (**a**). Once it is secured with silk over its groove, the redundant foreskin is excised (**b**). Final result of the procedure (**c**)

precise foreskin removal [53]. Surgeons can remove the foreskin with the clamp, which can lead to an optimal cosmetic outcome [57].

Selecting the appropriate surgical technique for circumcision depends on a variety of factors, including the age and size of the patient, the surgeon's experience and preferences, and the specific clinical circumstances. Regardless of the technique chosen, meticulous attention to detail, proper pain management, and adherence to sterile technique are essential to ensure a safe and successful outcome. Every clinician performing circumcision occasionally has concerns or questions regarding the procedure [52]. By anticipating potential difficulties and developing strategies for dealing with them, the practitioner can become more confident in his or her ability to provide safe, effective circumcision services [52]. Furthermore, regardless of the chosen method, controlling the amount of removed prepuce allows these devices to be employed even on smaller penises [54].

In some instances, a partial dorsal slit may be created to facilitate proper retraction of the foreskin, potentially accompanied by skin crushing for a short duration [61]. In addition, alternative techniques, along with specialized in situ devices that crush the foreskin while simultaneously ensuring hemostasis, have been developed to improve effectiveness and minimize the risk of complications [62].

Alternatives for Anesthesia and Pain Management in Neonatal Circumcision

Effective pain management is an essential component of circumcision, especially in the pediatric population. Neonates experience pain, and, therefore, anesthesia should be provided to all newborns undergoing circumcision, irrespective of the technique used [59]. Several methods of anesthesia and analgesia are available, including topical anesthetics, local anesthetic injections, and systemic analgesics [35].

Local Anesthesia

Penile block using local anesthetics represents a frequently employed method for pain control during circumcision. Lidocaine, with or without epinephrine, is commonly used for nerve blocks, administered approximately 5 minutes prior to the procedure [35].

A dorsal penile nerve block entails injecting 0.2 to 0.4 mL of lidocaine or bupivacaine subcutaneously at the base of the penis in the 10 and 2 o'clock positions to anesthetize both branches of the dorsal penile nerve [59].

A ring block involves injecting 0.8 mL of local anesthetic subcutaneously around the perimeter of the base of the penis [59]. Studies show that either a ring block or a dorsal penile nerve block is more effective than topical lidocaine/prilocaine alone [59, 63].

Topical Anesthetics

Topical anesthetics, such as lidocaine–prilocaine cream, can provide local analgesia when applied to the foreskin 30 to 60 minutes before the procedure [59]. While topical anesthetics are generally safe and well-tolerated, their efficacy may be limited by the depth of penetration and the duration of action.

The pain-relieving effects of EMLA cream (Eutectic Mixture of Local Anesthetics, containing lidocaine and prilocaine) have been demonstrated when used prior to newborn circumcision [59].

Systemic Analgesics

Systemic analgesics, such as acetaminophen or ibuprofen, may be administered preoperatively and postoperatively to alleviate pain and discomfort. Sucrose pacifiers are another possible analgesic option in neonatal circumcisions [59]. However, in certain instances, a combination of general anesthesia with a penile nerve block may be utilized to offer optimal postoperative pain relief and ensure child satisfaction [64]. Parents should be educated on the importance of administering pain medication as prescribed and monitoring for any adverse effects.

Pediatric and Adolescent Surgical Circumcision Techniques Beyond the Newborn Period

Surgical Excision

These techniques are familiar to most urologists as they are also those utilized in the adult population. Surgical excision of the foreskin is a technique that allows precise control over the amount of foreskin removed and can be tailored to address specific anatomical variations or underlying conditions [65]. Surgical excision may be the preferred approach in cases of pathologic phimosis, older children, or other foreskin abnormalities that require more extensive surgical intervention [24]. There are many surgical techniques described for circumcision. All techniques typically involve separating adhesions between the foreskin and glans, excising the foreskin, and achieving hemostasis [1]. Surgical approaches require more surgical skill and are usually performed in the operating room under general anesthesia, although consideration of sedation and proper local anesthetic techniques may be considered in selected patients. Circumcision devices used in newborns have occasionally been employed in older boys, but seem to be less adequate. As a result, most circumcisions are conducted by the sleeve or freehand techniques [24].

With the sleeve technique, the inner and outer layers of the foreskin are incised circumferentially, and the preputial skin is reapproximated using absorbable sutures following hemostasis (Fig. 3.8) [24]. Alternatively, the dorsal slit procedure entails making a longitudinal incision along the dorsal aspect of the foreskin to release the

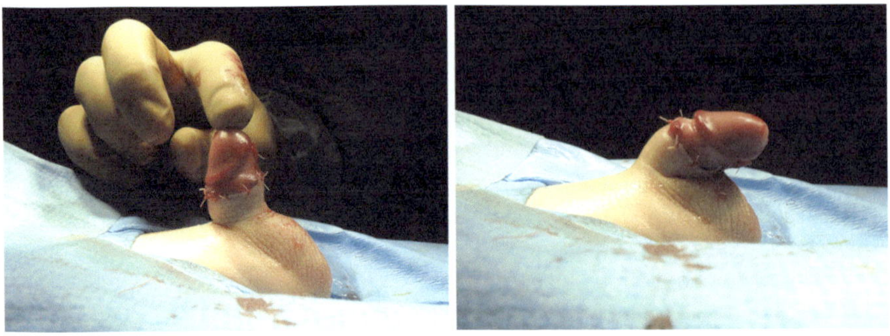

Fig. 3.8 Final result of circumcision using a sleeve technique

constriction and allow for foreskin retraction [60]. The relationship between circumcision and the incidence of complications remains controversial; however, some evidence suggests a positive correlation between increased complications and circumcisions performed after the neonatal period [66].

Complications following circumcision, although infrequent, can encompass a range of issues such as bleeding, infection, inadequate foreskin removal, meatal stenosis, and, in exceedingly rare instances, glans amputation [67, 68]. Overzealous circumcision may result in shaft skin excision, requiring surgical reconstruction using techniques such as full-thickness skin grafts or tissue expanders [67].

Regardless of the technique employed, meticulous surgical technique, proficient pain management, and thorough postoperative care are paramount to minimizing complications and ensuring patient satisfaction [35, 54, 67].

Potential Risks and Complications of Circumcision

While circumcision is generally considered a safe procedure, it is not without potential risks and complications, including fatalities [69]. Potential risks and complications include bleeding, infection, inadequate skin removal, pain, meatal stenosis, and injury to the glans, and fatalities have been reported. Hence, like any other intervention, appropriate informed consent must be obtained, and expectations of the family consenting must be understood [69].

Bleeding

Bleeding is the most common complication of circumcision, with an incidence of 1% in a large retrospective review, typically occurring within the first 24 hours after the procedure (Fig. 3.9) [70]. Careful attention to hemostasis during the procedure, along with allowing adequate time for skin edge compression during newborn circumcisions, are crucial steps that can prevent most bleeding cases. Despite these precautions, clot dislodgement or cautery eschar formation may still occur,

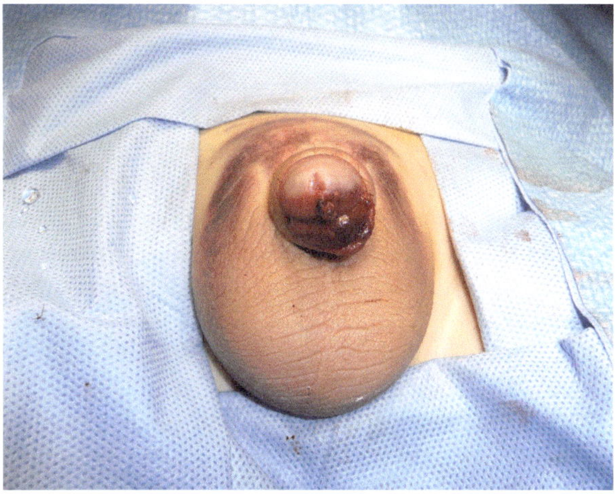

Fig. 3.9 Bleeding after circumcision. Note the hematoma that compromises the mucosa collar and penile shaft

potentially leading to bleeding complications [71]. In most cases, bleeding is minor and can be controlled with direct pressure or application of a topical hemostatic agent [34]. However, in rare instances, significant bleeding may require further intervention, such as sutures or electrocautery [71].

A hematologic workup is warranted only in patients who persistently bleed or bleed significantly. Any patient with a known bleeding disorder should have their circumcision delayed until they are medically cleared for surgery [72].

Infection

Infection is another potential complication of circumcision, although the risk is generally low when proper sterile technique is used [70]. Signs of infection may include increased pain, redness, swelling, pus, or fever. Topical or oral antibiotics are typically prescribed to treat infections, and in some cases, surgical drainage may be necessary [73].

To prevent infection, surgeons should adhere to strict sterile techniques during the procedure, using appropriate antiseptic solutions and sterile instruments. Parents should be educated on proper wound care, including keeping the area clean and dry, and changing dressings as directed. Parents should also be advised to watch for any signs of infection, such as increased redness, swelling, or discharge from the circumcision site, and seek medical attention promptly if any concerns arise [74].

Severe infections, such as necrotizing fasciitis, have been reported after Plastibell circumcision. Though rare, these infections highlight the need for meticulous surgical technique and vigilant aftercare. Signs and symptoms include pronounced redness, hardening, and disproportionate pain, accompanied by a rapid heart rate, elevated white blood cell count, or increased band cells. These infections are typically polymicrobial, necessitating broad-spectrum antibiotics effective against Gram-negative, Gram-positive, and anaerobic organisms. Prompt surgical assessment and debridement of necrotic tissue are critical to prevent further complications [75, 76].

Loss of Skin/Wound Dehiscence

Wound dehiscence and skin injuries of the shaft can occur with any of the surgical techniques described above. This can happen when an excess of penile skin is drawn into the clamp and then amputated. Less likely, improper determination of the amount of skin to remove during a surgical circumcision may occur. In addition, when there is a significant degree of penoscrotal webbing which is not recognized, ventral skin dehiscence may result. These types of injuries are treated with local wound care, allowing the penile skin and mucosa to heal by secondary intention (Fig. 3.10) [77]. In severe cases of significant skin loss, auto-grafting has shown good cosmetic and functional results [78, 79].

Trapped Penis

Trapped penis is a rare complication in which the penile shaft becomes trapped beneath the skin of the scrotum or suprapubic area (Fig. 3.11). This can occur if the

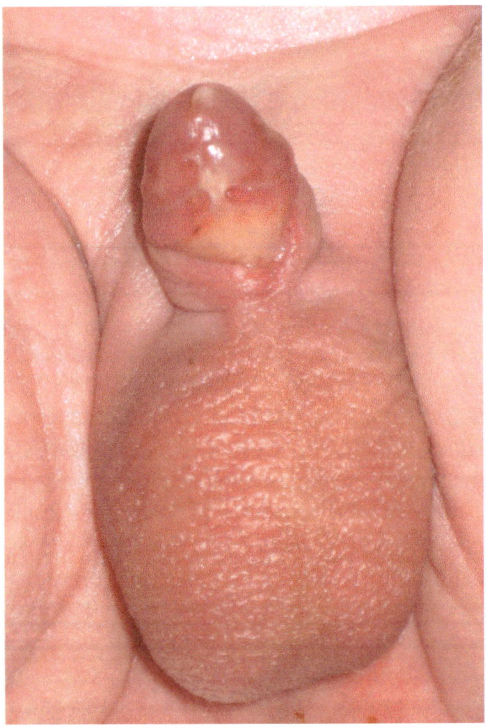

Fig. 3.10 Ventral dehiscence after neonatal circumcision

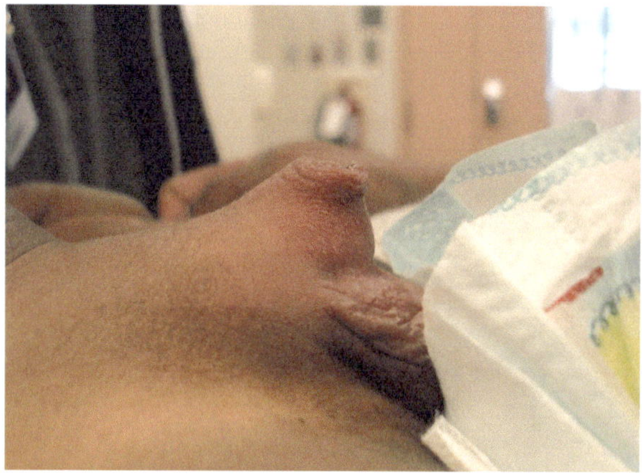

Fig. 3.11 Trapped penis following circumcision. Note the constricting scar ring over the glans, resulting in penile entrapment

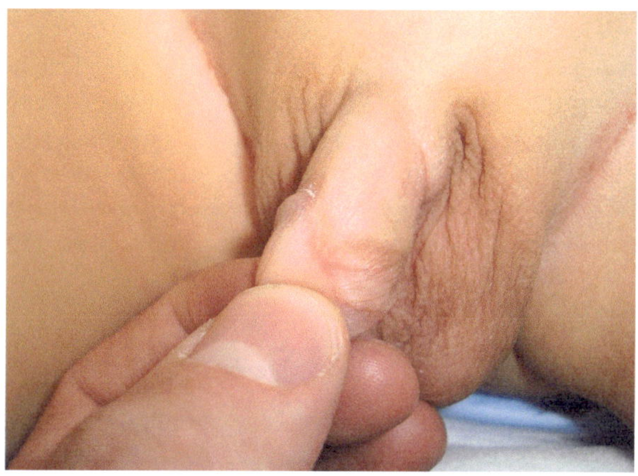

Fig. 3.12 Glanular adhesions after circumcision. Note the adherence of residual preputial skin to the glans penis

circumcision incision is made too close to the base of the penis, resulting in inadequate skin coverage and subsequent secondary phimosis from the progressive closure of the skin over the glans [80]. Compressing the suprapubic fat pad to best determine the amount of penile skin that can be removed during the procedure helps prevent this complication, underscoring the importance of precise surgical technique and a thorough understanding of penile anatomy during circumcision. In most situations, a trapped penis can be corrected with local tissue rearrangement or, in severe cases, with skin grafting [79, 81].

Glanular Adhesions and Skin Bridges

Glanular adhesions and skin bridges are relatively frequent complications following neonatal circumcision, especially if meticulous surgical technique and diligent post-operative care are not observed (Fig. 3.12) [77]. These adhesions commonly arise from either inadequate lysis of preputial adhesions before the procedure or distal migration of the skin due to a prominent suprapubic fat pad. Minor adhesions often resolve spontaneously or with gentle manual retraction. However, persistent or more substantial skin bridges may necessitate surgical lysis to mitigate potential complications, including pain, compromised hygiene, or sexual dysfunction (Fig. 3.13) [80]. This surgical procedure typically involves meticulous dissection and sharp division of the adhesions after a period of compression with a hemostatic instrument, followed by careful approximation of the skin edges using either skin glue or stitches to prevent recurrence [82].

Injury to the Glans

Injury to the glans penis is a rare but serious complication of circumcision. Glandular necrosis can occur as a result of cautery injury or from distal migration of an incorrectly sized Plastibell ring [71]. During circumcision, the glans penis is at risk of injury from direct trauma, excessive heat from cautery, or compression from instruments (Fig. 3.14). In severe cases, injury to the glans may require surgical repair or reconstruction [59, 83]. There have been rare descriptions of glans amputation resulting from the use of guillotine-type devices during circumcision. To minimize the risk of injury to the glans penis, surgeons should employ meticulous surgical techniques, ensuring adequate protection of the glans throughout the procedure and avoiding the application of excessive force or heat [55, 56].

Meatal Stenosis

Meatal stenosis, or narrowing of the urethral opening, is a relatively common late consequence of circumcision (Fig. 3.15). The etiology of meatal stenosis is thought to be due to the exposure of the glans to the ammonia in urine after the foreskin has

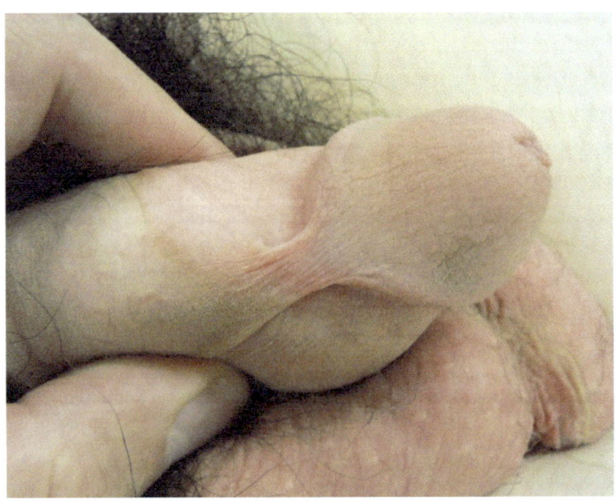

Fig. 3.13 The image demonstrates a fully epithelialized skin bridge extending over the glans penis

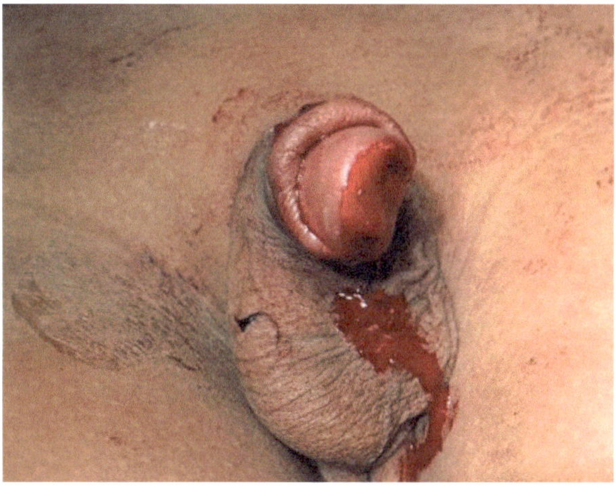

Fig. 3.14 Partial glans amputation following a clamp circumcision. Observe the loss of distal glans tissue consistent with device-related injury

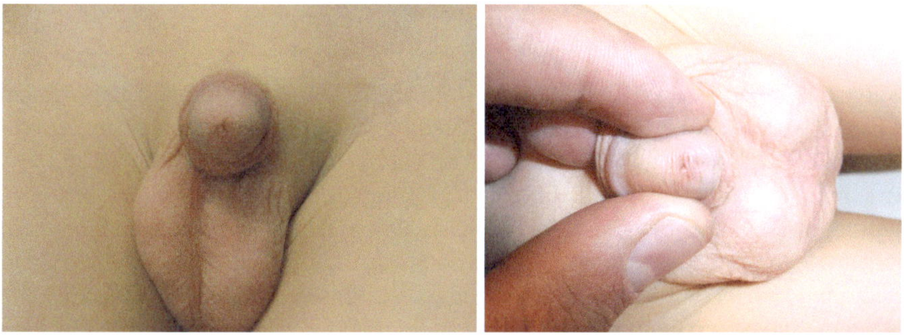

Fig. 3.15 Severe meatal stenosis. The image demonstrates a markedly narrowed, pinpoint external urethral opening

been removed or the ligation of the frenular artery [84]. While the meatus may appear small, it can open adequately during voiding; this explains why most children with meatal stenosis do not present it until after toilet training. In severe cases, meatal stenosis can cause difficulty with urination, a weak urinary stream, and pain [71].

Meatal stenosis is usually prevented by advising parents to apply petroleum jelly liberally to the glans postprocedure [35]. Treatment for meatal stenosis typically involves surgical meatal dilatation or meatotomy [71].

Fatalities After Neonatal Circumcision

Death resulting from circumcision is exceedingly rare [80]. A recent study from one institution describes seven boys ages 6–35 days who were admitted to the ICU as a result of severe bleeding or sepsis. Five infants out of the seven required ICU care for up to 18 days, and two patients died as a consequence of septic or hemorrhagic shock. The study authors estimated the annual incidence of severe complications necessitating hospitalization following neonatal circumcision to be 0.01%, with a 0.0012% fatality rate based on a 14-year review [69].

Circumcision in Different Age Groups

The risks and benefits of circumcision may vary depending on the age at which the procedure is performed [55]. Neonatal circumcision, performed within the first few weeks of life, is associated with a lower risk of complications, faster healing, and lower cost compared to circumcision performed later in life [85]. Neonates and infants experience fewer complications compared to older boys, likely due to the procedure's simplicity and the newborn's healing capabilities [84].

Neonatal Circumcision

Neonatal circumcision is commonly performed for cultural, religious, and medical reasons. Neonates have a lower risk of bleeding during circumcision due to several anatomical and physiological factors. In newborns, the foreskin is thinner and less vascularized, reducing the likelihood of significant bleeding during its removal. Furthermore, the penile blood vessels are smaller and less developed, making them less prone to injury and easier to seal. In addition, routine administration of vitamin K at birth enhances coagulation, providing an additional protective factor against bleeding in this population [35, 71]. One study reported that the ideal timeframe for a "pain-free" circumcision is during the first week of life [71]. The advantage of circumcision in the neonatal period is that it is associated with a lower risk of complications and faster healing. Circumcision performed in the neonatal period demonstrates superior cost-effectiveness compared to the procedure when performed later in life, primarily due to a reduced risk of complications and more rapid healing times in neonates [85].

Circumcision in Older Children and Adolescents

Circumcision performed in older children and adolescents is associated with a higher risk of complications, increased pain, and longer recovery times compared to neonatal circumcision [35]. Older children may also experience greater psychological distress related to the procedure, particularly if it is performed without adequate preparation and support. Furthermore, a study has shown that complications increase significantly when circumcision is performed after 1 year of age. When complications do occur, especially surgical complications, specialist referral may be required for evaluation and reoperation [71].

From a medical perspective, surgical intervention in older children and adolescents is typically considered only when the patient presents with recurring infections or a specific medical condition, such as phimosis, where circumcision is required as a therapeutic measure. Given the increased risks and potential for psychological distress associated with circumcision at this age, a thorough evaluation and discussion of alternative treatment options are warranted before proceeding with surgery [74, 84]. It is also essential to ensure that the child or adolescent is fully informed about the procedure and actively participates in the decision-making process.

Postoperative Care and Follow-Up

Proper postoperative care is essential for ensuring optimal healing and minimizing the risk of complications after circumcision. Parents should be provided with detailed instructions on wound care, pain management, and signs of potential complications.

Following circumcision, it is generally recommended to apply a sterile dressing or topical ointment to the surgical site to promote healing and prevent infection. A skin barrier, such as petroleum jelly, is recommended until the skin edge has fully healed, generally by 2 weeks [35]. Parents should be instructed to gently clean the area with mild soap and water during diaper changes and to avoid using harsh chemicals or scrubbing the wound vigorously. In addition, parents are advised to observe for signs of infection, such as increased redness, swelling, drainage, or fever, and to seek medical attention if any concerns arise [85].

Wound Care Instructions

Wound care instructions typically include keeping the area clean and dry, applying a topical ointment. For procedures employing the Plastibell device, application of a topical antimicrobial preparation, such as mupirocin, to the surgical site two to three times daily is recommended until the device undergoes spontaneous separation [58]. Parents should be instructed to gently clean the area with mild soap and water during diaper changes and to avoid using harsh chemicals or scrubbing the wound vigorously [85]. Parents should also be advised to avoid using baby wipes that contain alcohol or fragrances, as these may irritate the wound.

Signs of Infection

Parents should be educated on the signs of infection, such as increased redness, swelling, drainage, or fever. They should be instructed to seek medical attention promptly if any of these signs develop, as early intervention can prevent more serious complications [71].

Conclusion: A Balanced View on Circumcision

Circumcision in the pediatric population is a complex and controversial topic, with passionate advocates and detractors on both sides. Physicians should accurately and impartially present information about the potential benefits and risks of circumcision, and parents' decisions regarding the procedure should be respected [35]. Ultimately, the decision to circumcise a child is a personal one that should be made by the parents after careful consideration of all relevant factors.

Medical conditions of the foreskin or urinary tract infections can present during childhood and adolescence. Pediatricians and urologists should be knowledgeable about these conditions to offer families the most appropriate therapeutic options for their children. When medically indicated, circumcision can provide significant benefits, alleviating symptoms, preventing recurrent infections, and improving overall quality of life [86].

By providing comprehensive information and respecting parental autonomy, healthcare professionals can play a crucial role in supporting families as they navigate this complex and deeply personal decision [7, 87, 88]. It is also vital for all medical staff to be aware of the various operative techniques and their complications to cope with these consultations with an evidence base [89]. The debate around pediatric circumcision continues, highlighting the importance of understanding the procedure's history, benefits, and risks [90].

References

1. Abdulwahab-Ahmed A, Mungadi I. Techniques of male circumcision. J Surg Tech Case Rep [Internet]. 2013 [cited 2025 Jun 7];5(1):1. Available from: http://www.jstcr.org/text.asp?2013/5/1/1/118588.
2. Abusharaf RM. Virtuous cuts: female genital circumcision in an African ontology. Differences [Internet]. 2001;12(1):112–40. Available from: https://doi.org/10.1215/10407391-12-1-112.
3. Lebese RT, Mothiba TM, Mulaudzi MT, Mashau NS, Makhado L. Rite of passage: an African indigenous knowledge perspective. In: Working with indigenous knowledge: strategies for health professionals [Internet]; 2022. p. 51–68. Available from: https://doi.org/10.4102/aosis.2022.bk296.04.
4. Khademi G, Abbasi MA, Bahreini A, Saeidi M. Customs and desirable after childbirth, in Islam. DOAJ DOAJ Dir Open Access J [Internet]. 2016. Available from: https://doaj.org/article/1313e72880fd4753b439414893e99d00.
5. Shapiro E. American academy of pediatrics policy statements on circumcision and urinary tract infection. PubMed [Internet]. 1999;1(3):154–6. Available from: https://pubmed.ncbi.nlm.nih.gov/16985788.
6. Morris BJ, Krieger JN. The contrasting evidence concerning the effect of male circumcision on sexual function, sensation, and pleasure: a systematic review [Internet]. In: Sexual medicine, vol. 8. Elsevier BV; 2020. p. 577–98. Available from: https://doi.org/10.1016/j.esxm.2020.08.011.
7. Blank S, Brady MT, Buerk E, Carlo WA, Diekema DS, Freedman AL, et al. Male circumcision. Pediatrics [Internet]. 2012;130(3). Available from: https://doi.org/10.1542/peds.2012-1990.
8. Sarvestani AS, Bufumbo L, Geiger JD, Sienko KH. Traditional male circumcision in uganda: a qualitative focus group discussion analysis. PLoS ONE [Internet]. 2012;7(10). Available from: https://doi.org/10.1371/journal.pone.0045316.

9. Shezi MH, Tlou B, Naidoo S. Knowledge, attitudes and acceptance of voluntary medical male circumcision among males attending high school in Shiselweni region, Eswatini: a cross sectional study. BMC Public Health [Internet]. 2023;23(1). Available from: https://doi.org/10.1186/s12889-023-15228-3.
10. Medical Ethics, Human rights and law [Internet]. 2019. Available from: https://www.circinfo.org/ethics.html.
11. The Ethics of Circumcision [Internet]. 2022. Available from: https://www.researchgate.net/publication/360554804_The_Ethics_of_Circumcision.
12. Mwashambwa MY, Mwampagatwa I, Rastagaev A, Gesase AP. The male circumcision: the oldest ancient procedure, its past, present and future roles. [Internet]. Tanzan J Health Res. 2013;15. Available from: https://doi.org/10.4314/thrb.v15i3.8
13. Doyle D. Ritual male circumcision: a brief history. J R Coll Physicians Edinb [Internet]. 2005;35(3):279–85. Available from: https://doi.org/10.1177/1478271520053503005.
14. Dunsmuir WD, Gordon EM. The history of circumcision. BJU Int [Internet]. 1999;83:1–12. Available from: https://doi.org/10.1046/j.1464-410x.1999.0830s1001.x.
15. Anwar MS, Munawar F, Anwar Q. Circumcision: a religious obligation or 'the cruellest of cuts'? Br J Gen Pract [Internet]. 2009;60(570):59–61. Available from: https://doi.org/10.3399/bjgp10x482194.
16. Novik A. The rite of male circumcision among the Muslim population in the Western Balkans. Folk Electron J Folk [Internet]. 2020;80:151–68. Available from: https://doi.org/10.7592/fejf2020.80.novik.
17. Morris BJ, Wiswell TE. Circumcision and lifetime risk of urinary tract infection: a systematic review and meta-analysis [Internet]. J Urol. Lippincott Williams & Wilkins. 2012;189:2118–24. Available from: https://doi.org/10.1016/j.juro.2012.11.114.
18. Schoen EJ, Colby CJ, Ray GT. Newborn circumcision decreases incidence and costs of urinary tract infections during the first year of life. Pediatrics [Internet]. 2000;105(4):789–93. Available from: https://doi.org/10.1542/peds.105.4.789.
19. Winberg J, Gothefors L, Bollgren I, Herthelius M, Tullus K. The prepuce: a mistake of nature? The Lancet [Internet]. 1989;333(8638):598–9. Available from: https://doi.org/10.1016/s0140-6736(89)91619-x.
20. Allen T, Razavi SE, Court NB. Immunotherapy and penis cancer. Pharm Pharmacol Int J [Internet]. 2019;7(1). Available from: https://doi.org/10.15406/ppij.2019.07.00224.
21. Douglawi A, Masterson TA. Updates on the epidemiology and risk factors for penile cancer [Internet]. In: Translational andrology and urology, vol. 6. AME Publishing Company; 2017. p. 785–90. Available from: https://doi.org/10.21037/tau.2017.05.19.
22. Tseng HF, Morgenstern H, Mack TM, Peters R. Risk factors for penile cancer: results of a population-based case-control study in Los Angeles County (United States). Cancer Causes Control [Internet]. 2001;12(3):267–77. Available from: https://doi.org/10.1023/a:1011266405062s.
23. Blank S, Brady MT, Buerk E, Carlo WA, Diekema DS, Freedman AL, et al. Circumcision policy statement. Pediatrics [Internet]. 2012;130(3):585–6. Available from: https://doi.org/10.1542/peds.2012-1989.
24. Hayashi Y, Kojima Y, Mizuno K, Kohri K. Prepuce: phimosis, paraphimosis, and circumcision. Sci World J [Internet]. 2011 [cited 2025 Jun 7];11:289–301. Available from: http://www.hindawi.com/journals/tswj/2011/405910/abs/.
25. Shahid SK. Phimosis in children. ISRN Urol [Internet]. 2012;2012:1–6. Available from: https://doi.org/10.5402/2012/707329.
26. de Abreu MRP, Quezado MIM, Valdenize T, Moreno JH, de Amorim RFB. Experiences in the care and treatment of children and adolescents with phimosis. Arch Pediatr Surg [Internet]. 2021;5(1). Available from: https://doi.org/10.36959/472/365.
27. Salhadine YA, Teko DV, Kebalo SP, Donou AA, Sibabi-Akpo O, Sekoudji E, et al. Phimosis and paraphimosis in children: about 7 cases in the pediatric surgery Department of the Sylvanus Olympio University Hospital in Lomé (Togo). OALib [Internet]. 2022;9(12):1–5. Available from: https://doi.org/10.4236/oalib.1109499.

28. Pandya I, Shinojia M, Vadukul D, Marfatia YS. Approach to balanitis/balanoposthitis: current guidelines. Indian J Sex Transm Dis AIDS [Internet]. 2014;35(2):155. Available from: https://doi.org/10.4103/0253-7184.142415.
29. Shabbir M, Barod R, Hegarty PK, Minhas S. Primary prevention and vaccination for penile cancer. Ther Adv Urol [Internet]. 2012;5(3):161–9. Available from: https://doi.org/10.1177/1756287212465456.
30. Morris BJ, Krieger JN. Balanitis and related inflammatory conditions affecting the penis. 2018. Available from: https://books.publisso.de/en/publisso_gold/publishing/books/overview/52/22.
31. Prendergast MA. Prevalence of urinary tract infection in childhood: a meta-analysis. J Emerg Med [Internet]. 2009;36(1):101. Available from: https://doi.org/10.1016/j.jemermed.2008.09.011.
32. Robinson J, Finlay JC, Lang M, Bortolussi R. Urinary tract infections in infants and children: diagnosis and management. Paediatr Child Health [Internet]. 2014;19(6):315–9. Available from: https://doi.org/10.1093/pch/19.6.315.
33. Singh-Grewal D. Circumcision for the prevention of urinary tract infection in boys: a systematic review of randomised trials and observational studies [Internet]. Arch Dis Childhood. BMJ. 2005;90:853–958. Available from: https://doi.org/10.1136/adc.2004.049353.
34. Yang SSD, Hsieh CH, Chang SJ. Effects of circumcision on urinary tract infection and sexually transmitted disease. Tzu Chi Med J [Internet]. 2009;21(3):185–9. Available from: https://doi.org/10.1016/s1016-3190(09)60037-9.
35. Zeitler M, Rayala B. Neonatal circumcision. Prim Care Clin Off Pract [Internet]. 2021 Dec [cited 2025 Jun 7];48(4):597–611. Available from: https://linkinghub.elsevier.com/retrieve/pii/S0095454321016079.
36. Tewary K, Narchi H. Recurrent urinary tract infections in children: preventive interventions other than prophylactic antibiotics. World J Methodol [Internet]. 2015;5(2):13. Available from: https://doi.org/10.5662/wjm.v5.i2.13.
37. Pinto K. Circumcision controversies. Pediatr Clin North Am [Internet]. 2012 [cited 2025 Jun 7];59(4):977–86. Available from: https://linkinghub.elsevier.com/retrieve/pii/S0031395512000880.
38. Howe RSV. Sexually transmitted infections and male circumcision: a systematic review and meta-analysis [Internet]. ISRN Urol. Hindawi Publishing Corporation. 2013;2013:1–42. Available from: https://doi.org/10.1155/2013/109846.
39. Douglawi A, Masterson TA. Penile cancer epidemiology and risk factors: a contemporary review [Internet]. 2019. Available from: https://journals.lww.com/00042307-201903000-00014
40. Larke NL, Thomas SL, Dos Santos Silva I, Weiss HA. Male circumcision and penile cancer: a systematic review and meta-analysis. Cancer Causes Control [Internet]. 2011 Aug [cited 2025 Jun 7];22(8):1097–110. Available from: http://link.springer.com/10.1007/s10552-011-9785-9.
41. Schoen EJ. Should newborns be circumcised? Yes. PubMed [Internet]. 2007; Available from: https://pubmed.ncbi.nlm.nih.gov/18077736.
42. Bawazir OA, Alharbi I. Circumcision in hemophilia: a multicenter experience. J Pediatr Hematol Oncol [Internet]. 2021 Jan [cited 2025 Jul 6];43(1):e33–6. Available from: https://journals.lww.com/10.1097/MPH.0000000000001960.
43. Shearer MJ. Vitamin K deficiency bleeding (VKDB) in early infancy. Blood Rev [Internet]. 2009 Mar [cited 2025 Jul 9];23(2):49–59. Available from: https://linkinghub.elsevier.com/retrieve/pii/S0268960X08000520.
44. American Academy of Pediatrics Committee on Fetus and Newborn. Controversies concerning vitamin K and the newborn. American Academy of Pediatrics Committee on Fetus and Newborn. Pediatrics. 2003;112(1 Pt 1):191–2.
45. Cornelissen M, Von Kries R, Loughnan P, Schubiger G. Prevention of vitamin K deficiency bleeding: efficacy of different multiple oral dose schedules of vitamin K. Eur J Pediatr [Internet]. 1997 Jan 24 [cited 2025 Jul 9];156(2):126–130. Available from: http://link.springer.com/10.1007/s004310050570.

46. Alanis MC, Lucidi RS. Neonatal circumcision: a review of the world's oldest and most controversial operation. Obstet Gynecol Surv [Internet]. 2004 May [cited 2025 Jul 6];59(5):379–395. Available from: http://journals.lww.com/00006254-200405000-00026.
47. Slotkowski EL. Contraindications to neonatal circumcision. J Pediatr [Internet]. 1982 May [cited 2025 Jul 6];100(5):837. Available from: https://linkinghub.elsevier.com/retrieve/pii/S0022347682806124.
48. Task Force On Circumcision, Blank S, Brady M, Buerk E, Carlo W, Diekema D, et al. Circumcision policy statement. Pediatr Int 2012 Sep 1 [cited 2025 Jul 9];130(3):585–6. Available from: https://publications.aap.org/pediatrics/article/130/3/585/30235/Circumcision-Policy-Statement.
49. Stang HJ, Snellman LW. Circumcision practice patterns in the United States. Pediatr Int. 1998 Jun 1 [cited 2025 Jul 9];101(6):e5. Available from: https://publications.aap.org/pediatrics/article/101/6/e5/61768/Circumcision-Practice-Patterns-in-the-United.
50. Snodgrass WT, Khavari R. Prior circumcision does not complicate repair of hypospadias with an intact Prepuce. J Urol [Internet]. 2006 Jul [cited 2025 Jul 9];176(1):296–8. Available from: http://www.jurology.com/doi/10.1016/S0022-5347%2806%2900564-7.
51. Alter GJ, Horton CE, Horton CEJ. Buried penis as a contraindication for circumcision. J Am Coll Surg. 1994;178(5):487–90.
52. Peleg D, Steiner A. The Gomco circumcision: common problems and solutions. PubMed [Internet]. 1998;58(4):891–8. Available from: https://pubmed.ncbi.nlm.nih.gov/9767725.
53. Reynolds RD. Use of the Mogen clamp for neonatal circumcision. PubMed [Internet]. 1996;54(1):177–82. Available from: https://pubmed.ncbi.nlm.nih.gov/8677833.
54. Kaweblum YA, Press S, Kogan L, Levine M, Kaweblum M. Circumcision using the Mogen Clamp. Clin Pediatr (Phila) [Internet]. 1984;23(12):679–82. Available from: https://doi.org/10.1177/000992288402301204.
55. Salle JLP, de Jesus LE, Lorenzo AJ, Romao R, Figueroa V, Bägli D, et al. Glans amputation during routine neonatal circumcision: mechanism of injury and strategy for prevention. J Pediatr Urol [Internet]. 2012;9(6):763–8. Available from: https://doi.org/10.1016/j.jpurol.2012.09.012.
56. Strimling BS. Partial amputation of glans penis during Mogen Clamp circumcision. Pediatrics [Internet]. 1996;97(6):906–7. Available from: https://doi.org/10.1542/peds.97.6.906.
57. Peterson AC, Joyner BD, Allen RC. Plastibell template circumcision: a new technique. Urology [Internet]. 2001;58(4):603–4. Available from: https://doi.org/10.1016/s0090-4295(01)01308-5.
58. Pillai RG, Naieb ZA. Plastibell circumcision supported by a calcium-alginate fibre dressing to reduce bleeding. Arab J Urol [Internet]. 2015;13(3):179–81. Available from: https://doi.org/10.1016/j.aju.2015.04.001.
59. Omole F, Smith W, Carter-Wicker K. Newborn circumcision techniques. Am Fam Physician. 2020;101(11):680–5.
60. Güler Y. Comparison of a modified Mogen clamp and classic dorsal slit circumcision under local anesthesia: a clinical study. Curr Urol [Internet]. 2022;16(3):175–9. Available from: https://doi.org/10.1097/cu9.0000000000000083.
61. Luthra M, Gupta H. Plastibell circumcision in neonates: a review of procedure and analysis of complications [Internet]. Int J Paediatr Geriatrics. 2020;3:1–3. Available from: https://doi.org/10.33545/26643685.2020.v3.i1a.50.
62. Rosato E, Miano R, Germani S, Asimakopoulos AD. Phimosis in adults: narrative review of the new available devices and the standard treatments. Clin Pract [Internet]. 2024;14(1):361–76. Available from: https://doi.org/10.3390/clinpract14010028.
63. Soh CR, Ng SB, Lim SL. Dorsal penile nerve block. Pediatr Anesth [Internet] 2003;13(4):329–33. Available from: https://doi.org/10.1046/j.1460-9592.2003.01033.x.
64. Sharma NR, Timalsena P, Rai U. Penile nerve block at the base of penis in combination with intravenous ketamin plus midazolam versus general anaesthesia(GA) in children undergoing circumcision for post operative pain management in the Eastern Nepal. J Chitwan Med Coll [Internet]. 2014;4(1):33–6. Available from: https://doi.org/10.3126/jcmc.v4i1.10846.

65. Pietzsch TT. Fifty consecutive cases of circumcision with the "plastibell" circumcision device. Med J Aust [Internet]. 1971;1(26):1380–2. Available from: https://doi.org/10.5694/j.1326-5377.1971.tb50337.x.
66. Moosa S, Muhammad AA, Dogar S, Iftikhar S, Johnson W, Latif A, et al. Implementation of an infant male circumcision programme, Pakistan. Bull World Health Organ [Internet]. 2021 Apr 1 [cited 2025 Jul 5];99(4):250–8. Available from: https://www.ncbi.nlm.nih.gov/pmc/articles/PMC8085631/pdf/BLT.19.249656.pdf.
67. Harris T, Khandge P, Wu WJ, Barone AAL, Steinberg JP, Redett RJ, et al. Surgical approach to penile reconstruction for shaft skin excision from circumcision. Pediatr Surg Int [Internet]. 2023;39(1). Available from: https://doi.org/10.1007/s00383-023-05409-x.
68. Petrella F, Ammar S, El-Ghar MA, Capolicchio JP. Total glans amputation after neonatal circumcision. Urol Case Rep [Internet]. 2021;37:101624. Available from: https://doi.org/10.1016/j.eucr.2021.101624.
69. Schröder A, Farhat WA, Chiasson D, Wilson GJ, Koyle MA. Serious and fatal complications after neonatal circumcision. Eur Urol Focus [Internet]. 2022 Sep [cited 2025 Jun 17];8(5):1560–1563. Available from: https://linkinghub.elsevier.com/retrieve/pii/S2405456921003163.
70. Gee WF, Ansell JS. Neonatal circumcision: a ten-year overview: with comparison of the Gomco Clamp and the Plastibell Device. Pediatrics [Internet]. 1976;58(6):824–7. Available from: https://doi.org/10.1542/peds.58.6.824.
71. Williams N, Kapila L. Complications of circumcision [Internet]. Br J Surg. Oxford University Press. 1993;80:1231–6. Available from: https://doi.org/10.1002/bjs.1800801005.
72. Rodriguez V, Titapiwatanakun R, Moir C, Schmidt K, Pruthi RK. To circumcise or not to circumcise? Circumcision in patients with bleeding disorders. Haemophilia [Internet]. 2009;16(2):272–6. Available from: https://doi.org/10.1111/j.1365-2516.2009.02119.x.
73. Hutcheson JC. Male neonatal circumcision: indications, controversies and complications [Internet]. Urol Clin N Am. Elsevier BV. 2004;31:461–7. Available from: https://doi.org/10.1016/j.ucl.2004.04.011.
74. Iacob SI, Feinn R, Sardi LM. Systematic review of complications arising from male circumcision [Internet], vol. 3. BJUI Compass. Wiley; 2021. p. 99–123. Available from: https://doi.org/10.1002/bco2.123.
75. Bliss DP, Healey PJ, Waldhausen JHT. Necrotizing fasciitis after plastibell circumcision. J Urol [Internet]. 1998;159(4):1408. Available from: https://doi.org/10.1016/s0022-5347(01)63646-2.
76. Woodside JR. Necrotizing fasciitis after neonatal circumcision. Arch Pediatr Adolesc Med [Internet]. 1980;134(3):301. Available from: https://doi.org/10.1001/archpedi.1980.02130150055015.
77. Krill AJ, Palmer LS, Palmer JS. Complications of circumcision. Sci World J [Internet]. 2011 [cited 2025 Jun 19];11:2458–68. Available from: http://www.hindawi.com/journals/tswj/2011/373829/.
78. Diaz EC, Corcoran JF, Johnson EK. Pediatric penile reconstruction using autologous split-thickness skin graft. J Pediatr Urol [Internet]. 2016 Jun [cited 2025 Jun 19];12(3):185–6. Available from: https://linkinghub.elsevier.com/retrieve/pii/S1477513116300249.
79. Qiu L, Zhang X, Liu Y, Fu Y, Yuan X. A case series of penile skin grafting in children. Eur J Pediatr Surg Rep [Internet]. 2020 Jan [cited 2025 Jun 18];08(01):e77–80. Available from: http://www.thieme-connect.de/DOI/DOI?10.1055/s-0040-1716525.
80. Williams N, Kapila L. Complications of circumcision [Internet]. British J Surg. 1993;80:1231–6. Oxford University Press. Available from: https://doi.org/10.1002/bjs.1800801005.
81. Qaid S, Ahmed F, Al-shami E, Alyhari Q, Ghabisha S, Askarpour MR, et al. Repair of total penile skin loss after ritual circumcision using a scrotal flap: a case report. Pan Afr Med J [Internet]. 2022;42. Available from: https://doi.org/10.11604/pamj.2022.42.152.35813.
82. Kamal BA. Penile skin bridges: causes and prevention. Int Surg [Internet]. 2010;94(1):35–7. Available from: https://pubmed.ncbi.nlm.nih.gov/20099424/.

83. Gluckman GR, Stoller ML, Jacobs MM, Kogan BA. Pediatric urology: newborn penile glans amputation during circumcision and successful reattachment. J Urol [Internet]. 1995;153(3):778–9. Available from: https://doi.org/10.1016/s0022-5347(01)67718-8.
84. Weiss HA, Larke N, Halperin D, Schenker I. Complications of circumcision in male neonates, infants and children: a systematic review. BMC Urol [Internet]. 2010 Dec [cited 2025 Jun 7];10(1):2. Available from: https://bmcurol.biomedcentral.com/articles/10.1186/1471-2490-10-2.
85. Omole F, Smith W, Carter-Wicker K. Newborn circumcision techniques. Am Fam Physician [Internet]. 2020;101(11):680–5. Available from: https://pubmed.ncbi.nlm.nih.gov/32463643/.
86. Bawazir OA, Alsaiari WS. Plastibell circumcision: comparison between neonates and infants. Urol Ann [Internet]. 2020;12(4):347. Available from: https://doi.org/10.4103/ua.ua_146_19.
87. Bartman T. Newborn circumcision and urinary tract infections. Pediatrics [Internet]. 2001;107(1):210–4. Available from: https://doi.org/10.1542/peds.107.1.210b.
88. O'Grady J, Taugher CJ. Circumcision: ritual and surgery. Glob Libr Women Med [Internet]. 2008. Available from: https://doi.org/10.3843/glowm.10144.
89. Malone PS, Steinbrecher H. Medical aspects of male circumcision [Internet]. BMJ. 2007;335:1206–90. Available from: https://doi.org/10.1136/bmj.39385.382708.ad.
90. Prabhakaran S, Ljuhar D, Coleman RE, Nataraja R. Circumcision in the paediatric patient: a review of indications, technique and complications [Internet]. J Paediatr Child Health Wiley. 2018;54:1299–307. Available from: https://doi.org/10.1111/jpc.14206.

4 Pediatric Testis

Katherine M. Fischer and Thomas F. Kolon

Abnormalities or concerns about the testes are a common reason pediatric patients present for urologic evaluation. While testicular complaints and conditions are also common among adults, there are some key differences between adult and pediatric patients in terms of the common conditions they present with and how they are treated. The goal of this chapter is to provide an overview of the most common conditions of the pediatric testis that urologists may encounter so that they can feel comfortable with initial evaluation, workup, and treatment of these, even if ultimately the patient will be referred to a pediatric specialist. These conditions include undescended testis (UDT), hydroceles and hernias, testicular pain, and testicular masses.

Undescended Testis

Cryptorchidism or UDT is one of the most common pediatric disorders of the male endocrine glands and the most common genital disorder identified in male infants at birth. In 2014, the American Urological Association (AUA) published guidelines regarding the evaluation and treatment of cryptorchidism based upon an extensive review of the published literature [1]. These guidelines provide clear and concise recommendations and should be followed by any urologist seeing patients with

K. M. Fischer (✉)
Division of Urology, Assistant Professor of Surgery at the Children's Hospital of Philadelphia, Philadelphia, PA, USA
e-mail: fischerk@chop.edu

T. F. Kolon
Children's Hospital of Philadelphia, Division of Urology, Philadelphia, PA, USA

Perelman School of Medicine at the University of Pennsylvania, Philadelphia, PA, USA
e-mail: kolon@chop.edu

H.-Y. Wu et al. (eds.), *Pediatric Urology for the Adult Urologist*, https://doi.org/10.1007/978-3-032-10306-2_4

UDT. Cryptorchidism is defined as the failure of a testis to descend to a dependent scrotal position and is estimated to occur in 1–4% of full-term and up to 45% of preterm newborn males [1, 2]. Spontaneous descent of UDT observed at birth is relatively common and generally occurs prior to 6 months corrected age, with an estimated 1% of male infants still having UDT by 1 year of age [3]. Data regarding the incidence of UDT in postpubertal boys and adults are much more limited and heterogeneous than that for infants, but the incidence is estimated to be 0.79–2.2% based upon older cohort studies [3, 4].

Cryptorchidism can be further categorized as congenital, testes that are extra-scrotal from the time of birth, or acquired/ascending, which are testes that are present in the scrotum at birth but subsequently found to be in an extra-scrotal location on exam. The reason for testicular ascent is not fully understood, but several hypotheses exist. One theory is that ascent occurs secondary to poor fixation of the testis in the scrotum and abnormal gubernacular attachment, causing a testis to be palpated in a higher position as the child grows despite being in the scrotum at birth. Others have postulated that ascent occurs because of abnormal regression of the patent process vaginalis after testicular descent and that this leads to a fibrous remnant that restricts lengthening of the spermatic cord with somatic growth. There are also testicles that ascend secondary to entrapment or scarring after ipsilateral inguinal surgery [5].

The peak age of diagnosis of acquired UDT is 5–7 years of age. The majority of UDT are unilateral, with about 20–30% of cryptorchid patients having bilateral UDT [3]. Cryptorchid testes may be located in the abdomen, inguinal canal, superficial inguinal pouch, upper scrotum, or ectopic. Approximately 70% of UDT are palpable and of those testes that are non-palpable, approximately 30% will be in the inguinal scrotal region, 55% intra-abdominal, and 15% will be absent [6, 7]. It is important to remember that a phenotypic male newborn with bilateral, non-palpable testes could be a genetic female (46XX) with congenital adrenal hyperplasia, and, therefore, represents a potential emergency until proven otherwise and immediate consultation of appropriate specialists is necessary in this scenario [1].

In all patients presenting with UDT, the workup should begin with a good physical exam, as this is the cornerstone of initial diagnosis. Testicular exam in pediatric patients can be challenging for several reasons, including being limited by patient anxiety and cooperation, the smaller size of the testicles in childhood, and a higher likelihood of the testicles retracting outside of the scrotum prior to puberty. Infants and young children should be examined supine with a gentle frog leg, and examining on a parent's lap may be helpful. Older children can be examined supine or upright, cross-legged, and adolescents can typically be examined standing. For testicles not readily palpable in the scrotum, gentle downward pressure should be applied along the inguinal canal, starting at the anterior iliac spine and sweeping toward the scrotum to identify a testis within the canal and see how low it can be brought. Once the testis is palpated, it can be grasped with the dominant hand while the other hand continues to gently sweep along the inguinal canal to see if it can be manipulated into the scrotum. Retractile testis should be able to be brought into the scrotum with this technique and remain there after the cremasteric muscle has been fatigued. A warm room, distracting the patient to help relax them, and using lubricant or soap when sweeping in the inguinal canal to help feel the testicle "glide" within it can all be helpful for a difficult exam [1].

The AUA and EAU/ESPU guidelines and the Choosing Wisely Campaign all recommend that providers should not perform an initial ultrasound (US) or other imaging (MRI) in the evaluation of boys with cryptorchidism prior to referral, as these studies rarely assist in decision-making or change clinical outcomes [1, 8, 9]. The ideal imaging technique would accurately localize a viable testis requiring intervention, identify a vanishing or absent testis (this is further discussed in the acute scrotum section under neonatal torsion) that does not require intervention, and identify and localize testicular nubbins that may or may not require removal [10]. Such an imaging study would aid in presurgical planning and also allow some patients to forgo unnecessary surgery. Unfortunately, at this point, there is no imaging technique that is 100% sensitive for the presence of a testis, and therefore, diagnostic laparoscopy is considered the gold standard for localizing non-palpable testes. Laparoscopy offers the additional benefit of definitive intervention, should it be needed, at the time of diagnosis, further increasing its utility.

The goals of treating cryptorchidism include optimizing endocrine and reproductive function, decreasing testicular malignancy risk, permitting easy testicular self-exam, preventing testicular torsion, and correcting associated inguinal hernia. According to the AUA guidelines, providers should refer any infant that does not have spontaneous descent of the testis by 6 months corrected gestational age to a specialist, and surgery should be performed within the next year (by 18 months of age). Boys with the possibility of newly diagnosed (acquired/ascending) cryptorchidism after 6 months of age should be referred promptly to an appropriate surgical specialist [1].

Both endocrine and reproductive testicular functions are negatively impacted by delay or failure to correct UDT; however, reproductive function seems to be more susceptible to progressive damage. This is well illustrated by the fact that virtually all adult men with uncorrected bilateral cryptorchidism will have azoospermia and infertility, and only 49% of men with persistent unilateral cryptorchidism will have a normal sperm concentration. However, after orchiopexy in childhood, 71% of patients with unilateral and 28% of patients with bilateral cryptorchidism will have normal semen analysis parameters with essentially normal paternity rates for patients with a history of unilateral cryptorchidism (around 90%) versus 65% paternity for patients with corrected bilateral UDT [11–15].

Cryptorchidism is a well-known and long-accepted risk factor associated with testicular malignancy, and a history of UDT is associated with a two- to eightfold increase in risk of testicular germ cell tumor [2, 16]. Evidence suggests that performing orchiopexy prior to puberty does not eliminate but does lower this risk to about two to three times higher than the general population. This emphasizes the importance of education on self-examination at puberty, especially in those with a history of orchidopexy. Bilateral UDT and postpubertal or uncorrected UDT have all been found to carry an increased risk of malignancy [17].

The AUA guidelines recommend against the use of hormonal therapy to induce testicular descent, given low response rates and a lack of evidence for long-term efficacy. In boys with palpable UDT, scrotal or inguinal orchiopexy is the recommended treatment of choice [1]. Testes that are non-palpable may require an abdominal or laparoscopic approach. Some surgeons prefer a scrotal approach for testes that can be brought into the high scrotum on examination under anesthesia, particularly in older boys who are less likely to have a patent hernia sac [18].

Retractile testes differ from true UDT in that they can be brought into a satisfactory scrotal position on exam with fatigue of the cremasteric reflex. This is a common and normal finding in prepubertal boys and does not require surgery. However, because of the subtle difference in exam findings, these patients are often referred to a urologist. It is important that retractile testes are assessed with a physical exam at least annually, as a small percentage will become "ascended" as linear growth changes [1]. The AUA guidelines recommend that primary care providers palpable all boys' testes for quality and position at every well child visit [1]. However, if an exam is very difficult or concerns about the position persist from the PCP or family, it may be prudent for a urologist to follow these patients longitudinally.

Hydrocele/Hernias

In pediatric patients, inguinal hernias are almost always indirect, resulting from a patent processus vaginalis that extends distal to the internal inguinal ring and allows abdominal contents to pass into the canal or scrotum. The processus vaginalis forms during the third month of gestation when the peritoneum bulges into the inguinal canal, just prior to testicular descent. Once the testes are descended, the processus normally obliterates, and the part adjacent to the testes becomes the tunica vaginalis. This process continues postnatally, and failure to close results in the most common type of hernias and hydroceles seen in pediatric patients [18].

There are multiple types of hydroceles seen in pediatric patients, and understanding the differences is critical to appropriate management. A communicating hydrocele occurs via the same mechanism as an indirect inguinal hernia (a patent processus vaginalis), with the only difference being that the contents are peritoneal fluid only, as opposed to other abdominal contents such as bowel or omentum. A hydrocele of the spermatic cord is fluid contained within a closed segment of the processus vaginalis, which is obliterated both proximally and distally to the fluid. A scrotal or noncommunicating hydrocele occurs when fluid is contained within the tunica vaginalis that surrounds the testis without proximal communication (closed processus vaginalis); this is the type of hydrocele most often seen in adults. Finally, abdominoscrotal hydroceles are very large scrotal hydroceles that extend proximally across the internal inguinal ring and into the abdomen but are separate from the peritoneum and do not communicate with it [19].

Inguinal hernias affect 1–4% of full-term infants and up to 30% of premature neonates with decreased birth weight and increasing prematurity associated with increased risk. They are more common on the right than on the left side (estimated

75% vs. 25%) and are 10 times more common in boys than girls. Approximately one-third of inguinal hernias present before 6 months of age, and 15–20% of cases are bilateral [20–22]. The majority of new hydroceles that occur after birth but before puberty will be communicating (associated with a patent processus vaginalis). Noncommunicating hydroceles that spontaneously resolve are common, present in at least 5% of infants [23]. Postpubertal boys are also more likely to have noncommunicating hydroceles, but, similar to adults, the hydroceles do not always resolve without surgery [19].

Like UDT, the diagnosis and classification of hernias and hydroceles rely on physical exam. Both hernias and communicating hydroceles typically present as a painless bulge in either the groin or along the spermatic cord into the scrotum. Fluctuation of the bulge on exam or based on history is helpful in distinguishing communicating versus noncommunicating hydroceles. Physical exam done in a standing position and with increased intra-abdominal pressure, such as jumping, coughing, or straining, can be helpful to elicit a bulge if it is not readily appreciated on exam. If the bulge cannot be reproduced at the time of the exam, having a family member take photos has been found to be diagnostically reliable [24]. Although imaging is not typically needed, ultrasound can be useful in some scenarios, including: identifying and ensuring a testis that may not be palpable within a tense hydrocele is healthy and normal, confirming the diagnosis of incarcerated hernia with bowel, and distinguishing spermatic cord hydroceles from other types of paratesticular masses.

Typically, pediatric patients found to have non-incarcerated inguinal hernias or patients greater than 12 months of age with communicating hydroceles are scheduled for surgery on an elective basis at the time of presentation, even if they have no symptoms other than a palpable bulge on exam. The rationale for this is to decrease the risk of incarceration, which is most common in newborns, with reported rates up to 30% [25]. Those patients with bowel-containing hernias or hernias that have been difficult to reduce are thought to be at higher risk of incarceration and, therefore, are typically repaired soon after presentation. An incarcerated hernia that cannot be reduced is a true surgical emergency and should be treated as such.

In most cases, noncommunicating hydroceles in infants will resolve spontaneously, so they can be observed until at least 1 year of age and only operated on if they persist, fluctuate, or increase in size. While hydroceles of the cord typically do not resolve spontaneously, they also do not require urgent surgery and can be excised electively after 1 year of age. Noncommunicating hydroceles in older postpubertal boys can be managed in the same way as adult hydroceles with elective repair if they are very large in size, precluding palpation of the ipsilateral testis, increasing in size, or bothersome to the patient.

Standard inguinal hernia repair is done in an open manner via a groin incision with high ligation of the hernia sac [20]. Communicating hydroceles should be managed in the same manner as an indirect inguinal hernia via an inguinal incision and high ligation of the hernia sac, and are different than the scrotal hydroceles that adult urologists commonly encounter [20]. Noncommunicating hydroceles in older boys can be managed via a scrotal approach with excision of the redundant tunica vaginalis in the same way adult hydroceles are typically repaired. Laparoscopic hernia repair can also be performed via either intraperitoneal or extraperitoneal approaches to close the defect, though the recurrence rate has been reported to be higher (up to 4%) than traditional open approaches (0.5–1%) [19]. Routine examination of the contralateral internal ring is not recommended unless there is a history of prematurity, contralateral hydrocele, or ventriculo-peritoneal shunt. The incidence of contralateral inguinal hernia presentation after a unilateral hernia repair is only 9% [26].

The Acute Scrotum/Testicular Pain

The acute scrotum refers to a combination of new onset pain, swelling, and/or tenderness of the scrotal contents and is a common reason for pediatric male patients to present, particularly to an emergency department. The differential diagnosis includes appendage torsion, epididymitis, scrotal edema, orchitis, trauma, hernias/hydrocele, varicoceles, intrascrotal mass, musculoskeletal pain, referred pain (ex-, from a kidney stone), and testicular torsion, which is a time-sensitive surgical emergency [19]. For this reason, the differential, workup, and management of acute scrotal pain is important for all urologists to be familiar with, as they may need to evaluate these patients if no pediatric specialist is available.

Testicular torsion is one of the few true urologic emergencies and occurs when twisting of the spermatic cord impedes arterial inflow and venous outflow, causing ischemic changes. If not promptly corrected, torsion can lead to testicular infarction. Intravaginal torsion, where the spermatic cord twists within the tunica vaginalis, is most common between 12 and 16 years of age, with an annual incidence of 3.8 per 100,000 boys younger than 18 years. This accounts for 10–15% of presentations with acute scrotal pain in boys [19, 27–29]. There is no clear cause of intravaginal testicular torsion though there is believed to be an association with the bell clapper deformity, where the testicle lacks its normal posterior attachment to the scrotum, causing it to hang freely like a bell clapper. Other possible causes, such as cold weather or temperature changes activating the cremasteric reflex, rapid testicular growth, and UDT, have been evaluated without definite conclusions [19].

Patients with testicular torsion typically present with acute onset of scrotal pain without alleviating factors. A total of 10–60% of patients will have associated nausea and vomiting, and exam commonly reveals edema, erythema, tenderness, high-riding and/or horizontal orientation of the testis, and absent cremasteric reflex [19]. Patients with these signs and symptoms should have immediate scrotal ultrasound with color doppler, as this has high sensitivity and specificity for detecting testicular torsion. Ultrasound findings concerning testicular torsion include decreased or absent blood flow to the affected testis as detected by doppler, twisting of the spermatic cord, and heterogeneous appearance of the testicular parenchyma. If ultrasound is not readily available and would create a significant delay in care, immediate surgical exploration when torsion is suspected based on history and exam is reasonable.

Once diagnosed, testicular torsion is managed surgically with detorsion and bilateral septopexy. If the testis is not viable after detorsion, orchiectomy is performed. Testicular torsion is associated with an orchiectomy rate of 30–70% in children undergoing operative management [19]. In cases of questionable testicular viability, incising the tunica albuginea to check for arterial bleeding and to alleviate increased pressure and compartment syndrome can be useful. A tunica vaginalis flap is used to cover the albuginea incision if there is bleeding from the tubules and they appear viable [30]. Three critical components to maximize the likelihood of testicular salvage in cases of testicular torsion are early presentation, accurate diagnosis, and prompt treatment. It is recognized that minimizing the time from onset of ischemia to surgery maximizes the likelihood of testicular preservation; detorsion within 8–10 hours of symptom onset is generally accepted as the optimal timeframe for testicular salvage [31–33]. It should be stressed that while manual detorsion can restore blood flow to the testis and alleviate symptoms, it may fail to completely correct torsion in up to one-third of cases, so it should not preclude the need for surgical management [19]. One-third of cases have exhibited external/lateral torsion rather than the usual internal/medial torsion.

Intermittent testicular torsion, characterized by episodes of acute scrotal pain that resolve within minutes to hours, may precede acute testicular torsion requiring surgical management in 30–50% of patients [19]. This is a difficult diagnosis to make as it relies primarily on patient history unless a patient happens to have acute pain that resolves during exam or ultrasound, with improvement in blood flow seen on ultrasound after resolution of symptoms. If intermittent torsion is suspected, patients can be offered elective bilateral septopexy.

Aside from teenagers, the other age group that most often experiences testicular torsion is neonates. These patients typically have extravaginal torsion with twisting of the entire cord, including the tunica vaginalis, as the event occurs prior to the fixation of the tunica vaginalis to the dartos of the scrotum. Perinatal torsion is estimated to occur in 6.1 per 100,000 births and most commonly occurs well before the patient is born, resulting in a "vanishing testis" or testicular nubbin [34]. Torsion occurring later in gestation can result in a hard, painless, and enlarged testis at birth associated with overlying erythema or scrotal skin changes. Rarely, an infant will be noted to have an acute change in exam and found to have acute testicular torsion.

Scrotal ultrasound is helpful in confirming the diagnosis, and if acute torsion is suspected after a change in a previously normal newborn exam, emergency surgery should be performed. In most cases, the torsion event will have occurred well before birth, and the affected testis will not be salvageable, and in these cases, management is controversial. Some pediatric urologists advocate prompt surgical management to avoid the potential for bilateral torsion, which is a devastating event and has been reported in 5–22% of cases [19]. Others advocate delayed surgery as the affected testis is highly unlikely to be salvaged, and delaying surgery can decrease the anesthetic risks associated with neonatal surgery. It is important to consider the clinical scenario, ability to continue to monitor with serial exams, and the overall health of the newborn relative to anesthesia risk when making this decision. In addition, one must take into consideration the expertise of local anesthesiologists in managing the newborn. A full discussion with the parents, outlining all risks and benefits concerning surgery in a newborn and long-term outcomes, is warranted.

Appendix testis or appendix epididymis torsion is the most common cause of acute scrotum pain in prepubertal boys, with a peak occurrence at 7 to 12 years of age, and occurs with torsion of either the appendix testis or appendix epididymis, which are both embryologic remnants without function [19]. There is no known cause, and the presentation can be quite similar to testicular torsion with acute onset of pain as the primary complaint, though pain is often improved at rest. An exam can reveal a "blue dot sign"—discoloration at the superior aspect of the testis representing the ischemic appendage that is seen through the scrotal skin. Ultrasound is the most reliable way to differentiate this from testicular torsion, as both testes will have adequate, symmetric blood flow, and often the affected appendage can be seen as well. Treatment is conservative with rest, anti-inflammatory medications, and ice.

Epididymitis, inflammation of the epididymis, can be infectious or noninfectious in pediatric patients and is another common cause of the acute scrotum. Symptoms are often more insidious in onset but otherwise similar and can include pain, swelling, and erythema. On exam, the cremasteric reflex is typically intact. Ultrasound typically shows increased blood flow to the ipsilateral epididymis and/or testis. In boys who are not sexually active and do not have any other urinary tract abnormalities (ectopic ureter, hypospadias, etc.), epididymitis is most often noninfectious and can be treated conservatively with rest, anti-inflammatory medications, and ice, and does not require antibiotics. Sexually transmitted infections should be considered in sexually active boys and tested/treated as indicated. In boys with atypical presentation, associated urinary tract infection and/ or repeated episodes, imaging of the kidneys and bladder should be considered to rule out anatomic abnormalities, and antibiotics may be needed [19].

Testicular Masses

Prepubertal testicular tumors are different from those in postpubertal and adult males in that a benign etiology is more common. In addition, malignant tumors in prepubertal boys tend to have a more favorable prognosis. It is estimated that testicular tumors comprise 1% of pediatric solid tumors, with an incidence of 0.5 to 2 per 100,000 [35]. Mature teratoma is the most common benign lesion and is more common than yolk sac tumor, which is the most common malignant tumor in boys [36].

Like adults, pediatric testicular tumors often present as a painless mass, however, they can also be found incidentally on imaging obtained to evaluate swelling or pain. Ultrasound has a near 100% sensitivity for detecting testicular tumors, and there are some findings that can be used to suggest a specific pathology. However, imaging cannot reliably differentiate benign from malignant lesions, and therefore, surgery is almost always indicated. Teratomas most often appear as heterogenous and complex lesions with both cystic and solid components and sometimes contain calcifications as well. Epidermoid cysts classically have an "onion skin" appearance with concentric rings. Yolk sac tumors are usually well-circumscribed and heterogenous in appearance [35].

When a diagnosis of testicular tumor is suspected based on exam and/or imaging, serum biomarkers (β-hCG, AFP, and LDH) should be obtained as in adults. These play an important role in management as benign lesions are often treated with testis-sparing surgery and should not have elevated biomarkers. AFP is elevated in yolk sac tumors, but is also physiologically elevated in children <1 year of age, so it is important to keep in mind when interpreting lab results. If a malignant lesion is suspected based on elevated tumor markers, cross-sectional imaging of the abdomen and chest with CT or MRI can be obtained preoperatively, but otherwise, this can be obtained postoperatively only if malignant pathology is found [35].

A special population that needs to be considered in pediatrics is those patients with Differences of Sex Development (DSD) and dysgenetic gonads. Patients with DSD with Y chromosome material have an increased incidence of tumors, and for this reason, prophylactic gonadectomy is often recommended. However, this is a nuanced decision based upon the endocrine and reproductive potential of the gonad, likelihood of malignancy in the specific clinical situation, location of the gonad, and whether it can be easily monitored on exam [37].

Surgical management of a pediatric testicular mass is based on the suspected pathology. In prepubertal boys where teratoma is suspected, partial orchiectomy is the preferred and safe management, as these almost always contain mature elements only [38]. This is different in postpubertal boys, where teratoma should be managed in the same manner as adults, with radical inguinal orchiectomy. Because most lesions in prepubertal boys are benign, masses that are not believed to be yolk sac tumors can be treated with testis-sparing surgery. This should be done via an inguinal incision with control of the spermatic cord, and the mass and margins should be sent for frozen pathologic analysis with a plan to convert to radical orchiectomy if a malignant diagnosis is found. If the lesion is not easily palpable and/or small and central on ultrasound, intraoperative ultrasound is useful in localizing the lesion and ensuring complete excision. In contrast, suspected yolk sac tumor (elevated AFP) should be treated with radical inguinal orchiectomy [34].

Paratesticular rhabdomyosarcoma (RMS) accounts for 7–10% of GU RMS with a bimodal age distribution that peaks at less than 1 year and 16 years of age [37]. This typically presents as a painless, firm mass that may or may not be distinct from the testis on exam. Ultrasound most often will show a hyperechoic, heterogenous, solid mass. These patients should have tumor markers checked and should also have cross-sectional imaging performed to evaluate for metastases to the lungs and/or retroperitoneal lymph nodes, which are positive in up to 20% of patients. Radical inguinal orchiectomy is recommended with spermatic cord ligation with permanent suture in case retroperitoneal lymph node dissection (RPLND) is necessary in the future. In rare cases, the tumor may be safely excised from the testis and cord with negative margins [39]. The management of the retroperitoneum is unique in paratesticular RMS. Patients less than 10 years old who are clinical group 1 (complete resection with negative margins on orchiectomy and negative imaging) do not require RPLND, whereas those over 10 years always should undergo ipsilateral RLPND because of the high rate of positive lymph nodes [37].

Summary

- Undescended testis (UDT) occurs in approximately 1% of boys and should be corrected surgically if the testis is not in a scrotal position by 6 months of age. Reasons for correction include optimizing endocrine and reproductive function and minimizing the risk of malignancy.
- Most hydroceles in prepubertal pediatric patients are communicating hydroceles resulting from a patent process vaginalis. This is the same pathology that causes indirect inguinal hernias, and these hydroceles should be treated in the same way as hernias with high ligation of the patent process vaginalis.
- Testicular torsion, epididymitis/orchitis, and torsion of testicular appendages can all present similarly with acute onset, severe testicular pain with swelling and erythema. Only testicular torsion is a surgical emergency, and testicular ultrasound is very helpful in differentiating these diagnoses to allow for prompt and appropriate treatment.
- Unlike postpubertal males, most testicular tumors in prepubertal boys will be benign. For this reason, testis-sparing surgery can often be performed safely with favorable outcomes and should be considered when appropriate.

References

1. Kolon TF, Herndon CA, Baker LA, et al. Evaluation and treatment of cryptorchidism: AUA guideline. J Urol. 2014;192(2):337.
2. Barthold JS, Hagerty JA. Etiology, diagnosis, and management of the undescended testis. In: Wein AJ, Kavoussi LR, Partin AW, et al., editors. Campbell-Walsh urology. 12th ed. Philadelphia: Elsevier; 2020. p. 949. Ch. 46.
3. Sijstermans K, Hack WW, Meijer RW, Voort-Doedens LV. The frequency of undescended testis from birth to adulthood: a review. Int J Androl. 2008;31(1):1.
4. Baumrucker GO. Incidence of testicular pathology: bulletin of the US Army Medical Department. United States Army Medical Department. 1946;5:312.
5. Alchoikani N, Ashour K. Ascending testis: a congenital predetermined condition. J Pediatr Urol. 2021;17(2):192-e1.
6. Smolko MJ, Kaplan GW, Brock WA. Location and fate of the nonpalpable testis in children. J Urol. 1983;129(6):1204.
7. Denes FT, Saito FJ, Silva FA, et al. Laparoscopic diagnosis and treatment of nonpalpable testis. Int Braz J Urol. 2008;34(3):329.
8. Radmayr C, Dogan HS, Hoebeke P, et al. Management of undescended testes: European association of urology/European society for paediatric urology guidelines. J Pediatr Urol. 2016;12(6):335.
9. Don't routinely perform ultrasound on boys with cryptorchidism. Retrieved from http://www.choosingwisely.org/clinician-lists/american-urological-association-ultrasounds-on-boys-with-cryptorchidism. 2017.

10. Eggener SE, Lotan Y, Cheng EY. Magnetic resonance angiography for the nonpalpable testis: a cost and cancer risk analysis. J Urol. 2005;173(5):1745.
11. Virtanen HE, Bjerknes R, Cortes D, et al. Cryptorchidism: classification, prevalence and long-term consequences. Acta Paediatr. 2007;96(5):611.
12. Lee PA, Coughlin MT. Fertility after bilateral cryptorchidism. Evaluation by paternity, hormone, and semen data. Horm Res. 2001;55(1):28.
13. Miller KD, Coughlin MT, Lee PA. Fertility after unilateral cryptorchidism. Paternity, time to conception, pretreatment testicular location and size, hormone and sperm parameters. Horm Res. 2001;55(5):249.
14. Coughlin MT, O'Leary LA, Songer NJ, et al. Time to conception after orchidopexy: evidence for subfertility? Fertil Steril. 1997;67(4):742.
15. Virtanen HE, Toppari J. Cryptorchidism and fertility. Endocrinol Metab Clin N Am. 2015;44(4):751.
16. Kim SO, Hwang EC, Hwang IS, et al. Testicular catch up growth: the impact of orchiopexy age. Urology. 2011;78(4):886.
17. Wood HM, Elder JS. Cryptorchidism and testicular cancer: separating fact from fiction. J Urol. 2009;181(2):452.
18. Gordon M, Cervellione RM, Morabito A, Bianchi A. 20 years of transcrotal orchidopexy for undescended testis: results and outcomes. J Pediatr Urol. 2010;6(5):506–12.
19. Palmer LS, Palmer JS. Management of abnormalities of the external genitalia in boys. In: Wein AJ, Kavoussi LR, Partin AW, et al., editors. Campbell-Walsh urology. 12th ed. Philadelphia: Elsevier; 2020. p. 871. Ch. 44.
20. Lao OB, Fitzgibbons RJ, Cusick RA. Pediatric inguinal hernias, hydroceles, and undescended testicles. Surg Clin. 2012;92(3):487–504.
21. Ein SH, Njere I, Ein A. Six thousand three hundred sixty-one pediatric inguinal hernias: a 35-year review. J Pediatr Surg. 2006;41(5):980–6.
22. Brandt ML. Pediatric hernias. Surg Clin N Am. 2008;88(1):27–43.
23. Osifo OD, Osaigbovo EO. Congenital hydrocele: prevalence and outcome among male children who underwent neonatal circumcision in Benin city, Nigeria. J Pediatr Urol. 2008;4:178–82.
24. Kawaguchi AL, Shaul DB. Inguinal hernias can be accurately diagnosed using the parent's digital photographs when the physical examination is non- diagnostic. J Pediatr Surg. 2009;44(12):2327–9.
25. Rosenberg J. Pediatric inguinal hernia repair—a critical appraisal. Hernia. 2008;12(2):113–5.
26. Tackett LD, Breuer CK, Luks FI, Caldamone AA, Breuer JG, DeLuca FG, Caesar RE, Efthemiou E, Wesselhoeft JCW. Incidence of contralateral inguinal hernia: a prospective analysis. J Pediatr Surg. 1999;34(5):684–8.
27. Zhao LC, Lautz TB, Meeks JJ, Maizels M. Pediatric testicular torsion epidemiology using a national database: incidence, risk of orchiectomy and possible measures toward improving the quality of care. J Urol. 2011;186:2009–13. https://doi.org/10.1016/j.juro.2011.07.024.
28. Barbosa JA, Tiseo BC, Barayan GA, Rosman BM, Torricelli FCM, Passerotti CC, et al. Development and initial validation of a scoring system to diagnose testicular torsion in children. J Urol. 2013;189:1859–64. https://doi.org/10.1016/j.juro.2012.10.056.
29. Liang T, Metcalfe P, Sevcik W, Noga M. Retrospective review of diagnosis and treatment in children presenting to the pediatric department with acute scrotum. AJR Am J Roentgenol. 2013;200:W444–9. https://doi.org/10.2214/AJR.12.10036.
30. Kutikov A, Casale P, White MA, Meyer WA, Chang A, Gosalbez R, Canning DA. Testicular compartment syndrome: a new approach to conceptualizing and managing testicular torsion. Urology. 2008;72(4):786–9.
31. Frohlich LC, Paydar-Darian N, Cilento BG, Lee LK. Prospective validation of clinical score for males presenting with an acute scrotum. Acad Emerg Med. 2017;24:1474–82. https://doi.org/10.1111/acem.13295.
32. Kapoor S. Testicular torsion: a race against time: testicular torsion. Int J Clin Pract. 2008;62:821–7. https://doi.org/10.1111/j.1742-1241.2008.01727.x.

33. Sessions AE, Rabinowitz R, Hulbert WC, Goldstein MM, Mevorach RA. Testicular torsion: direction, degree, duration and disinformation. J Urol. 2003;169:663–5. https://doi.org/10.1097/01.ju.0000047381.36380.0e.
34. John CM, Kooner G, Mathew DE, et al. Neonatal testicular torsion—a lost cause? Acta Paediatr. 2008;97:502–4.
35. Ferrer FA. Pediatric urologic oncology: bladder and testis. In: Wein AJ, Kavoussi LR, Partin AW, et al., editors. Campbell-Walsh urology. 12th ed. Philadelphia: Elsevier; 2020. p. 1111. Ch. 54.
36. Pohl HG, Shukla AR, Metcalf PD, et al. Prepubertal testis tumors: actual prevalence rate of histological types. J Urol. 2004;172(6 Pt1):2370–2.
37. Kathrins M, Kolon TF. Malignancy in disorders of sex development. Transl Androl Urol. 2016;5(5):794–8.
38. Shukla AR, Woodard C, Carr MC, et al. Experience with testis sparing surgery for testicular teratoma. J Urol. 2004;171(1):161–3.
39. Ahmed HU, Arya M, Muneer A, et al. Testicular and paratesticular tumours in the prepubertal population. Lancet Oncol. 2010;11(5):476–83.

Evaluation and Management of Pediatric Patients with Urinary Tract Infection and Vesicoureteral Reflux for the Adult Urologist

5

Olamide Olawoyin and Angela M. Arlen

Introduction

Urinary tract infection (UTI) refers to the presence of bacteria in the urinary tract and includes asymptomatic bacteriuria, infection of the bladder (cystitis), and infection of the upper tract (pyelonephritis). Incidence and prevalence of UTI in the pediatric population depend on a given child's age, sex, race/ethnicity, and circumcision status. There is an estimated 8% incidence of at least one UTI by age 7 in females and 2% in males in the United States annually [1, 2]. First time, symptomatic occurrences are more common in boys (3.7%) during the first year of life compared to girls (2%) [3, 4]. This trend reverses after the first year of life, with prevalence in females peaking during the toddler years/toilet training and again in adolescence, presumably due to the short urethra length, vaginal pH, and increased colonization of enteric organisms [5–7]. Symptomatic UTI in children often warrants further investigation as infection may be the first sign of a congenital anomaly of the kidneys and urinary tract (CAKUT), including vesicoureteral reflux (VUR), neurogenic bladder, and bladder and bowel dysfunction (BBD) that may lead to considerable morbidity [1]. Obstructive anomalies are found in 4% and VUR in up to 40% of children following evaluation of initial febrile UTI. Furthermore, approximately 15% of these children, especially those <12 months of age, will have evidence of renal parenchymal injury/scarring at diagnosis [8, 9]. Early diagnosis and treatment of UTI and screening for VUR by providers, including pediatricians, urologists, and emergency medicine physicians, is essential. In here, we present current decision-making considerations for evaluation and management of pediatric urinary tract infection and vesicoureteral reflux.

O. Olawoyin · A. M. Arlen (✉)
Department of Urology, Yale University School of Medicine, New Haven, CT, USA
e-mail: olamide.olawoyin@yale.edu; angela.arlen@yale.edu

H.-Y. Wu et al. (eds.), *Pediatric Urology for the Adult Urologist*,
https://doi.org/10.1007/978-3-032-10306-2_5

Diagnosis of Urinary Tract Infection in Children

Signs and symptoms of UTI vary depending on age. In children younger than 2 years, fever may be the only symptom. Other possible symptoms include irritability, malodorous urine, gastrointestinal symptoms, and lower urinary tract symptoms. As presentation may be non-specific, clinicians must have a high index of suspicion. Clinical evaluation of UTI should include a history and physical examination focusing on the presence and/or duration of fever and other symptoms, as well as prior personal and family urologic history. Evaluation for anatomic abnormalities and other sources of fever is paramount.

Definite diagnosis requires both microscopic analysis and urine culture. Catheterized urine samples should be collected in non-toilet-trained children; clean-catch may be acceptable for toilet-trained children [10]. Suprapubic aspiration may also be considered in rare circumstances. Bagged samples are unacceptable, given the high false-positive culture rate [10]. Urine testing is indicated for all infants younger than 3 months presenting with fever ≥38 °C. For the evaluation of febrile UTI in children 2–24 months old, the now-retired 2011 American Academy of Pediatrics (AAP) guidelines recommend testing based on risk factors, including age < 12 months, sex, race, temperature ≥ 39 °C, fever for at least 2 days, and absence of another source of infection [10–12]. This version was modified by the University of Pittsburgh to exclude race as a risk factor and include a history of prior UTI [13]. Given the risk of renal scarring associated with urogenital anomalies such as VUR, the AAP suggests obtaining a renal–bladder ultrasound (RBUS) in children aged 2–24 months after the first febrile UTI [10, 14, 15]. Voiding cystourethrogram (VCUG) should be obtained in cases of recurrent UTIs or if RBUS reveals an anomaly such as collecting system dilation or parenchyma scarring [10]. In children aged ≥24 months, lower urinary tract symptoms, including dysuria, frequency, new-onset incontinence, abdominal or flank pain, and fever ≥39 °C, warrant obtaining a urine sample (Fig. 5.1).

The AAP requires >50,000 colony-forming units per mL of uropathogen per mL of urine from a catheterized sample [10]. Lower uropathogen criteria, presence of pyuria ≥5 WBC/HPF, and/or bacterial growth is acceptable for diagnosis in catheterized specimens from febrile infants, which is consistent with the recommendation by the European Society of Pediatric Urology (ESPU) [16].

Treatment and Further Workup of Urinary Tract Infections in Children

Objectives for UTI management include resolution of acute symptoms, elimination of infection, avoidance of urosepsis, and prevention of recurrence and renal scarring [10, 17]. The presence of fever and systemic signs of infection is critical in determining the route and duration of antibiotics, treatment setting, and need for additional workup. Urinalysis and urine culture should be obtained before the initiation of empiric therapy. The algorithm described in Fig. 5.2 and results from urinalysis

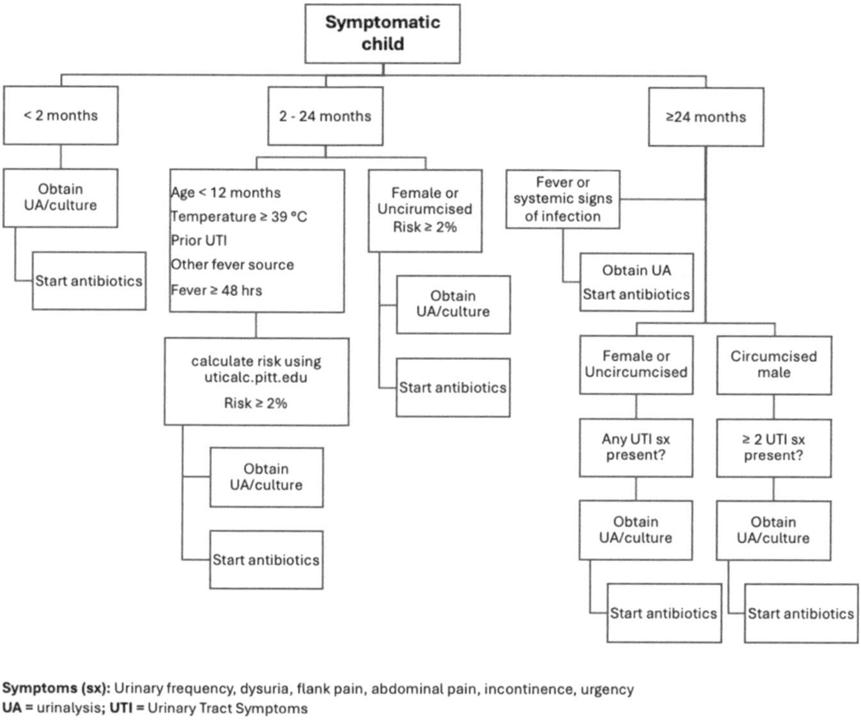

Fig. 5.1 Algorithm for evaluation of UTIs in children based on AAP guidelines [10–16]

(presence of leukocytes, nitrites, pyuria, and bacteria) can be used to determine the probability of UTI prior to urine culture results.

Empiric antibiotics based on local resistance patterns for *Escherichia coli* (*E. coli*), the most common pathogen causing 75–90% of UTIs, should be initiated early if high suspicion to prevent complications and reduce risks of scarring [10]. Antimicrobials should also be based on prior culture sensitivities [18]. Second- or third-generation cephalosporins (Cefixime 8 mg/kg once/day or Cefuroxime axetil 20–30 mg/day, divided into two doses) are recommended as the oral agent of choice in the outpatient management of pyelonephritis, given lower resistance patterns when compared to amoxicillin–clavulanate and trimethoprim–sulfamethoxazole (TMP–SMX) [6, 19, 20]. First-generation cephalosporins are preferred in some studies over second or third generation given narrower spectrum of activity, lower rate of resistance, and similar bioavailability [13]. While nitrofurantoin can be considered in the management of simple cystitis, it has limited therapeutic concentrations in serum and should not be used in treating upper tract infections [6]. Third-generation cephalosporin (ceftriaxone 50 mg/kg once/day) is recommended for parenteral management; a renal-dosed aminoglycoside can be used in the presence of cephalosporin allergies. Empiric coverage of other pathogens, including Klebsiella, Proteus, Enterococcus, Pseudomonas, Staphylococcus saprophyticus

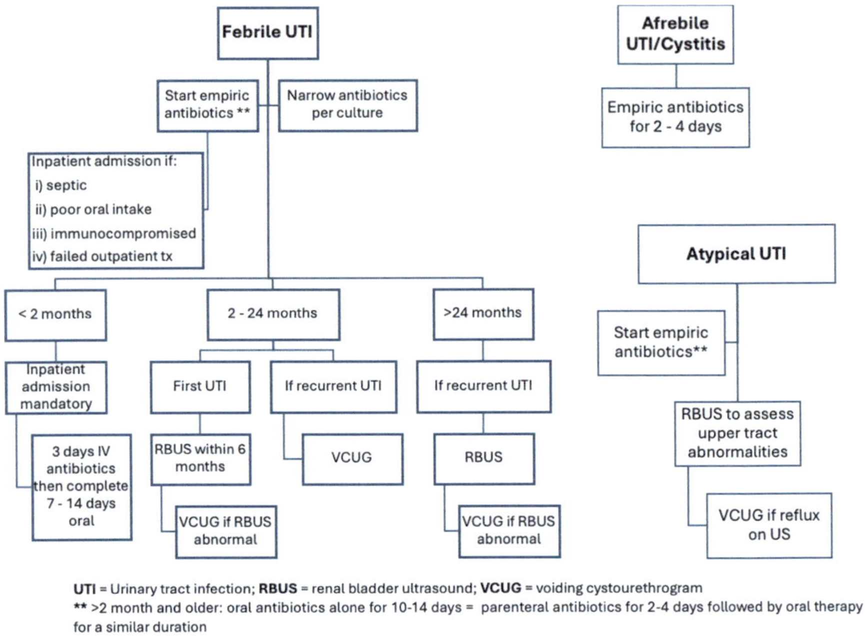

Fig. 5.2 Treatment algorithm for UTI in children [10, 13, 22–28]

especially among female adolescents, and Group B Streptococcus, especially among neonates should be considered based on recent hospitalizations and prior infection patterns [21]. Notably, Enterococcus and Pseudomonas do not have susceptibility to commonly used cephalosporins.

Children with afebrile UTI/simple cystitis can be treated with empiric antibiotics covering common pathogens for 2 to 4 days [13, 22]. Inpatient hospitalization is usually indicated in infants <2 months old, given that fever is common. There is limited high-evidence data on the appropriate duration of antibiotics in this cohort. The AAP suggests completing a 7–14 day antibiotic with future studies investigating shorter duration [23]. A systematic retrospective review and meta-analysis by the INSIGHTSCOPE TEAM concluded that there is no difference in clinical outcomes with a shorter duration (≤3 days) of parenteral antibiotics in infants <2 months old [24]. There was also no difference in recurrence between the total duration of ≤10 vs. >10 days. Earlier transition to oral antibiotics based on local sensitivity and shorter antibiotic courses was associated with reduced antibiotic resistance, shorter length of stay, and lower health care costs [24].

In children older than 2 months, the route of administration should be based on practical considerations. A 2014 Cochrane review identified that in children >1 month old and without grades III to IV VUR with acute pyelonephritis, oral antibiotics given alone for 10 to 14 days are as effective as parenteral antibiotics for 2 to 4 days followed by oral therapy for a similar duration [25]. Parenteral antibiotics should be considered in children who are toxic appearing, immunocompromised, unable to tolerate oral medications, or fail to respond to outpatient therapy [26, 27].

The AAP and AUA recommend that a renal ultrasound should be obtained within 6 months in children <24 months with a first febrile UTI, in older children with recurrent UTIs, and immediately in children with recurrent or atypical UTI (severe illness, kidney injury, poor-treatment response, or non-*E.coli* pathogens) to rule out renal abscess, obstruction, or anatomic abnormalities. VCUG should be obtained if RBUS findings show evidence of VUR or signs of renal scarring. A VCUG should also be considered in cases of repeated febrile infections with a normal sonogram, given increased likelihood of reflux [10, 26, 28].

Modifiable Risk Factors and Epidemiology of UTI in Children

The pathogenesis of UTI begins with colonization of the usually sterile periurethral mucosa by uropathogenic enteric organisms [29]. Host defenses that induce bacterial elimination, immune cell recruitment, and activation reduce the risks for UTI and prevent ascending infections. Factors that increase periurethral mucosa colonization and impair the host defenses increase the risks for UTI [30]. The inability to empty the bladder completely, anatomic anomalies, neurogenic bladder, BBD, and VUR impair natural host defenses [6]. Foreskin in male infants, short urethral length in females, meatal abnormalities, and sexual activity may increase periurethral mucosa colonization [31].

During the first year of life, there is an estimated ten-fold increase in UTI in uncircumcised males compared to circumcised infants. UTI prevalence in the first 3 months has been reported as 2.4% in circumcised boys, 20.1% in uncircumcised boys and 7.5% in girls [16, 32]. AAP recommends consideration of circumcision in newborns with significant perinatal hydronephrosis or reflux—otherwise, routine circumcision is based on family preference [31]. Beyond infancy, the incidence of UTI remains higher in females [3].

Pediatric Primary Vesicoureteral Reflux

Congenital kidney and urinary tract anomalies increase the risk for UTI. VUR is the most common urological abnormality in children [33]. Primary VUR occurs when closure of the intramural ureter fails to occur despite bladder filling and micturition, facilitating retrograde flow of urine from the bladder into the upper tract [6]. A deficiency of longitudinal muscle of the submucosal ureter causes shortening of the intramural portion of the ureter as it transverses the bladder wall, resulting in VUR [6]. Secondary VUR occurs when high voiding bladder pressure results in failure of the closure of the ureterovesical junction (UVJ) during bladder contraction or in the presence of a primary abnormality of the UVJ, such as a diverticulum or ureterocele. The AAP developed a grading system to standardize the severity of VUR based on the retrograde fill and degree of dilation demonstrated on VCUG (Fig. 5.3). VUR

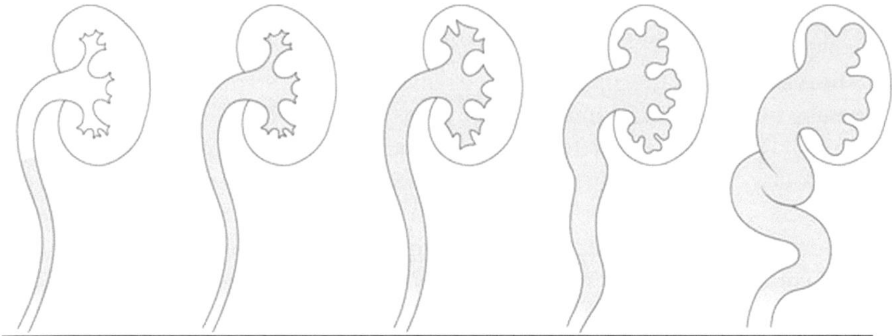

Grade I	Grade II	Grade IIII	Grade IV	Grade V
Reflux into a ureter without dilatation	Reflux into the renal pelvis and calyces without dilation	Mild dilation of the ureter, renal pelvis, and calyces with minimal blunting of the fornices	Moderate ureteral tortuosity and dilation of the renal pelvis and calyces	Gross dilation of the ureter, pelvis, and calyces with loss of papillary impression and ureteral tortuosity

International Reflux Classification

Fig. 5.3 Demonstration of vesicoureteral reflux on voiding cystourethrogram. (Adapted from Lebowitz et al. [62])

increases the risk for pyelonephritis and renal scarring, putting affected patients at risk of developing hypertension, proteinuria, and progression to renal disease.

Guidelines on Management of Pediatric Primary Vesicoureteral Reflux

There has been an evolution in the evaluation and management of VUR since the American Urological Association (AUA) updated their guidelines in 2010 to reflect new research evidence, current practice, and panel consensus. The guidelines were further amended in 2017. Guidelines focused on the evaluation and management of VUR in infants and children over 1 year, the management of children with VUR and BBD, screening of infants with prenatal hydronephrosis, and screening of siblings of patients with VUR [28]. The goal of management of VUR is to prevent recurrent UTIs and renal scarring while limiting treatment-associated morbidity and health-care cost burden [34].

Initial evaluation consists of a thorough medical assessment, including height, weight, blood pressure, screening for BBD, and serum creatinine if bilateral renal parenchymal abnormalities are detected. AUA recommends obtaining a urinalysis to evaluate for proteinuria and bacteriuria with reflex culture as indicated [28]. RBUS should be obtained in infants diagnosed with hydronephrosis in utero and after initial febrile UTI to identify structural abnormalities, including hydronephrosis [6, 10, 28]. Published reports have demonstrated 11% to 67% of screened siblings have VUR; however, the clinical significance of sibling VUR, and the potential benefit of screening siblings to identify it, is unclear [35].

VUR management depends on patient age, reflux grade, and clinical course (Fig. 5.4). In children <1 with grades III–V VUR, the AUA recommends continuous antibiotic prophylaxis (CAP) [28]. For those >1 year old, CAP is recommended if there is clinical evidence of BBD or evidence of renal scarring. Observation without CAP may be considered in the absence of BBD, recurrent febrile UTIs, or renal parenchymal abnormalities [28]. Endoscopic or open surgery may be considered in severe cases and may reduce the incidence of febrile UTIs. Given that there are limited prospective clinical trials on the management of VUR in children, the overall clinical picture of the patient and shared decision discussing benefits and risks with the parents/guidelines should be taken into consideration.

Continued close monitoring to assess for new or progressive renal injury is critical. The AUA recommends annual BP monitoring, height, weight, and urinalysis for proteinuria and bacteriuria [28]. RBUS is recommended annually to assess renal growth and parenchymal scarring. VCUG should be obtained every 12–24 hours in patients with higher grades of VUR (grades III–V), BBD, and older age, with a lower likelihood of spontaneous resolution. Dimercaptosuccinic acid (DMSA) is considered if high concern for renal scarring. For patients with either spontaneous or surgical resolution of VUR, blood pressure, height, weight, and urinalysis are recommended annually through adolescence only if RBUS or DMSA scan demonstrates abnormalities [28]. The risks of continued chronic kidney disease should be discussed with these patients.

Management of Bladder and Bowel Dysfunction

Bladder and bowel dysfunction is a combination of lower urinary tract symptoms (LUTS) and bowel symptoms, including overactive/underactive bladder, incontinence, enuresis, frequency, voiding postponement, straining, constipation, and encopresis in patients without known neurological abnormalities. BBD may lead to incomplete bladder emptying, which provides a nidus for bacterial adherence, replication and increased UTI risk [36]. Rates of recurrent UTIs can be as high as 51% in children with BBD [37]. Concurrent VUR and BBD increase the risk of febrile UTI as well as renal injury. BBD also affects the likelihood of spontaneous reflux resolution, efficacy of CAP, and success of anti-reflux surgery. VUR resolution of rate is 31% in those with BBD vs. 61% in those without [28]. Similarly, in children undergoing endoscopic surgery, a 50% resolution rate has been reported in children with BBD compared to 89% in children without [28].

Standardized questionnaires such as the Dysfunctional Voiding Scoring System and the Vancouver Symptom Score for Dysfunctional Elimination Syndrome can be used to screen for BBD [38]. A spinning top urethra may be seen during voiding on VCUG. Stool burden may also be evaluated on a scout film on VCUG. Treatment of BBD should be prioritized before any surgical intervention for VUR is performed [28]. Management should include the reduction of constipation and LUTS with behavioral modifications such as timed voiding, biofeedback, and alpha blockers.

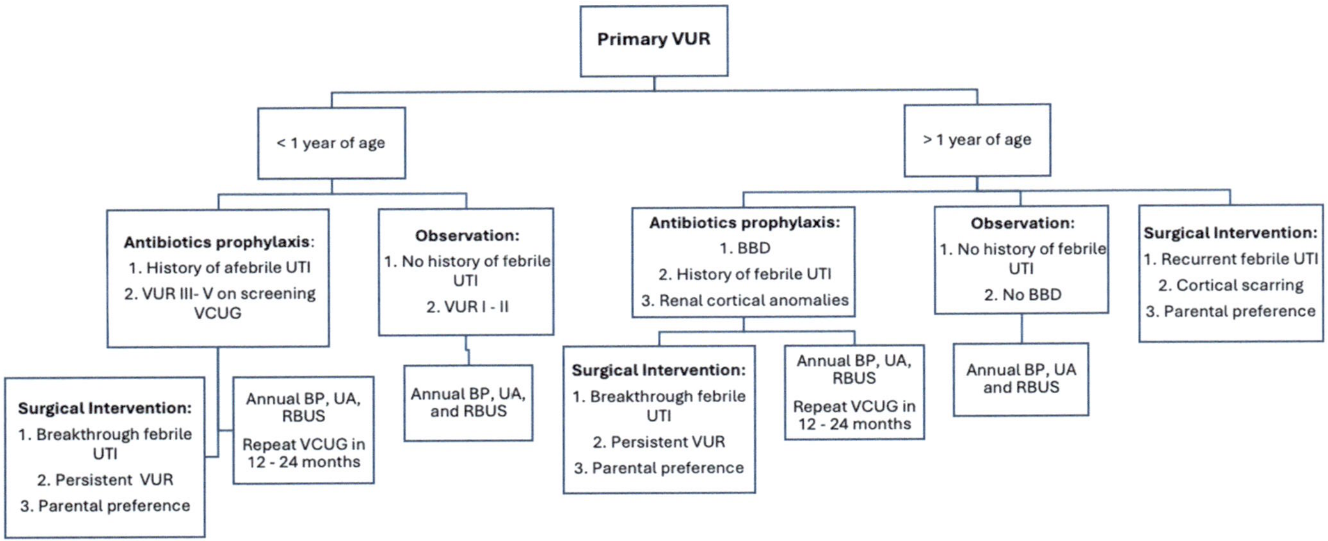

VUR = Vesicoureteral reflux; **UTI** = Urinary Tract Infection; **BBD** = Bowel Bladder Dysfunction; **UA** = Urinalysis; **BP** = Blood pressure; **RBUS** = Renal Bladder Ultrasound; **VCUG** = Voiding Cystourethrogram

Fig. 5.4 Management algorithm for primary vesicoureteral reflux. (Adapted from AUA Update Series Lesson 9, Vol 39, Arlen AM, Cooper CS, 2020)

Anticholinergic agents may be considered in children with an overactive bladder [39].

Role of Continuous Antibiotic Prophylaxis

The role of CAP in the reduction of UTI and renal scarring in children with VUR is controversial and the focus of extensive research. Theoretically, CAP sterilizes urine and promotes the reflux of sterile urine into the upper tracts, therefore preventing recurrent infection and renal scarring. Several studies have demonstrated that CAP prevents renal scarring, while others have reported that CAP has a limited effect on scarring [40–44]. Randomized Intervention for Children with Vesicoureteral Reflux (RIVUR) trial and the Prevention of Urinary Tract Infection in Children with Vesicoureteral and Normal Renal Tracts (PRIVENT) trial are the largest such studies. RIVUR trial was a double-blind, placebo-controlled trial involving children diagnosed with VUR after febrile or symptomatic UTI. It concluded that CAP was associated with a 45% reduced risk of UTI recurrence but not prevention of scarring [42]. Similarly, the PRIVENT trial reported an association with decreased number of UTIs without impact on the rate of renal damage in the CAP group [45]. Children with any degree of VUR and BBD were identified to have the highest risk of recurrent UTI in the Careful Urinary Tract Infection Evaluation (CUTIE) study, and CAP and treatment of BBD were protective in these children [43]. However, a randomized trial by Pennesi et al. reported that CAP was ineffective at reducing UTI risks and preventing renal damage in children <30 months with VUR grades II–IV [46]. Hari et al. reported a 14.8% increased risk of symptomatic UTI with CAP compared to placebo in grades I–IV VUR [47]. These studies were heterogenous, some inadequately powered, especially to detect renal scarring, and some conclusions were not generalizable.

Given conflicting data, the AUA and AAP recommend the selective use of antibiotic prophylaxis to prevent UTIs. Specifically, CAP is recommended for children <1 year old with VUR and a history of febrile UTI or with grades III–V VUR in the absence of febrile UTI who are at greatest risk of UTI and renal scarring [10, 28]. For children >1 year old, the guidelines recommend CAP for the child with BBD and VUR due to the increased risk of UTI while BBD is present [28].

A major concern of CAP is the development of multidrug-resistant (MDR) infection. A meta-analysis by Selekman et al. concluded that CAP increased the risk of MDR—they reported 1 MDR for every 21 VUR patients on CAP [44]. The PRIVENT and RIVUR trials also reported a 2- to 3-fold increase in resistance to trimethoprim-sulfamethoxazole in the CAP compared to the placebo group [42, 45]. Early CAP use, within the first few years of a child's life has also been associated with increase in body mass index and obesity later in life. This has been hypothesized to likely be secondary to the alteration of the gut microbiota by bacteria, which may predispose to obesity later in life [48]. Probiotics have been proposed as adjuvants to modulate the gut microbiota [49]. Other adverse effects, including side effects of antibiotics, parental compliance, and health care costs should also be considered.

Shared decision-making with parents/guardians, risk of recurrent febrile UTIs, and likelihood of spontaneous resolution of VUR should be determined when considering CAP. Patients most likely to benefit from CAP are those with high-grade reflux (grades III–V), children with febrile UTI before toilet training, low-grade VUR with preexisting kidney scarring or congenital anomaly and all patients with BBD regardless of VUR severity who are at highest risk of recurrent UTIs [28]. Surveillance remains an option for patients who prefer observation and are compliant with regular follow-up [28].

Surgical Management of Pediatric Vesicoureteral Reflux

VUR often resolves. Rate of spontaneous resolution has been reported to be 82% in grade I VUR, 30% in grade IV and 13% in grade V over a 5-year period [50]. The incidence of recurrent UTI and renal scarring is similar with medical versus surgical treatment of VUR [51]. As such, most children with VUR can be managed conservatively. Surgical intervention is reserved for patients with severe VUR, older children who are unlikely to have spontaneous resolution, febrile breakthrough UTI despite CAP and optimization of BBD, high risk of pyelonephritis, history of renal scarring, and/or impaired renal function [52]. AUA advocates both open and endoscopic methods for VUR correction [28]. VUR resolution rate with endoscopic surgery after a single bulking agent injection is 83% compared to 98% for open surgery [28, 53]. The incidence of postoperative adverse effects is low and strongly associated with preoperative UTI and BBD. The management of BBD is strongly recommended prior to any surgical intervention and should be continued postoperatively [28].

Endoscopic treatment of VUR is a minimally invasive method that involves performing subureteric injection of bulking agents such as dextranomer/hyaluronic acid (Dx/HA). The gradual absorption of these agents forms a collagen agent that buttresses the distal ureter and narrows the ureterovesical junction (UVJ), preventing reflux without causing obstruction. The most common method is the double hydrodistension implantation technique (Double HIT), which includes the submucosal injection at the distal ureter and hydrodistension of the ureter with fluid, which allows for improved visualization and success rate (Fig. 5.5). Dx/HA is FDA approved for the treatment of grades II to IV VUR, although there are limited studies for approval for Grade V VUR [54].

The Swedish Reflux Trial in Children compared the outcomes of CAP, endoscopic treatment, or surveillance alone in children with grade III or IV. A total of 71% of patients who underwent endoscopic treatment had resolved or diminished VUR on VCUG at 2 years compared to 47% in the surveillance group [55]. Success rate is as high as 89% in grade I VUR and 71% in grade III VUR, compared to almost 98% in open ureteral reimplantation, as already mentioned [56]. Adverse effects are very low, the most concerning is postoperative obstruction, reported to be 0.7% [54]. Given the higher likelihood of recurrence of reflux with endoscopic

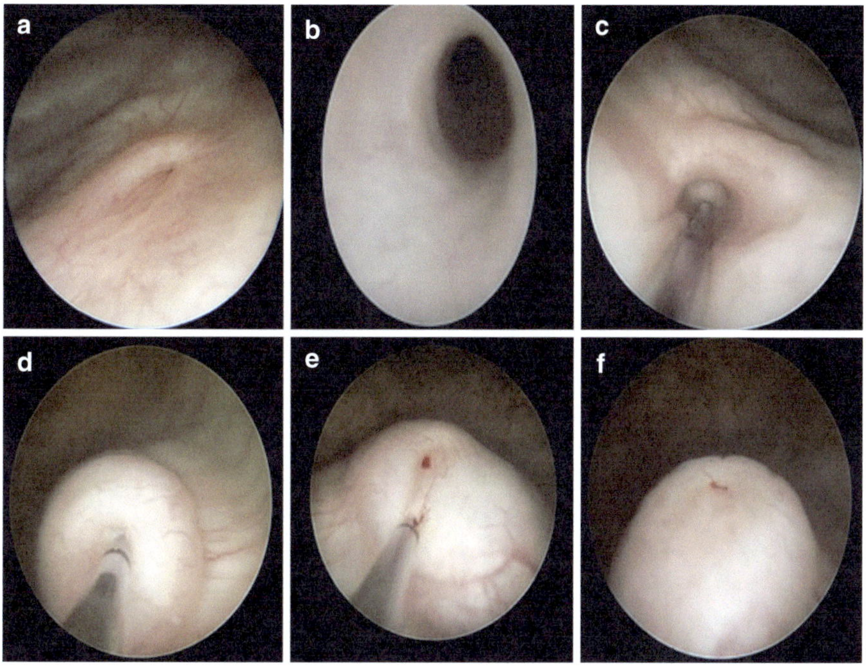

Fig. 5.5 Double HIT Method. Bladder is drained and ureteral orifice visualized (**a**), followed by hydrodistension with the extramural ureter visualized (**b**). Proximal HIT is then performed with the needle inserted into the mid-ureteral tunnel at the 6 o'clock position (**c**). Sufficient bulking agent is injected to produce a bulge which coapts the tunnel (**d**). Distal HIT is subsequently performed (**e**) and leading to coaptation of the ureteral orifice (**f**). (Photo from AUA Update Series Lesson 9, Vol 39, Arlen AM, Cooper CS, 2020, used with permission from author)

treatment compared to open surgery, children are maintained on antibiotic prophylaxis until reflux resolution is confirmed on follow-up VCUG in 3 months. The AUA recommends postoperative RBUS to assess for obstruction and VCUG to assess for resolution [28]. Second injections may be considered if a first injection fails; however, the success rate decreases to 50% [54]. Open surgical approaches should be considered in patients with persistent reflux.

Ureteral reimplantation involves creation of a ureteroneocystostomy which increases intravesical ureteral length and facilitates compression of the ureter against the detrusor muscle, preventing reflux. With a 98% success rate for grades I–IV VUR, open ureteral reimplantation remains the gold standard treatment [56]. The Cohen cross-trigonal reimplantation, an intravesical technique, is utilized most frequently due to its generalizability and reliability (Fig. 5.6) [57, 58].

Given the high-resolution rate of VUR with open ureteral reimplantation, the AUA recommends that obtaining a postoperative VCUG is optional and dependent on the patient's postoperative course [28]. Compared to the endoscopic approach, open ureteral reimplantation is associated with more morbidity, most commonly UTI. Postoperative UTI was reported to be as high as 21.8% and pyelonephritis in

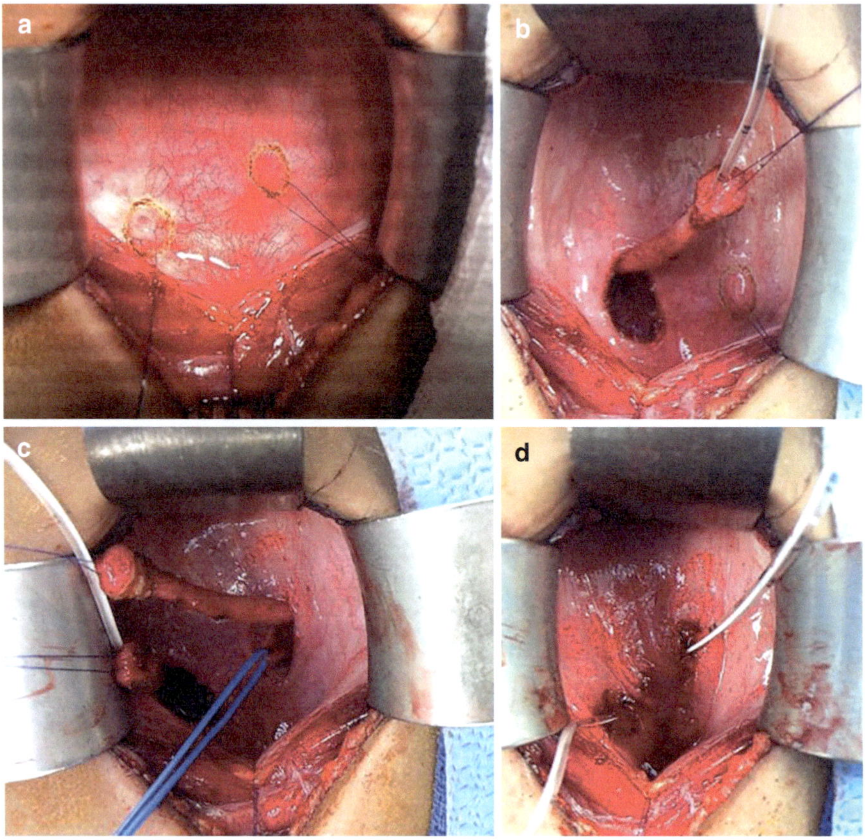

Fig. 5.6 Bilateral Cohen cross-trigonal reimplant. Ureteral orifices are tagged and needlepoint cautery is utilized to circumscribe the orifices (**a**). The ureter is mobilized to ensure the tunnel length is five times the ureteral diameter (**b**). In boys, it is important to ensure preservation of the vas deferens (encircled with blue vessel loop) (**c**). After the creation of tunnels, the ureters are approximated to the neo-orifices bilaterally, and feeding tubes temporarily passed to ensure there is no obstruction (**d**). (Photo from AUA Update Series Lesson 9, Vol 39, Arlen AM, Cooper CS, 2020, used with permission from author)

up to 6.5% of patients at a median follow-up of 2.9 years [59]. VCUG should be obtained in cases of recurrent UTIs, and this risk should be discussed with family and caregivers [57].

Robotic-assisted laparoscopic ureteral reimplantation has been gaining popularity over the past decade with increased popularity of the robotic technology, which allows for superior stereoscopic visualization. Multi-institutional retrospective studies have reported radiographic reflux resolution rate of 87.9–93.8% and clinical success rate of 91.9% [60, 61]. Compared to the open approach, robotic reimplantation is associated with less morbidity, earlier ambulation, shorter hospital length of stay, lower postoperative pain, and analgesic requirements [57]. These advantages are more relevant in older children. The robotic approach is usually extravesical. Clinical course, severity of VUR, treatment goals, and surgeon training must be taken into consideration to determine the most appropriate intervention for each patient.

Clinical Pearls

- UTI diagnosis requires UA and culture with >50,000 CFU; lower counts are acceptable if associated with fever.
- Catheterized specimens are necessary in children who are unable to provide a clean catch sample.
- Empiric antibiotic choice should be based on prior cultures and the hospital antibiogram.
- RBUS should be obtained in children with febrile UTI; VCUG should be obtained if recurrent febrile UTI or an anomaly is noted on US.
- Children with UTI, particularly those who are toilet-trained, should be screened for BBD.
- BBD must be addressed prior to any surgical intervention for reflux and continued postoperatively.
- CAP should be considered in children with high-grade reflux, febrile UTI before toilet training, low-grade VUR with preexisting kidney scarring or congenital anomaly, and all patients with BBD, regardless of VUR severity, who are at the highest risk of recurrent UTIs.
- Surgical management of VUR should be reserved for children with high-grade VUR, febrile breakthrough UTI despite CAP and optimization of BBD, high risk of pyelonephritis, presence of renal scarring, and/or impaired renal function—best approach is individualized.

References

1. Daniel M, Szymanik-Grzelak H, Sierdzinski J, Podsiadly E, Kowalewska-Mlot M, Panczyk-Tomaszewska M. Epidemiology and risk factors of UTIs in children-a single-center observation. J Pers Med. 2023;13(1) https://doi.org/10.3390/jpm13010138.
2. Conway PH, Cnaan A, Zaoutis T, Henry BV, Grundmeier RW, Keren R. Recurrent urinary tract infections in children: risk factors and association with prophylactic antimicrobials. JAMA. 2007;298(2):179–86. https://doi.org/10.1001/jama.298.2.179.
3. Shaikh N, Morone NE, Bost JE, Farrell MH. Prevalence of urinary tract infection in childhood: a meta-analysis. Pediatr Infect Dis J. 2008;27(4):302–8. https://doi.org/10.1097/INF.0b013e31815e4122.
4. Leung AKC, Wong AHC, Leung AAM, Hon KL. Urinary tract infection in children. Recent Patents Inflamm Allergy Drug Discov. 2019;13(1):2–18. https://doi.org/10.2174/1872213X13666181228154940.
5. Tullus K, Shaikh N. Urinary tract infections in children. Lancet. 2020;395(10237):1659–68. https://doi.org/10.1016/S0140-6736(20)30676-0.

6. Schlager TA. Urinary tract infections in infants and children. Microbiol Spectr. 2016;4(5) https://doi.org/10.1128/microbiolspec.UTI-0022-2016.
7. Atay N, Uslu GA. Evaluation of urinalysis and urine culture in children with first-time urinary tract infection. Turk J Urol. 2021;47(3):242–7. https://doi.org/10.5152/tud.2020.20387.
8. Piepsz A, Tamminen-Mobius T, Reiners C, et al. Five-year study of medical or surgical treatment in children with severe vesico-ureteral reflux dimercaptosuccinic acid findings. International Reflux Study Group in Europe. Eur J Pediatr. 1998;157(9):753–8. https://doi.org/10.1007/s004310050929.
9. Shaikh N, Craig JC, Rovers MM, et al. Identification of children and adolescents at risk for renal scarring after a first urinary tract infection: a meta-analysis with individual patient data. JAMA Pediatr. 2014;168(10):893–900. https://doi.org/10.1001/jamapediatrics.2014.637.
10. Subcommittee on Urinary Tract Infection SCoQI, Management, Roberts KB. Urinary tract infection: clinical practice guideline for the diagnosis and management of the initial UTI in febrile infants and children 2 to 24 months. Pediatrics. 2011;128(3):595–610. https://doi.org/10.1542/peds.2011-1330.
11. Shaikh N, Hoberman A, Hum SW, et al. Development and validation of a calculator for estimating the probability of urinary tract infection in young febrile children. JAMA Pediatr. 2018;172(6):550–6. https://doi.org/10.1001/jamapediatrics.2018.0217.
12. O'Brien K, Edwards A, Hood K, Butler CC. Prevalence of urinary tract infection in acutely unwell children in general practice: a prospective study with systematic urine sampling. Br J Gen Pract. 2013;63(607):e156–64. https://doi.org/10.3399/bjgp13X663127.
13. Veauthier B, Miller MV. Urinary tract infections in young children and infants: common questions and answers. Am Fam Physician. 2020;102(5):278–85. https://www.ncbi.nlm.nih.gov/pubmed/32866365.
14. Gorelick MH, Hoberman A, Kearney D, Wald E, Shaw KN. Validation of a decision rule identifying febrile young girls at high risk for urinary tract infection. Pediatr Emerg Care. 2003;19(3):162–4. https://doi.org/10.1097/01.pec.0000081238.98249.40.
15. Shaw KN, Gorelick M, McGowan KL, Yakscoe NM, Schwartz JS. Prevalence of urinary tract infection in febrile young children in the emergency department. Pediatrics. 1998;102(2):e16. https://doi.org/10.1542/peds.102.2.e16.
16. Stein R, Dogan HS, Hoebeke P, et al. Urinary tract infections in children: EAU/ESPU guidelines. Eur Urol. 2015;67(3):546–58. https://doi.org/10.1016/j.eururo.2014.11.007.
17. Larcombe J. Urinary tract infection in children. Clin Evid. 2005;13:444–57. https://www.ncbi.nlm.nih.gov/pubmed/16135271.
18. Subcommittee On Urinary Tract I. Reaffirmation of AAP clinical practice guideline: the diagnosis and management of the initial urinary tract infection in febrile infants and young children 2-24 months of age. Pediatrics. 2016;138(6) https://doi.org/10.1542/peds.2016-3026.
19. Bryce A, Hay AD, Lane IF, Thornton HV, Wootton M, Costelloe C. Global prevalence of antibiotic resistance in paediatric urinary tract infections caused by Escherichia coli and association with routine use of antibiotics in primary care: systematic review and meta-analysis. BMJ. 2016;352:i939. https://doi.org/10.1136/bmj.i939.
20. Yakubov R, van den Akker M, Machamad K, Hochberg A, Nadir E, Klein A. Antimicrobial resistance among uropathogens that cause childhood community-acquired urinary tract infections in Central Israel. Pediatr Infect Dis J. 2017;36(1):113–5. https://doi.org/10.1097/INF.0000000000001373.
21. Edlin RS, Shapiro DJ, Hersh AL, Copp HL. Antibiotic resistance patterns of outpatient pediatric urinary tract infections. J Urol. 2013;190(1):222–7. https://doi.org/10.1016/j.juro.2013.01.069.
22. Michael M, Hodson EM, Craig JC, Martin S, Moyer VA. Short compared with standard duration of antibiotic treatment for urinary tract infection: a systematic review of randomised controlled trials. Arch Dis Child. 2002;87(2):118–23. https://doi.org/10.1136/adc.87.2.118.

23. Chang PW, Wang ME, Schroeder AR. Diagnosis and management of UTI in febrile infants age 0-2 months: applicability of the AAP guideline. J Hosp Med. 2020;15(2):e1–5. https://doi.org/10.12788/jhm.3349.
24. Nama N, Donken R, Pawliuk C, et al. Treatment of UTIs in infants <2 months: a living systematic review. Hosp Pediatr. 2021;11(9):1017–30. https://doi.org/10.1542/hpeds.2021-005877.
25. Strohmeier Y, Hodson EM, Willis NS, Webster AC, Craig JC. Antibiotics for acute pyelonephritis in children. Cochrane Database Syst Rev. 2014;2014(7):CD003772. https://doi.org/10.1002/14651858.CD003772.pub4.
26. Zorc JJ, Kiddoo DA, Shaw KN. Diagnosis and management of pediatric urinary tract infections. Clin Microbiol Rev. 2005;18(2):417–22. https://doi.org/10.1128/CMR.18.2.417-422.2005.
27. Jones ME, Karlowsky JA, Draghi DC, Thornsberry C, Sahm DF, Bradley JS. Rates of antimicrobial resistance among common bacterial pathogens causing respiratory, blood, urine, and skin and soft tissue infections in pediatric patients. Eur J Clin Microbiol Infect Dis. 2004;23(6):445–55. https://doi.org/10.1007/s10096-004-1133-5.
28. Peters CA, Skoog SJ, Arant BS Jr, et al. Summary of the AUA guideline on management of primary vesicoureteral reflux in children. J Urol. 2010;184(3):1134–44. https://doi.org/10.1016/j.juro.2010.05.065.
29. Bollgren I, Winberg J. The periurethral aerobic bacterial flora in healthy boys and girls. Acta Paediatr Scand. 1976;65(1):74–80. https://doi.org/10.1111/j.1651-2227.1976.tb04410.x.
30. Ballek NK, McKenna PH. Lower urinary tract dysfunction in childhood. Urol Clin North Am. 2010;37(2):215–28. https://doi.org/10.1016/j.ucl.2010.03.001.
31. Shapiro E. American academy of pediatrics policy statements on circumcision and urinary tract infection. Rev Urol. 1999;1(3):154–6. https://www.ncbi.nlm.nih.gov/pubmed/16985788.
32. Gondim R, Azevedo R, Braga A, Veiga ML, Barroso U Jr. Risk factors for urinary tract infection in children with urinary urgency. Int Braz J Urol. 2018;44(2):378–83. https://doi.org/10.1590/S1677-5538.IBJU.2017.0434.
33. Naseri M, Tafazoli N, Tafazoli N. Prevalence of vesicoureteral reflux in children with urinary tract infection. Saudi J Kidney Dis Transpl. 2022;33(Supplement):S111–20. https://doi.org/10.4103/1319-2442.384183.
34. Mattoo TK. Selective antimicrobial prophylaxis for vesicoureteral reflux. N Engl J Med. 2023;389(11):1043–4. https://doi.org/10.1056/NEJMe2308885.
35. Nelson CP, Finkelstein JA, Logvinenko T, Schuster MA. Incidence of urinary tract infection among siblings of children with vesicoureteral reflux. Acad Pediatr. 2016;16(5):489–95. https://doi.org/10.1016/j.acap.2015.11.003.
36. Chang SJ, Yang SS, Chiang IN. Large voided volume suggestive of abnormal uroflow pattern and elevated post-void residual urine. Neurourol Urodyn. 2011;30(1):58–61. https://doi.org/10.1002/nau.20901.
37. Shaikh N, Hoberman A, Keren R, et al. Recurrent urinary tract infections in children with bladder and bowel dysfunction. Pediatrics. 2016;137(1) https://doi.org/10.1542/peds.2015-2982.
38. Afshar K, Mirbagheri A, Scott H, MacNeily AE. Development of a symptom score for dysfunctional elimination syndrome. J Urol. 2009;182(4 Suppl):1939–43. https://doi.org/10.1016/j.juro.2009.03.009.
39. Santos JD, Lopes RI, Koyle MA. Bladder and bowel dysfunction in children: an update on the diagnosis and treatment of a common, but underdiagnosed pediatric problem. Can Urol Assoc J. 2017;11(1-2Suppl1):S64–72. https://doi.org/10.5489/cuaj.4411.
40. Williams G, Craig JC. Long-term antibiotics for preventing recurrent urinary tract infection in children. Cochrane Database Syst Rev. 2019;4(4):CD001534. https://doi.org/10.1002/14651858.CD001534.pub4.
41. Larcombe J. Urinary tract infection in children: recurrent infections. BMJ Clin Evid. 2015:2015. https://www.ncbi.nlm.nih.gov/pubmed/26067232.
42. Investigators RT, Hoberman A, Greenfield SP, et al. Antimicrobial prophylaxis for children with vesicoureteral reflux. N Engl J Med. 2014;370(25):2367–76. https://doi.org/10.1056/NEJMoa1401811.

43. Keren R, Shaikh N, Pohl H, et al. Risk factors for recurrent urinary tract infection and renal scarring. Pediatrics. 2015;136(1):e13–21. https://doi.org/10.1542/peds.2015-0409.
44. Selekman RE, Shapiro DJ, Boscardin J, et al. Uropathogen resistance and antibiotic prophylaxis: a meta-analysis. Pediatrics. 2018;142(1) https://doi.org/10.1542/peds.2018-0119.
45. Craig JC, Simpson JM, Williams GJ, et al. Antibiotic prophylaxis and recurrent urinary tract infection in children. N Engl J Med. 2009;361(18):1748–59. https://doi.org/10.1056/NEJMoa0902295.
46. Pennesi M, Travan L, Peratoner L, et al. Is antibiotic prophylaxis in children with vesicoureteral reflux effective in preventing pyelonephritis and renal scars? A randomized, controlled trial. Pediatrics. 2008;121(6):e1489–94. https://doi.org/10.1542/peds.2007-2652.
47. Hari P, Hari S, Sinha A, et al. Antibiotic prophylaxis in the management of vesicoureteric reflux: a randomized double-blind placebo-controlled trial. Pediatr Nephrol. 2015;30(3):479–86. https://doi.org/10.1007/s00467-014-2943-z.
48. Rawat SS, Narain NP, Marathe SM, Sonawale SB, Veligandla KC. Early-life antibiotics and childhood obesity: yeast probiotics as a strategy to modulate gut microbiota. Cureus. 2023;15(3):e36795. https://doi.org/10.7759/cureus.36795.
49. Neut C, Mahieux S, Dubreuil LJ. Antibiotic susceptibility of probiotic strains: is it reasonable to combine probiotics with antibiotics? Med Mal Infect. 2017;47(7):477–83. https://doi.org/10.1016/j.medmal.2017.07.001.
50. Shaikh N, Ewing AL, Bhatnagar S, Hoberman A. Risk of renal scarring in children with a first urinary tract infection: a systematic review. Pediatrics. 2010;126(6):1084–91. https://doi.org/10.1542/peds.2010-0685.
51. Weiss R, Duckett J, Spitzer A. Results of a randomized clinical trial of medical versus surgical management of infants and children with grades III and IV primary vesicoureteral reflux (United States). The International Reflux Study in children. J Urol. 1992;148(5 Pt 2):1667–73. https://doi.org/10.1016/s0022-5347(17)36998-7.
52. Marsh MC, Junquera GY, Stonebrook E, Spencer JD, Watson JR. Urinary Tract infections in children. Pediatr Rev. 2024;45(5):260–70. https://doi.org/10.1542/pir.2023-006017.
53. Hunziker M, Mohanan N, Puri P. Dextranomer/hyaluronic acid endoscopic injection is effective in the treatment of intermediate and high grade vesicoureteral reflux in patients with complete duplex systems. J Urol. 2013;189(5):1876–81. https://doi.org/10.1016/j.juro.2012.11.048.
54. Diamond DA, Mattoo TK. Endoscopic treatment of primary vesicoureteral reflux. N Engl J Med. 2012;366(13):1218–26. https://doi.org/10.1056/NEJMct1108922.
55. Holmdahl G, Brandstrom P, Lackgren G, et al. The Swedish reflux trial in children: II. Vesicoureteral reflux outcome. J Urol. 2010;184(1):280–5. https://doi.org/10.1016/j.juro.2010.01.059.
56. Routh JC, Inman BA, Reinberg Y. Dextranomer/hyaluronic acid for pediatric vesicoureteral reflux: systematic review. Pediatrics. 2010;125(5):1010–9. https://doi.org/10.1542/peds.2009-2225.
57. Kirsch AJ, Arlen AM. Evolving surgical management of pediatric vesicoureteral reflux: is open ureteral reimplantation still the 'gold standard'? Int Braz J Urol. 2020;46(3):314–21. https://doi.org/10.1590/S1677-5538.IBJU.2020.99.05.
58. Sung J, Skoog S. Surgical management of vesicoureteral reflux in children. Pediatr Nephrol. 2012;27(4):551–61. https://doi.org/10.1007/s00467-011-1933-7.
59. Nelson CP, Hubert KC, Kokorowski PJ, et al. Long-term incidence of urinary tract infection after ureteral reimplantation for primary vesicoureteral reflux. J Pediatr Urol. 2013;9(1):92–8. https://doi.org/10.1016/j.jpurol.2011.12.009.

60. Grimsby GM, Dwyer ME, Jacobs MA, et al. Multi-institutional review of outcomes of robot-assisted laparoscopic extravesical ureteral reimplantation. J Urol. 2015;193(5 Suppl):1791–5. https://doi.org/10.1016/j.juro.2014.07.128.
61. Boysen WR, Ellison JS, Kim C, et al. Multi-institutional review of outcomes and complications of robot-assisted laparoscopic extravesical ureteral reimplantation for treatment of primary vesicoureteral reflux in children. J Urol. 2017;197(6):1555–61. https://doi.org/10.1016/j.juro.2017.01.062.
62. Lebowitz RL, Olbing H, Parkkulainen KV, et al. International reflux study in children: international system of radiographic grading of Vesico-ureteral reflux: International Reflux Study in Children. Pediatr Radiol. 1985;15:105.

6 Urinary Incontinence

Hsi-Yang Wu

This chapter provides a practical approach to treating non-neurogenic pediatric urinary incontinence. The main differences between pediatric and adult urinary incontinence are that there are two main causes of functional urinary incontinence in children, and a child's symptoms do not correlate well with the underlying problem, leading to more emphasis being placed on functional studies.

Urinary incontinence is sometimes treated by pediatric nephrologists or pediatricians (more so in Europe), but it represents 20% of outpatient pediatric urology visits in the United States. The reason that urologists became involved in treating incontinence was due to the rare girl who presented with continuous urinary incontinence from an ectopic ureter draining into the vagina, or the boy who presented late with posterior urethral valves. While both conditions are on the differential diagnosis, most neurologically normal patients with urinary continence have a functional rather than an anatomical problem.

Girls usually toilet train at age 2 years, and boys at 3 years. Many daycare centers will help out with the toilet training process by taking all the children at regular intervals to the toilet. Parents will often seek medical help at age 5, before their children enter kindergarten. About 15% of children will still have nocturnal enuresis at age 5 years [1].

Daytime Incontinence

By the time patients are referred to a urologist for daytime urinary incontinence, the pediatrician will have usually checked a urinalysis for infection or diabetes, and ordered a renal bladder ultrasound to look for hydronephrosis suggestive of an

H.-Y. Wu (✉)
Surgery, Division of Urology, Alpert Medical School of Brown University, Providence, RI, USA

H.-Y. Wu et al. (eds.), *Pediatric Urology for the Adult Urologist*, https://doi.org/10.1007/978-3-032-10306-2_6

ectopic ureter or posterior urethral valves. If these screening tests have not been done, they should be obtained to rule out anatomical conditions that would require surgery. Prior treatments that the parents have already tried, such as timed voiding, limiting of bladder irritants, and treatment of constipation should be reviewed, to decide how the treatment plan can be advanced [2].

When I first meet a patient with urinary incontinence, I try to decide whether the patient has overactive bladder (OAB) or dysfunctional voiding (DV). Dysfunctional voiding is a specific condition where the external urethral sphincter and pelvic floor do not relax when the child tries to void. While "voiding dysfunction" is used in urology, it leads to confusion as to whether the child has OAB or DV. Since the treatment of OAB and DV are different, I prefer to use the specific condition when describing daytime incontinence [3].

The normal maturation of the lower urinary tract during toilet training follows a typical pattern: stool continence, urinary continence during the day, and then finally urinary continence at night. The infant's bladder has a small capacity, and the infant's external urethral sphincter does not relax appropriately to allow the bladder to empty completely. Children start toilet training by tightening their pelvic floor to hold their urine until they can get to the toilet. As they hold their urine, the bladder increases in volume. Failure to develop a normal bladder capacity leads to OAB. The second step in toilet training is learning how to relax the pelvic floor and external urethral sphincter to allow the bladder to empty completely. Failure to relax the pelvic floor leads to DV. Our treatments are aimed at getting children to complete the toilet training process, so that coordinated and complete bladder emptying can occur [1].

History The age at toilet training can give some idea of how difficult it was for the child to do toilet train. Getting a baseline of how may days and nights out of a week the child is wet will set the expectation for how much treatment will be needed. A detailed voiding history will suggest whether the child is holding their urine for long periods [2]. As children will often give a random number when asked how often they void during the day, I ask a series of questions:

"Do you urinate before school?"

"How many times do you urinate at school (at lunch or recess)?"

"How many times do you urinate between getting home at dinner?"

"Do you urinate before going to bed?"

I then ask about holding, urgency, hesitancy, abdominal straining, interruption of the stream, incomplete emptying, and post-void dribbling. These symptoms don't necessarily correlate with OAB or DV, but it does tell me what their most bothersome symptom is. Children should void five to seven times during the day.

UTI's can worsen daytime incontinence, and even without vesicoureteral reflux, I will offer daily antibiotic prophylaxis to children who have UTI's every month to calm the bladder down, so that they can work on getting the bladder to store properly.

Constipation can worsen incontinence by decreasing the storage capacity of the bladder or producing an urge to void that is not due to the bladder itself. Effective treatment of constipation will often improve urinary continence. In addition, another reason I look for constipation is to decide if I should avoid anticholinergics in a child with OAB, as medications will make their constipation worse.

Dietary causes of incontinence can be due to excess intake of sugary drinks (soda, sweetened juices), caffeine, or even excess water.

If the diagnosis is clear at the initial visit, I will start treatment. However, if after checking a post-void residual (PVR), there seems to be a mixed picture of OAB and DV, I will ask the parents to carry out a 48-hour voiding diary. This is best done when the child is at home for the entire day. I ask parents to record the time that the child voids and the volume voided. The goal is to make sure that the child is not polyuric and to get an accurate idea of what the child's typical bladder capacity is. The age expected bladder capacity is calculated as (age in years +2) × 30 in mL [4]. To get an accurate PVR, the child's bladder should be between 50% and 115% of age expected capacity prior to voiding [3]. If the parents wish to record an intake diary as well, the daily expected fluid intake in mL (on top of a regular diet) is calculated as the child's weight in kg × 30. The calculated normal daily urine output in mL is the weight in kg × 24.

Physical Examination Checking for a distended bladder or sigmoid can be done on abdominal exam. I also check leg strength and gait to look for subtle signs of tethered cord. I examine the lower back to check for a deep sacral dimple or a tuft of hair. A genital exam to look for tight phimosis or labial adhesions is done if there is post-void dribbling. However, I rarely check a bulbocavernosus reflex as this is difficult for children to tolerate [2].

Functional Studies The renal ultrasound sometimes includes a bladder ultrasound, but often the bladder is not full enough to get an accurate post-void residual. A post-void residual of >10% of the age expected bladder capacity suggests incomplete emptying, possibly due to DV. If I am considering sending a child to physical therapy for pelvic floor biofeedback, I will have them do a uroflow with pelvic floor EMG to show that the problem is indeed the pelvic floor. I rarely perform urodynamics in neurologically normal children with daytime incontinence, as this is reserved for those who are refractory to treatment or who have other evidence of a neurogenic bladder [3].

Imaging I only order an MRI of the lumbar spine to look for a tethered cord in patients who are refractory to treatment or have a clearly abnormal lower extremity examination. Shallow sacral dimples without hair are fairly normal and by themselves are not a reason to get an MRI. VCUG is reserved for younger children with recurrent febrile UTI or abnormal kidneys.

Treatment OAB patients will have urinary frequency and a small bladder capacity. In such situations, I will start with an anticholinergic medication such as oxybutynin 0.1 mg/kg given twice a day. If they do not respond, I will try a β3 agonist at the appropriate dose. For mirabegron, the dose for 11–21 kg is 24 mg (3 mL), 22–34 kg is 32 mg (4 mL), and >35 kg is 48 mg (6 mL). If the OAB does not improve then I will discuss bladder botulinum toxin injection, limited to 100 U, as long as the parent and child are aware of the risk for urinary retention and possible urethral catheter placement [5].

Patients with constipation will need treatment with polyethylene glycol or senna so that they have regular bowel movements daily.

DV patients tend to have infrequent voids with an elevated PVR. I start out with a timed voiding schedule every 3 hours during the day and double voiding (10 minutes after they void), done at least three times a day when they are at home. If the PVR is not improved after 3 months, and the child is too young for biofeedback, then I will use tamsulosin 0.4 mg for children >4 years, and 0.2 mg for children <4 years. Sometimes, the younger children cannot swallow the tamsulosin capsule, so I ask their parents to open the capsule and put the contents into food. The other alternative is terazosin, which has a liquid formulation. For children >8 years who are motivated to do physical therapy, I will have them start PT without starting an alpha blocker. If the child is developing hydronephrosis, then I will move on to external urethral sphincter botulinum toxin injection (100 U) [6]. For the child who fails a sphincter botulinum toxin injection, then I will discuss teaching them clean intermittent catheterization, which is difficult in sensate children.

Less common causes for daytime incontinence are giggle incontinence and stress urinary incontinence in very active athletic girls. Giggle incontinence is often mixed with OAB or dysfunctional voiding, so treatment for those two conditions should be started first [7]. True isolated giggle incontinence responds well to methylphenidate at 5–20 mg [8]. Stress urinary incontinence can occur in girls who participate in high-impact sports such as gymnastics [9]. As a suburethral sling is too aggressive in teenagers, injection of a urethral bulking agent is a reasonable choice. Although it does not cause incontinence, extraordinary urinary frequency causes significant daytime frequency without nocturia and does not respond to anticholinergics. As long as the renal bladder ultrasound is normal, no treatment is needed, as it spontaneously resolves within a year [10].

Special Populations Children with ADHD or autism are harder to get dry, because it is harder for them to comply with behavioral therapies such as timed voiding, and their visceral sensation can be poor. The treatments for daytime incontinence are the same as those for other children [11]. I have seen some patients who were not making progress with treatment of their daytime incontinence improve rapidly when they were started on treatment for ADHD, since they could finally concentrate on what was going on with their bodies.

Nocturnal Enuresis

Bedwetting is due to an interaction of three factors: fluid intake, bladder capacity, and the child's ability to detect a full bladder while they are sleeping [12]. I tend to use the voiding diary for most patients with nocturnal enuresis because I want to know if their bladder capacity is normal. Desmopressin works better in children with normal to large bladder capacities. The voiding diary also allows me to see if they are drinking too close to bedtime, with the goal of stopping fluid intake 3 hours before bedtime. If the child has a small bladder capacity, I will start them on an anticholinergic medication. If they have difficulty sensing that their bladder is full during the day and have daytime incontinence as well, it will be hard for them to use the bedwetting alarm to achieve continence.

History Aside from the history obtained for daytime urinary incontinence, the relevant history for nocturnal enuresis should include a family history of nocturnal enuresis. The age at which other relatives had spontaneous resolution of nocturnal enuresis will suggest when the child may expect to become dry. I also ask if the child has sports activities late in the afternoon or at night, which would lead them to drink more water before going to bed. I then ask when the child goes to bed and when they wake up, and compare that with their daytime voiding pattern to decide if their bladder capacity is adequate for overnight storage. Parents may have tried waking the child up at night before they go to bed. If they have tried this, they will know if the child has one or multiple accidents at night, which may suggest a small bladder capacity. Finally, I ask how the child wakes up in the morning. If they sleep through their alarm and require their parents to wake them, the likelihood that they will wake up to a bedwetting alarm is low.

Physical Examination This is the same as for daytime incontinence.

Functional Studies I check a PVR during the clinic visit to make sure that the child is emptying their bladder correctly. Those who had a small bladder capacity on voiding diary but have a PVR are not good candidates for anticholinergic medications.

Imaging For isolated nocturnal enuresis, no imaging is needed, as a PVR will be obtained during the initial visit.

Treatment Nocturnal enuresis in older children can be associated with significant guilt and/or low self-esteem. It is important to defuse these feelings by emphasizing the frequency of the problem in other children, which they are not likely to be aware of. The voiding diary will give an indication if the patient is drinking the normal amount of fluid. Parents will likely have already tried fluid restriction, but they need to be told that stopping fluids 1 hour before bedtime is not adequate. If the child has sports in the afternoon or night, they need to try to front-load their fluid intake earlier in the day. For properly motivated children and families, the bedwetting alarm has a durable 50–70% cure rate [12]. Unfortunately, sometimes the parents are motivated, but the child is not, so treatment with desmopressin is the other first-line therapy. Children with a normal bladder capacity are more likely to respond to desmopressin. I usually start desmopressin at 0.2 mg × 3 at dinner for 1 month to see if it is effective. If the child remains completely wet after 2 weeks, they should stop the desmopressin. If the child is dry, then I have them drop the dose down to two tablets for 2 weeks, then one tablet for 2 weeks to determine the minimum dose that is needed. If they are partially improved, then I will add oxybutynin.

For children who have a small bladder capacity on the voiding diary, I will start with oxybutynin at 0.1 mg/kg at dinner to see if that is enough to get them dry. If there is some improvement, then I will add desmopressin. If there is no response to oxybutynin and desmopressin, then I will switch them from oxybutynin to imipramine, as there seems to be a better effect from the combination of imipramine and desmopressin [13]. Parents are often reluctant to start imipramine since it is thought of as an antidepressant medication. For imipramine, I start at 10 mg and work up to 25 or 50 mg as needed. Finally, there are some children where the bedwetting is due to excess sodium intake (fast food or snacks). If they continue to have bedwetting despite cutting down on their salt intake, I will try them on indomethacin to decrease their solute excretion at night. These children will need a metabolic panel to make sure that their renal function is normal before starting indomethacin. I start with 25 mg and go up to 50 mg, if the child cannot swallow the capsule, I ask them to open the capsule and sprinkle it into food [12].

Summary

1. Daytime incontinence is mainly due to an overactive bladder or dysfunctional voiding.
2. History, voiding diary, and post-void residual are the main tools in deciding what is causing the daytime incontinence.
3. Nocturnal enuresis is due to an interaction of nocturnal urine production, bladder capacity, and the ability to wake up when the bladder is full.
4. Patients with both daytime incontinence and nocturnal enuresis benefit by starting treatment of their daytime symptoms first.

References

1. Wu HY. Achieving urinary continence in children. Nat Rev Urol. 2010;7:1–7.
2. Hoebeke P, Bower W, Combs A, et al. Diagnostic evaluation of children with daytime incontinence. J Urol. 2010;183:699–703.
3. Austin PF, Bauer SB, Bower W, et al. The standardization of terminology of lower urinary tract function in children and adolescents: update report from the standardization committee of the International Children's Continence Society. J Urol. 2014;191(6):1865.e1–1865.e13.
4. Koff SA. Estimating bladder capacity in children. Urology. 1983;11(3):248.
5. Chang SJ, van Laecke E, Bauer SB, et al. Treatment of daytime urinary incontinence: a standardization document from the International Children's Continence Society. Neurourol Urodyn. 2017;3:43–50.
6. 't Hoen LA, van den Hoek J, Wolffenbuttel KP, et al. Breaking the vicious cycle: onabotulinum toxin A in children with therapy-refractory dysfunctional voiding. J Pediatr Urol. 2015;11:119.e1–6.

7. San ST, Barnes EH, Caldwell PHY. Urinary incontinence during laughter in children: is it giggle incontinence? J Pediatr Child Health. 2021;57:1971–5.
8. Svendsen AKM, Kamperis K, Hagstroem S, et al. The effect of methylphenidate for giggle incontinence in children. Neurourol Urodyn. 2023;42:1470–5.
9. Logan BL, Foster-Johnson L, Zotos E. Urinary incontinence among adolescent female atheletes. J Pediatr Urol. 2018;14:241.e1–9.
10. Koff SA, Byard MA. The daytime urinary frequency syndrome of childhood. J Urol. 1988;140(5):1280–1.
11. Von Gontard A, Hussong J, Yang SS, et al. Neurodevelopmental disorders and incontinence in children and adolescents: attention-deficit/hyperactivity disorder, autism disorder, and intellectual disability – a consensus document of the International Children's Continence Society. Neurourol Urodyn. 2022;41:102–14.
12. Neveus T, Fonseca E, Franco I, et al. Management and treatment of nocturnal enuresis – an updated standardization document from the International Children's Continence Society. J Pediatr Urol. 2020;16:10–9.
13. Shain S, Gitlin J, Pantazis A, et al. Management of the refractory nocturnal enuresis patient to desmopressin in a pediatric population: desmopressin + oxybutynin vs. desmopressin + imipramine. J Pediatr Urol. 2024;20:603.e1–8.

7 Neurogenic Bladder and Exstrophy Epispadias Complex (EEC)

Courtney K. Rowe and Anne G. Dudley

Key Points

- Most patients with open or closed neural tube conditions are diagnosed in infancy; in older children, symptoms of bladder/bowel incontinence, back pain, gait changes, or atypical patterns may prompt evaluation.
- The Urologic Management to Preserve Initial Renal Function or UMPIRE protocol is used to guide care for newborns with spina bifida.
- When a baby is born with Exstrophy Epispadias Complex (EEC), the exposed bladder plate is covered with plastic film such as Tegaderm or Saran Wrap, and a silk tie is used on the umbilicus to avoid irritation of the exposed bladder.
- Surgical closure for classic bladder exstrophy is typically done after the neonatal period, so there is ample time to refer to the family to a center experienced in closure.

Neurogenic Bladder: Initial Evaluation

Neurogenic bladder, or neuropathic bladder dysfunction may result from an abnormality of spinal cord development (spinal dysraphism) or other neurologic insult to the bladder, such as spinal cord injury or malignancy, or anorectal malformation. Spinal dysraphism includes myelomeningocele or spina bifida, lipomyleomeningocele or spinal lipoma, and other less common neural tube conditions. Spinal dysraphism occurs in about 1–3 in 1000 live births, with myelomeningocele occurring every 1 in 2875 live births in the United States [1, 2]. Presentation may be prenatal

C. K. Rowe (✉) · A. G. Dudley
Connecticut Children's, Hartford, CT, USA

UConn School of Medicine, Farmington, CT, USA
e-mail: crowe@connecticutchildrens.org; adudley@connecticutchildrens.org

H.-Y. Wu et al. (eds.), *Pediatric Urology for the Adult Urologist*, https://doi.org/10.1007/978-3-032-10306-2_7

or postnatal as advances in the detection of in utero conditions progress forward. Prenatal myelomeningocele repair is an option for some expectant mothers, depending on eligibility criteria.

Initial presentation depends on the type and level of a child's condition; however, does not always follow motor activity. The Spina Bifida Association refers to Spina Bifida as "The Snowflake Condition" as each child is unique in their presentation, and bladder function does not reliably follow motor function. Bladder characteristics may change over time, and this requires ongoing monitoring to determine clinical impact.

Most patients are diagnosed in infancy, with a finding of either an open or closed neural tube condition, such as spina bifida, or with some stigmata of spinal cord findings: a fatty mass, hair tuft, or other finding that prompts further workup. Open neural tube variants often require prompt intervention from a neurosurgical standpoint, and bladder management is initiated after the procedure. Close monitoring of bladder emptying and imaging of upper tracts with screening renal/bladder ultrasound will help define any underlying urologic concerns at baseline. For children with a closed neural tube variation, typical presentation includes screening renal/bladder ultrasound and often an ultrasound of the spine. Additionally, spinal MRI will further characterize neurosurgical findings and assist with planning for surgical intervention if indicated.

In older children, symptoms of bladder/bowel incontinence, back pain, gait changes, or atypical patterns may prompt evaluation and spinal imaging, highlighting a potential neurologic etiology for presenting symptoms. Injury to the spinal cord may occur from trauma, infection, inflammation, or due to mass effect from malignancy. Any of these conditions may lead to a later diagnosis of neurogenic bladder in some children or adolescents.

Neurogenic Bladder: Goals of Management

Neurogenic bladder may negatively impact the upper tracts and progress to chronic kidney disease. Goals of management primarily include the protection and preservation of renal function, optimizing continence, and minimizing comorbid conditions such as urinary tract infections. Proactive management is generally accepted as the preferred approach, as delayed management has higher rates of renal injury, urinary tract infections, and upper tract deterioration, despite limitations in historic data [3].

The Urologic Management to Preserve Initial Renal Function or UMPIRE protocol was an outgrowth of the CDC National Spina Bifida Patient Registry Urologic Protocol, beginning in 2015 (Figs. 7.1 and 7.2) [4]. This protocol has published initial baseline data and refined risk categorization of bladder characteristics from urodynamics [5]. Guidelines from the Spina Bifida Association, the CDC Urologic Protocol/UMPIRE, and ESPU guidelines have similar approaches, with key significant differences highlighted across childhood [4, 6, 7].

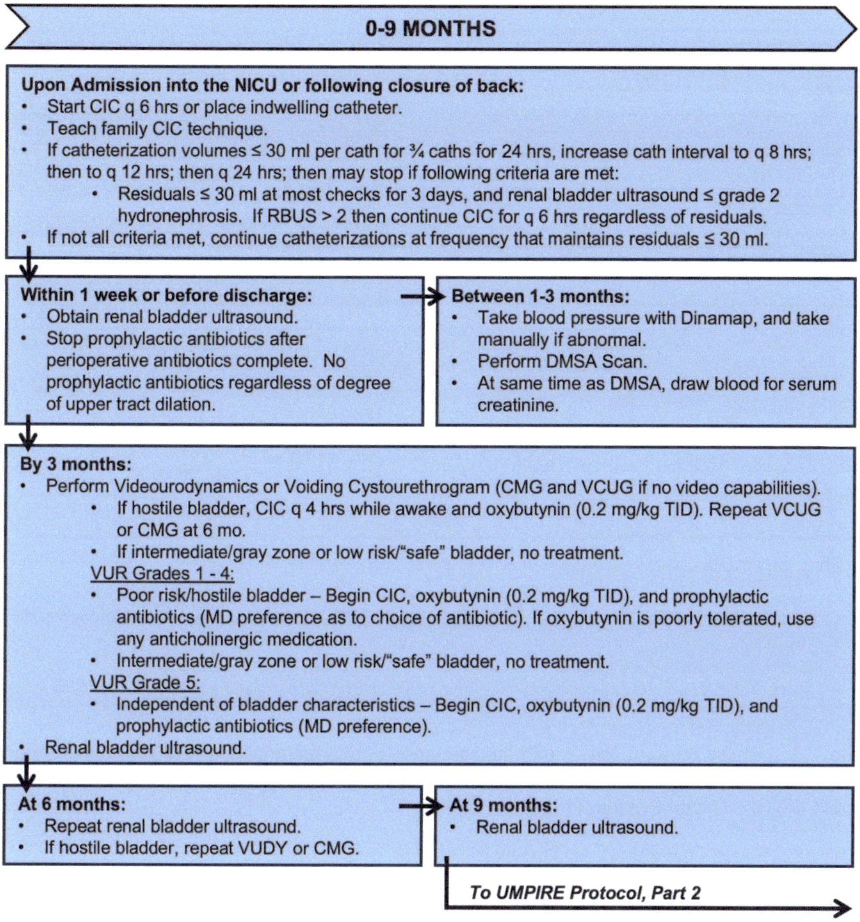

Fig. 7.1 Umpire Protocol, Part 1. *BP* blood pressure, *Cath* catheterization, *CMG* cystometrogram, *NICU* neonatal intensive care unit, *q* every, *TID* three times daily, *VCUG* voiding cystourethrogram, *VUDY* videourodynamics [4]

Neonatal Course

At birth, typical proactive management consists of monitoring of post-void residuals and understanding baseline bladder function. A regimen of intermittent catheterization with measurement of volumes is carried out as outlined in the NSBPR CDC Urologic/UMPIRE Protocol [4]. Infants who empty fully and who do not have significant hydronephrosis on imaging are weaned from catheterization, but teaching is completed for parents, as future dependence on catheterization is likely. Catheterization is continued for infants who have higher residual volumes and/or moderate or high-grade hydronephrosis (SFU Grade 2 or higher) until urodynamic testing is completed.

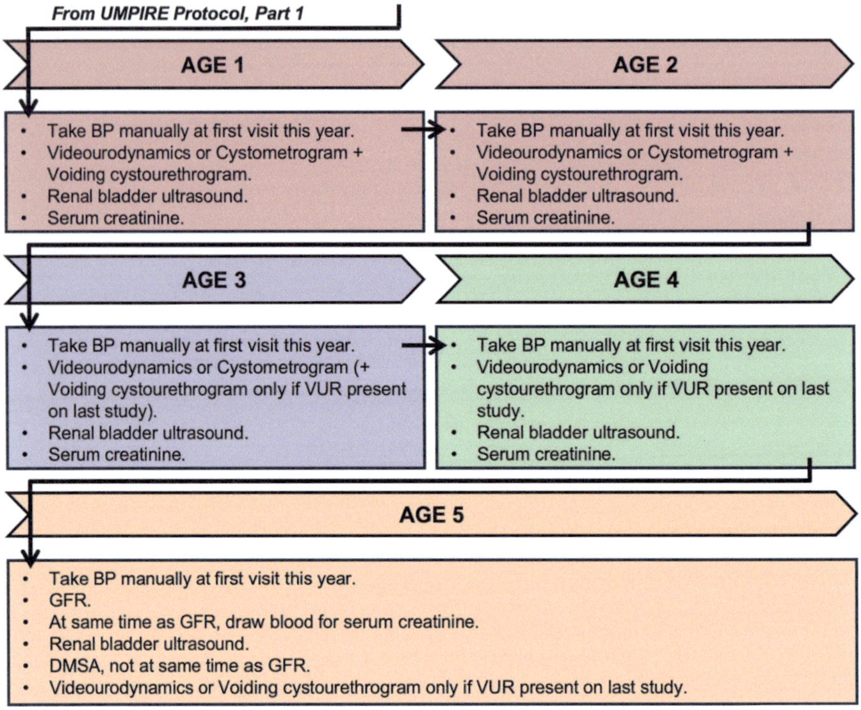

Fig. 7.2 Umpire Protocol, Part 2. *BP* blood pressure, *Cath* catheterization, *CMG* cystometrogram, *NICU* neonatal intensive care unit, *q* every, *TID* three times daily, *VCUG* voiding cystourethrogram, *VUDY* videourodynamics [4]

Baseline bladder function is assessed by urodynamics, ideally early in infancy, with goal completion by 3 months of age. Fluoroscopic urodynamics can be utilized, or a saline study paired with VCUG to assess vesicoureteral reflux status. Intermittent catheterization is utilized for those with high-risk parameters (Detrusor leak point pressure > 40, detrusor overactivity). Previous literature additionally included detrusor sphincter dyssynergia as a high-risk feature, though current UMPIRE protocols exclude this due to variability in reporting reliability. Categorization of risk levels is assigned based on urodynamic variables, as shown in Table 7.1 [5].

Catheterization permits medical therapy with oral medications, most commonly anticholinergics such as oxybutynin, with the goal of improving bladder compliance and treating detrusor overactivity. A paired approach of anticholinergic therapy and catheterization treats both bladder concerns: outlet and reservoir. Anticholinergic therapy is used to reduce high-risk filling pressures to safer levels and, when paired with catheterization, ensures complete emptying at low bladder pressures. Education and support are given to families to permit safe catheterization by caregivers.

If reflux is noted on VCUG or VUDS, antibiotic prophylaxis should be considered on a risk-stratified basis. Antibiotic prophylaxis is indicated for infants with

Table 7.1 Bladder risk categories

Low	Bladder capacity can be normal, low, or high. Compliance is normal or mildly decreased, but the end filling pressure or DLPP must be <25 cm H_2O. Leakage may be present. Detrusor overactivity should not be present on CMG.
Intermediate	This category is a grey zone for bladders that are neither safe nor hostile (see below). Bladder capacity may be low, normal, or high. Compliance is reduced with end filling pressure (measured prior to DO or voiding contraction if present) or DLPP of 25–39 cm H_2O. Detrusor overactivity (≥2 contractions of ≥15 cm H_2O over baseline) or voiding contractions may be present.
High risk	The bladder has poor compliance with end filling pressure or DLPP ≥40 cm H_2O.

high-risk bladder characteristics on urodynamics and VUR (Grades I–IV) and in all infants with high-grade reflux (Grade V) regardless of bladder characteristics. If bladder characteristics are safe or intermediate, observation is recommended without prophylaxis. Wallis and colleagues examined UMPIRE data and noted a low risk of culture proven symptomatic urinary tract infection in infancy at 4% of children [8]. The data indicate that infants with myelomeningocele do not require routine prophylaxis, but those with high-grade hydronephrosis, could benefit as their risk was higher (relative risk of 10.1). Their study confirmed that utilization of routine antibiotic prophylaxis for neurogenic bladder is discouraged, as colonization is common and antibiotic resistance may occur with prolonged use.

Both UMPIRE and ESPU guidelines include a baseline DMSA scan to assess for renal scars, though the benefit of these scans may be limited in the absence of a febrile UTI, known vesicoureteral reflux, or an ultrasound abnormality of the renal parenchyma [9].

Subtle differences in protocols exist across ESPU, UMPIRE, and SBA guidelines. For example, all children remain on intermittent catheterization after birth, with anticholinergic treatment added if detrusor overactivity is noted on urodynamics. SBA guidelines encourage serum laboratory values of creatinine prior to 1 year of age, while supporting early urodynamics and serial renal ultrasounds to guide treatment.

Pediatric Management

Routine follow-up visits in a multidisciplinary clinic are advised, with regular evaluation of upper tracts via ultrasound, and urodynamics with serum laboratories for monitoring renal function. Regular (yearly) urodynamics are utilized during early childhood, along with clinical examinations to assess changes in bladder function. Children with high-risk features undergo repeat testing to confirm the efficacy of regimen changes or the need for escalation of treatment.

A proactive approach, with early medical treatment of the bladder and catheterization, is utilized, as data have shown increased secondary reflux and renal deterioration with a delayed or reactive treatment plan, where upper tract changes or infections prompt intervention [3]. Current UMPIRE data suggests most children are born with normal kidneys, further strengthening the role of urologic management to preserve and maintain this normal renal function [10]. Recent data from the UMPIRE group highlighted the poor sensitivity of upper tract changes, such as hydronephrosis, to detect decline in renal function, showing only 25% sensitivity for CKD detection [11]. This report reinforces the need for routine monitoring, urodynamic testing, and renal function monitoring in childhood.

Adolescent Management

The adolescent individual with neuropathic bladder dysfunction often presents a challenge for multidisciplinary care and caregivers. Adolescents may increasingly desire independence and transitional care, while balancing increasing medical needs and limitations from both a medical and physical standpoint.

From a urologic perspective, adolescence is a critical time for monitoring renal function, as increased growth may unmask renal insufficiency not previously evident. Consistent use of renal serum studies and input from specialty care, such as nephrology, is advised if CKD is suspected or detected. Given atypical muscle mass and body habitus, individuals with spina bifida are at risk for underestimation of renal insufficiency by typical creatinine-based formulas and may benefit from cystatin C (muscle-independent protein produced by nucleated cells, degraded by proximal-tubule cells) based renal assays [12]. However, due to the variability of assays and formulas, consistency is key to detect changes. Bowen and colleagues [13] demonstrated a 22–27% difference in median eGFR when utilizing adult compared with pediatric equations in both creatinine and cystatin C-based equations, with potential to down stage CKD over time across transition from 16 to 18 years of age (pediatric to adult) despite unchanged renal function They suggest utilizing the same equation/assay for eGFR calculation during adolescence and emerging adulthood, even plotting both pediatric/adult values until transition is well established.

Transitional support and policies should be introduced as recommended by Got Transition at age 12. The focus on independence and optimization of self-directed care can be balanced by caregiver support and monitoring for completion of daily tasks. At times, adolescent compliance can be a challenge, and support such as social work, medical coping clinic, and nursing reinforcement can overcome hurdles of poor adherence and stress on family dynamics.

Typical visits will continue surveillance with renal function testing, bladder and kidney ultrasound, and may detect bladder stones, especially in the setting of augmentation cystoplasty or nephrolithiasis. Focusing on healthy behaviors, weight management, and nutrition can positively impact early adult lives, as obesity and metabolic syndrome are risk factors in a population that is not very mobile. Physical therapy, exercise prescriptions, and nutrition support can all be helpful, but patterns of reward-based eating and limited mobility can challenge even highly motivated individuals. Maintenance of a healthy weight can promote ongoing mobility and independence, permitting transfers and at-home ambulation, even if use of wheelchair assistance is needed in the community. Mental health support is linked strongly to independence, mobility and strength of community, and support groups have been highlighted as useful social outlets for many individuals and families.

Education regarding sexual health, reproductive potential, and discussion of contraception and erectile dysfunction is important in the adolescent and young adult population. Streur has published several studies indicating this is a critical aspect of care for individuals, and they desire education, assistance, and support while navigating sexuality and medical needs [14].

Exstrophy Epispadias Complex (EEC): Initial Evaluation

Exstrophy Epispadias Complex (EEC) refers to a group of midline defects. The mildest is Epispadias (2.4 per 100,000 live births), while the most common is classic bladder exstrophy (2.1 to 4.0 per 100,000 live births; Fig. 7.3) [15]. The most severe form of this complex is Cloacal Exstrophy (0.5 to 1 per 200,000 live births), which is also referred to as OEIS (omphalocele, exstrophy, imperforate anus, and spinal defects) complex [16].

Most cases of EEC are diagnosed with prenatal imaging [17]. After delivery, the exposed bladder plate and cecal plate are covered with plastic film such as Tegaderm or Saran Wrap. If a plastic clamp was used on the umbilicus, it should be switched to a silk tie to avoid irritation of the exposed bladder. A renal ultrasound is performed to screen for associated anomalies, and an abdominal plain film is used to measure the pubic diastasis. Prophylactic antibiotics are typically not given prior to bladder closure. A pathway for postnatal management for classic bladder exstrophy

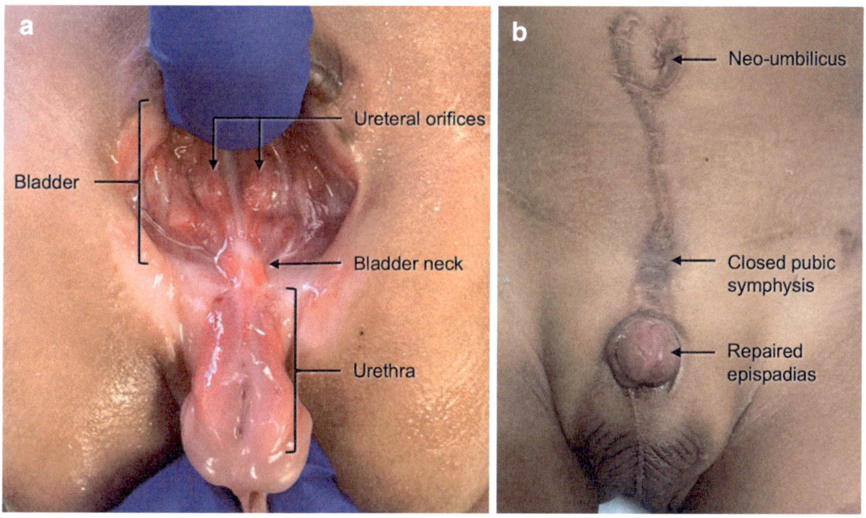

Fig. 7.3 Classic bladder exstrophy in a male patient before (**a**) and after (**b**) closure

that includes educational handouts for families about EEC and bladder plate care can be found at Seattle Children's Hospital (Fig. 7.4) [18]. While the sex of a child with EEC is typically clear with a thorough examination, a karyotype can be performed if there are questions.

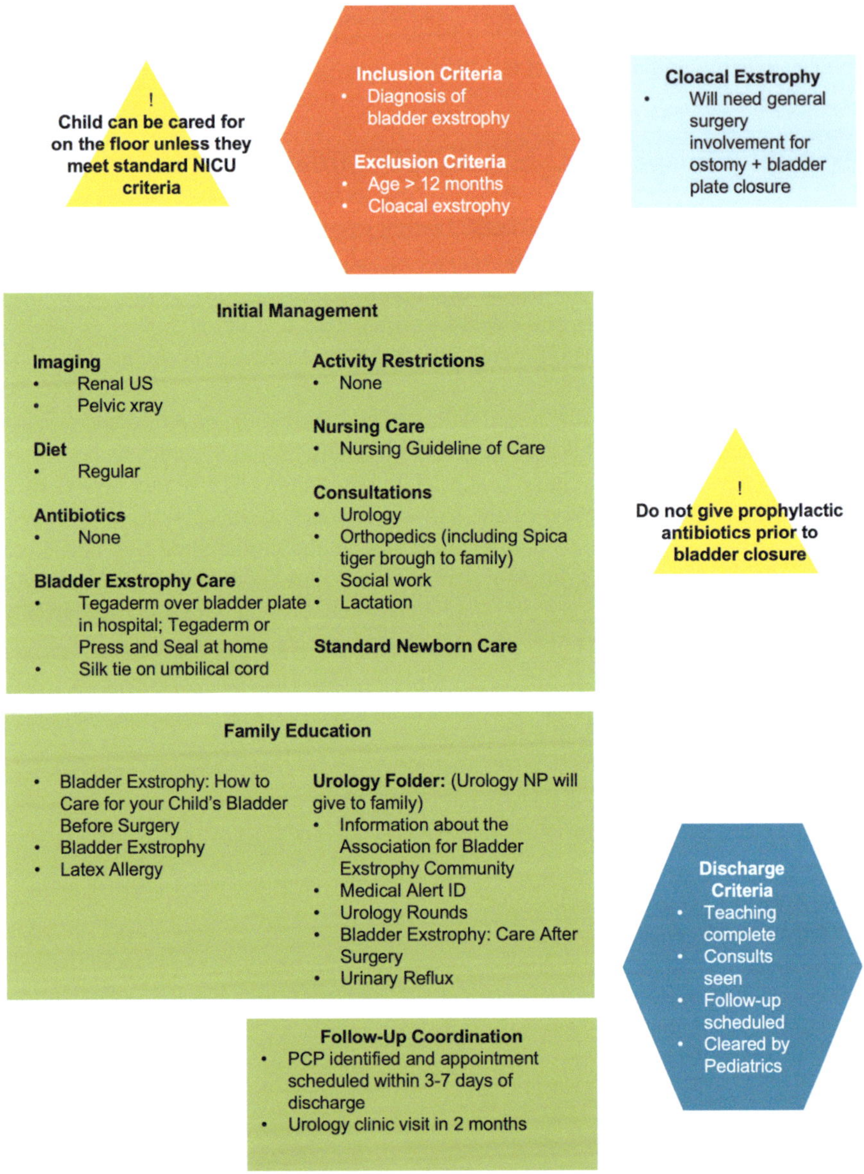

Fig. 7.4 Bladder exstrophy pathway from Seattle Children's: Neonatal management [18]

It is no longer common to perform immediate neonatal surgical closure for classic bladder exstrophy, so there is ample time to refer the family to a center experienced in closure.

Surgical diversion for cloacal exstrophy is performed more urgently, though it should also be performed at an experienced center. Separation of the urologic from the gastrointestinal systems is typically performed in the first 48–72 hours, though it can be safe to delay this for premature patients or those with pulmonary compromise [19].

When patients present after initial closure, it can be difficult to determine which condition was present at birth. Patients and families may be unsure of surgical details, and hospital records may be difficult to obtain, incomplete, or contain misinformation that has been perpetuated. A physical examination can often answer this initial question. While there are exceptions to any rule, patients with isolated epispadias are generally born with a typical umbilicus, while those with bladder exstrophy have had one surgically created. Patients with cloacal exstrophy will typically have evidence of a prior colostomy, with or without subsequent take-down.

A detailed surgical history is important for these complex patients and can also be difficult to obtain. Initial repair of classic bladder exstrophy is typically performed in one or two stages, while cloacal exstrophy is often repaired in two to three stages. Repair of isolated epispadias can include urethral and genital reconstruction alone or along with bladder neck reconstruction. Bilateral pelvic osteotomies may have been performed; in the vast majority of cases, this can be identified by scars at the hips. Inguinal hernias are often present after birth and may or may not have been repaired. Vesicoureteral reflux is also universally present after bladder closure and may or may not have been corrected. Girls with EEC have a bifid clitoris, which may have been left bifid or brought together in the midline. While the pubic symphysis is also typically brought together during initial bladder closure, there is universal recurrence of pubic diastasis over time.

The majority of patients with EEC have undergone multiple surgeries due to their diagnosis, with most having 10+ surgeries in their lifetime [20, 21]. These interventions can include bladder neck repair or closure, augmentation cystoplasty, Mitrofanoff or Monti, artificial urinary sphincter, orchiopexy, hernia repair, revision phalloplasty, vaginoplasty, or monsplasty.

There are number of associated conditions with EEC. Patients have an increased incidence of renal anomalies such as a solitary, pelvic, or horseshoe kidney [22] and EEC in boys is associated with undescended testicles [23]. Patients with OEIS have bowel and spinal defects that are often repaired in infancy but continue to impact their quality of life. Many patients with EEC report hip pain, and this seems to be independent of whether they underwent osteotomies at the time of bladder closure [24].

Exstrophy Epispadias Complex (EEC): Goals of Management

Urinary continence is a main focus for patients with EEC, with only about 20% expected to void volitionally through the urethra long term [25]. Continence rates do slowly increase through the teen years and are higher for isolated epispadias than classic bladder exstrophy [26]. Many centers use pelvic floor physical therapy in childhood to improve dry intervals. Given some chance of continence after initial bladder closure, surgical interventions for continence are typically performed in later childhood or teen years. There is no consensus on optimal timing or approach to continence; the most common approaches are bladder neck reconstruction or bladder neck closure along with ileal augmentation cystoplasty and Mitrofanoff [27]. Infections and stones are common after these procedures, similar to those patients with reconstruction for a neurogenic bladder.

References

1. Venkataramana NK. Spinal dysraphism. J Pediatr Neurosci. 2011;6(Suppl 1):S31–40.
2. Stallings EB, Isenburg JL, Rutkowski RE, et al. National population-based estimates for major birth defects, 2016-2020. Birth Defects Res. 2024;116(1):e2301.
3. Li Y, Stern N, Wang PZ, Braga LH, Dave S. Systematic review and meta-analysis to study the outcomes of proactive versus delayed management in children with a congenital neurogenic bladder. J Pediatr Urol. 2023;19(6):730–41.
4. Routh JC, Cheng EY, Austin JC, et al. Design and methodological considerations of the centers for disease control and prevention urologic and renal protocol for the newborn and young child with spina bifida. J Urol. 2016;196(6):1728–34.
5. Tanaka ST, Yerkes EB, Routh JC, et al. Urodynamic characteristics of neurogenic bladder in newborns with myelomeningocele and refinement of the definition of bladder hostility: findings from the UMPIRE multi-center study. J Pediatr Urol. 2021;17(5):726–32.
6. Joseph DB, Baillie S, Baum MA, Frimberger DC, Khavari R, Misseri R, Tanaka ST, Wood H, Yerkes EB. Guidelines for the care of people with spina bifida: urology guideline. https://www.spinabifidaassociation.org/wp-content/uploads/Urology-May-2023.pdf. Published 2023. Accessed 2025.
7. Stein R, Bogaert G, Dogan HS, et al. EAU/ESPU guidelines on the management of neurogenic bladder in children and adolescent part I diagnostics and conservative treatment. Neurourol Urodyn. 2020;39(1):45–57.
8. Wallis MC, Paramsothy P, Newsome K, et al. Incidence of urinary tract infections in newborns with spina bifida-is antibiotic prophylaxis necessary? J Urol. 2021;206(1):126–32.
9. Cascio S, Doyle M, Mahon OM, Kelly G. Urinary tract imaging in infants with spina bifida: a selective approach to a baseline DMSA. J Pediatr Urol. 2021;17(3):396.e391–6.
10. Tanaka ST, Paramsothy P, Thibadeau J, et al. Baseline urinary tract imaging in infants enrolled in the UMPIRE protocol for children with spina bifida. J Urol. 2019;201(6):1193–8.
11. Chu DI, Liu T, Williams T, et al. Diagnostic test characteristics of ultrasound-based hydronephrosis for chronic kidney disease in children and adolescents with myelomeningocele: results from the UMPIRE and National Spina Bifida Patient Registry Cohort Studies. J Urol. 2025;213(3):341–9.
12. Fox JA, Dudley AG, Bates C, Cannon GM Jr. Cystatin C as a marker of early renal insufficiency in children with congenital neuropathic bladder. J Urol. 2014;191(5 Suppl):1602–7.

13. Bowen DK, Balmert LC, Meyer T, et al. Variability in kidney function estimates in emerging adults with spina bifida: implications for transitioning from pediatric to adult care. Urology. 2021;148:306–13.
14. Streur CS, Sandberg DE, Kalpakjian CZ, Wittmann DA, Quint EH. How to discuss sexual health with girls and young women with spina bifida: a practical guide for the urologist. Urology. 2021;151:72–8.
15. Ebert AK, Reutter H, Ludwig M, Rösch WH. The exstrophy-epispadias complex. Orphanet J Rare Dis. 2009;4:23.
16. Bursac D, Bojanic K, Zmijanac Partl J, Lucic D, Duic Z, Horvat M. OEIS complex-using MRI in diagnostic: two case reports. Radiol Case Rep. 2023;18(1):364–7.
17. Lee T, Weiss D, Roth E, et al. Prenatal diagnosis of bladder exstrophy and OEIS over 20 years. Urology. 2023;172:174–7.
18. Seattle Children's Hospital MP, Rowe C, Dearn J, Herrman A, McMannis N, Nelson V, Popalisky J, Sheets E, Turner A, Villavicencio C. Bladder Exstrophy Pathway. https://www.seattlechildrens.org/globalassets/documents/healthcare-professionals/clinical-standard-work/bladder-exstrophy-org-pathway.pdf. Published 2018. Accessed 2025.
19. Ostertag-Hill CA, Delaplain PT, Lee T, Dickie BH. Updates on the Care of Cloacal Exstrophy. Children (Basel). 2024;11(5):544.
20. Rowe CK, Shnorhavorian M, Block P, Ahn J, Merguerian PA. Using social media for patient-reported outcomes: a study of genital appearance and sexual function in adult bladder exstrophy patients. J Pediatr Urol. 2018;14(4):322:e321–322 e326.
21. Canalichio K, Ahn J, Artigas P, et al. Patient-reported outcomes in adult females with bladder exstrophy: a study of long-term sexual, reproductive and urinary outcomes using social media. J Pediatr Urol. 2020;16:567.e1.
22. Stec AA, Baradaran N, Gearhart JP. Congenital renal anomalies in patients with classic bladder exstrophy. Urology. 2012;79(1):207–9.
23. Cheng W, Mya GH, Saing H. Associated anomalies in patients with undescended testes. J Trop Pediatr. 1996;42(4):204–6.
24. Promm M, Hofbauer R, Brandl R, et al. Long-term orthopaedic and radiological outcomes of symphysis approximation without osteotomy in primary bladder exstrophy repair. Eur J Pediatr Surg. 2024;35:195.
25. Weiss DA, Shukla AR, Borer JG, et al. Evaluation of outcomes following complete primary repair of bladder exstrophy at three individual sites prior to the establishment of a multi-institutional collaborative model. J Pediatr Urol. 2020;16:435.e1.
26. Taskinen S, Suominen J, Mäkelä E. Development of late continence in bladder exstrophy and epispadias patients. Urology. 2020;144:194–7.
27. Maruf M, Manyevitch R, Michaud J, et al. Urinary continence outcomes in classic bladder exstrophy: a long-term perspective. J Urol. 2020;203(1):200–5.

Hematuria in Children: Evaluation and Management

8

Robin Kremsdorf

Gross Hematuria

Gross hematuria is frequently an alarming symptom for children and their parents, which usually leads to prompt evaluation. During assessment, gross hematuria must be distinguished from conditions that cause urine discoloration without the presence of red blood cells (myoglobinuria, beeturia, rifampin, phenazopyridine exposure). It must also be distinguished from bleeding from outside of the urinary tract (vagina, rectum, skin). Gross hematuria can be a factitious symptom.

Common causes of gross hematuria in children include cystitis, pyelonephritis, irritation of the urethral meatus or perineum, and trauma. Nephrolithiasis, glomerulonephritis, papillary necrosis in sickle cell disease, primary vascular disorders, and coagulopathy can cause gross hematuria but are much less common. Most children with gross hematuria can be diagnosed through history, physical examination, lab evaluation, and imaging, and can be managed without cystoscopy. Cystoscopy is reserved for children with abnormal imaging, with bleeding due to traumatic injury, or with chronic sterile cystitis.

It is critical to elicit urine color in assessing gross hematuria. Red or pink urine is most commonly from lower urinary tract bleeding, while brown-/tea-/Coca-Cola-colored urine is typically from renal parenchymal disease. Discrete hematuria at the beginning or end of the urine stream is more likely from a structural or lower urinary tract source, whereas blood that appears throughout the urine stream is more likely to originate in the kidney. Gross hematuria during an illness may signify the presence of chronic microhematuria when well, as can occur with chronic glomerular disease.

R. Kremsdorf (✉)
The Warren Alpert Medical School of Brown University, Hasbro Children's Hospital, Providence, RI, USA
e-mail: rkremsdorf@brownhealth.org

H.-Y. Wu et al. (eds.), *Pediatric Urology for the Adult Urologist*,
https://doi.org/10.1007/978-3-032-10306-2_8

The preferred imaging modality in a child with suspected lower urinary tract bleeding is a kidney and bladder ultrasound. Ultrasound will detect most kidney stones, all hydronephrosis caused by stones, and some solid lesions. If clinical concern for kidney stone remains high and ultrasound is normal, CT may detect small non-obstructing stones missed on ultrasound. CT may also be indicated in the setting of traumatic hematuria and suspected renal vascular injury.

In neonates, gross hematuria raises concern for renal vein thrombosis, an acute and critical diagnosis. Late diagnosis can result in loss of kidney function. It can be readily diagnosed by a Doppler ultrasound. Treatment is usually supportive.

Gross hematuria can be associated with the passage of a kidney stone. While this is usually accompanied by dysuria, it is painless in some children. Children with self-limited gross hematuria and normal imaging are sometimes assumed to have passed a kidney stone. While this may be true, it also likely leads to overdiagnosis of kidney stones and risks over-medicalization of these patients.

Bacterial and viral cystitis can present with gross hematuria. There is usually associated dysuria and urinary frequency. While bacterial cystitis is usually identified by the presence of nitrates and white blood cells in the urine and a positive urine culture, viral pathogens are not routinely identified with usual diagnostic testing. With more focused testing, up to 42% of children with hemorrhagic cystitis were found to have adenovirus in the urine [1]. Children with transient, self-limited gross hematuria and a normal ultrasound are frequently assumed to have had adenoviral cystitis.

While older adults without a clear reason to have hematuria should be evaluated for bladder cancer with cystoscopy, this is not necessary in children. Bladder cancer is largely a disease of older adults, with an average age of diagnosis of 73 [2]. Bladder cancer is conceptualized as a condition where toxic exposures increase the risk of carcinogenesis over decades, which, by definition, will not have the opportunity to occur in childhood [3]. While bladder cancer in children can occur, it is extraordinarily rare [4]. In the absence of other abnormal findings (ultrasound abnormalities, failure to thrive), children with hematuria do not need to have a cystoscopy to evaluate for bladder cancer.

Teenagers and young adults who are carriers of sickle cell anemia have a risk of renal medullary carcinoma. This is an aggressive and treatment-refractory cancer with a poor prognosis. Most patients have metastatic disease at the time of diagnosis. Gross hematuria is the most common presenting symptom of renal medullary carcinoma [5]. This is a reason to obtain ultrasound imaging in patients with hemoglobinopathies who present with gross hematuria.

Patients with terminal gross hematuria or passage of blood in between voids may have idiopathic hemorrhagic urethritis of childhood (IHU) [6]. This condition has also been called idiopathic urethrorrhagia, idiopathic urethritis, bulbar urethritis, and anterior urethritis of adolescence. This is a condition sometimes associated with dysuria and voiding dysfunction. It is most commonly described in peri-pubertal and adolescent males. Cystoscopy frequently shows friable mucosa in the bulbar urethral (though cystoscopy is not indicated for the suspected diagnosis of IHU). Evidence is limited to case series, but up to one-third of patients develop chronic symptoms. It is typically managed with noninvasive urodynamics (flowmetry)and treatment of voiding dysfunction. Patients have a risk of urethral stenosis, depending on the duration of symptoms. Because of this risk, invasive evaluations and therapies are avoided whenever possible.

Microscopic Hematuria

Microscopic hematuria is, by definition, asymptomatic and thus diagnosed only in the evaluation of other symptoms or through surveillance practices. In the past, screening urinalysis was part of pediatric preventative care, with the goal of identifying kidney and urinary tract disease when intervention would be beneficial. However, evidence of benefit for this practice is lacking. The presence of hematuria in otherwise healthy children is often transient, and the risk of underlying kidney disease is small [7]. In 2007, the American Academy of Pediatrics stopped recommending surveillance urinalysis in the setting of well-child care [8]. Urinalysis in the outpatient setting is used primarily for the evaluation of urinary tract symptoms, abdominal symptoms, and fever.

Microscopic hematuria can originate in the kidneys, the lower urinary tract, or outside the urinary tract. Dipsticks used in outpatient offices are very sensitive, and there is a risk of false-positive testing. Hemoglobinuria (in the setting of chronic hemolysis, such as sickle cell disease) and myoglobinuria (in the setting of rhabdomyolysis or metabolic muscle disease) can cause an office-based dipstick to test positive in the absence of RBCs. Thus, a dipstick showing microscopic hematuria must be further evaluated with microscopy to determine if RBCs are truly present in the urine. Microscopy can be performed in a clinical laboratory or directly by a physician. The urologist must look for evidence of a kidney source of blood in the urine in order to refer patients with kidney disease to the appropriate care setting.

Microscopic hematuria can be a symptom of systemic illness that involves the kidney, such as lupus, ANCA vasculitis, Henoch–Schoenlein purpura, or anti-glomerular basement membrane disease. As such, evaluation of microhematuria should include assessment of systemic symptoms such as rash, joint pain, hair loss, epistaxis, and hemoptysis.

Hypertension in a patient with microscopic hematuria raises the suspicion of a primary kidney problem. Blood pressure in healthy young children is expected to be lower than in adults and is evaluated based on height, sex, and age. Blood pressure in adolescents aged 13 and older is evaluated by the same criteria as adults [9]. Hypertension in a child or adolescent with hematuria raises concern for acute glomerulonephritis or for chronic kidney disease. Children with microscopic hematuria and elevated blood pressure should have a prompt evaluation by a pediatric nephrologist or primary care pediatrician.

The presence of protein in the urine is a specific indicator of kidney pathology. If the dipstick that tests positive for blood also tests positive for protein, further evaluation of the kidneys is indicated. The urine protein:creatinine ratio provides information about the quantity of protein loss from the kidneys that is more precise than information from a dipstick. A urine protein:creatinine ratio greater than 0.2 mg/mg (200 mg/g) should prompt further evaluation by a nephrologist. In the presence of more severe proteinuria, renal biopsy may be required for definitive diagnosis.

Assessment of renal function by measuring serum creatinine is frequently part of the evaluation of microscopic hematuria Creatinine is a compound produced by muscle tissue, filtered by the glomeruli of the kidneys, and excreted into the urine. Infants and young children typically have very low serum creatinine. The normal value of serum creatinine rises slowly through childhood. Average serum creatinine for a healthy infant is 0.25 mg/dL, whereas it is 0.64 mg/dL for an 18 yo female and 0.84 mg/dL for an 18 yo male [10]. Many laboratories do not take patient age into account when providing normal values for serum creatinine. Thus, a small child with moderate kidney dysfunction may not have a serum creatinine value that flags as abnormal in a lab report.

Some of the most common causes of microscopic hematuria in children are familial. Alport nephropathy is caused by mutations in the COL4A3, COL4A4, or COL4A5 genes and can be inherited in an X-linked, autosomal dominant, or autosomal recessive pattern. It is associated with a variable (but significant) risk of chronic kidney disease and kidney failure during adolescence. Thus, a child with microscopic hematuria should have a thorough family history. Parents can even be screened for hematuria during their children's medical appointments! Genetic testing offers a definitive diagnosis of Alport nephropathy. Patients with Alport nephropathy benefit from chronic medical therapy with ACE inhibitor medication, which delays or prevents the onset of kidney failure [11].

The most common chronic glomerulonephritis in children (and adults) is IgA nephropathy. This condition is characterized by chronic microscopic hematuria, worsening to gross hematuria during periods of illness. IgA nephropathy requires a renal biopsy for definitive diagnosis. Patients with IgA nephropathy and proteinuria benefit from chronic medical therapy with an ACE inhibitor medication, which slows the progression of kidney function [12].

The coexistence of microhematuria and pyuria raises the concern for cystitis, pyelonephritis, and exudative glomerulonephritis. While cystitis and pyelonephritis are typically accompanied by urinary tract symptoms, glomerulonephritis is not. It is important to consider the diagnosis of glomerulonephritis in a child with hematuria and pyuria, particularly if evaluation for infection is normal or if hematuria persists after treatment for infection.

Hypercalciuria is frequently diagnosed in the evaluation of children with microscopic hematuria [13]. It is associated with kidney stone risk and with voiding dysfunction [14]. Children with hypercalciuria and voiding dysfunction are expected to have an excellent response to behavioral therapy and management with anticholinergic medication. For convenience, urine calcium assessment is performed on a spot urine specimen, rather than a 24-hour urine collection. For children over 2 years of age, a urine calcium:creatinine ratio < 0.2 mg/mg is normal.

In summary, children with microhematuria on a single evaluation should have a repeat evaluation to determine if microhematuria is persistent. If it is, they should be evaluated for hypertension, proteinuria, renal dysfunction, and high calcium excretion. A family history of hematuria and kidney problems should be elicited. If any of these problems are identified, a pediatric nephrologist should evaluate the child.

Take Home Points

- Gross hematuria in children is most commonly caused by UTI, irritation of the urethral meatus or perineum, or trauma.
- Ultrasound is the preferred imaging modality of the kidney and urinary tract in children.
- Microscopic hematuria in children should prompt an assessment for hypertension, proteinuria, renal dysfunction, and hypercalciuria. All of these symptoms indicate a need for nephrology evaluation.
- Cystoscopy for hematuria in children is reserved for the evaluation of bladder masses and chronic bladder inflammation. Most children with gross hematuria and microscopic hematuria do not require cystoscopy.

References

1. Lee HJ, et al. Isolation of adenovirus type 7 from the urine of children with acute hemorrhagic cystitis. Pediatr Infect Dis J. 1996;15(7):633–4.
2. Siegel RL, Miller KD, Jemal A. Cancer statistics, 2019. CA Cancer J Clin. 2019;69(1):7–34.
3. Saginala K, et al. Epidemiology of bladder cancer. Med Sci (Basel). 2020;8(1):15.
4. Galiya R, et al. Pediatric urothelial bladder neoplasm. J Pediatr Urol. 2022;18(6):833 e1–4.
5. Blas L, et al. Renal medullary carcinoma: a report of the current literature. Curr Urol Rep. 2019;20(1):4.
6. Eyer de Jesus L, et al. Idiopathic hemorrhagic urethritis of childhood. J Pediatr Urol. 2020;16(5):690–9.
7. Kaplan RE, Springate JE, Feld LG. Screening dipstick urinalysis: a time to change. Pediatrics. 1997;100(6):919–21.
8. Filice CE, et al. Pediatric screening urinalysis: a difference-in-differences analysis of how a 2007 change in guidelines impacted use. BMC Pediatr. 2014;14:260.
9. Flynn JT, et al. Clinical practice guideline for screening and management of high blood pressure in children and adolescents. Pediatrics. 2017;140(3).
10. Chuang GT, Tsai IJ, Tsau YK. Serum creatinine reference limits in pediatric population-a single center electronic health record-based database in Taiwan. Front Pediatr. 2021;9:793446.
11. Savige J, et al. Guidelines for genetic testing and management of Alport Syndrome. Clin J Am Soc Nephrol. 2022;17(1):143–54.
12. Vivarelli M, et al. IPNA clinical practice recommendations for the diagnosis and management of children with IgA nephropathy and IgA vasculitis nephritis. Pediatr Nephrol. 2025;40(2):533–69.
13. Garcia CD, Miller LA, Stapleton FB. Natural history of hematuria associated with hypercalciuria in children. Am J Dis Child. 1991;145(10):1204–7.
14. Parekh DJ, et al. The role of hypercalciuria in a subgroup of dysfunctional voiding syndromes of childhood. J Urol. 2000;164(3 Pt 2):1008–10.

Pediatric Nephrolithiasis

9

Shannon Cannon and Stephen Y. Nakada

Introduction

While less common in the pediatric population, nephrolithiasis represents a burden for patients and their families, as well as an increasing financial burden for the health care system. Annual expenditures related to acute care for pediatric stone disease has been estimated to be around $375 million [1]. Long-term preventive care, surveillance imaging, and medical treatment may further increase this cost. Unique considerations for the pediatric stone-former impact the approach to care, as pediatric-specific risk factors contribute to stone disease, clinical presentation, and differences in medical, surgical, and preventive care. This chapter presents a comprehensive overview of the current literature focused on pediatric nephrolithiasis and provides comparisons to adult stone disease trends and management. The chapter also highlights areas of management where care for the pediatric patient may differ from adult care.

Epidemiology

Compared to adults, few studies have specifically characterized the incidence of stone disease in children. However, several epidemiological studies suggest that the incidence of pediatric nephrolithiasis is on the rise [2–6], particularly among adolescents [2, 5]. A study of South Carolina emergency room visits identified a rise in unique cases of nephrolithiasis from 7.9 per 100,000 in 1997 to 18.5 per 100,000 in 2007, with the largest increase among girls and children aged 14–18 years [4].

S. Cannon (✉) · S. Y. Nakada
Department of Urology, University of Wisconsin School of Medicine and Public Health, Madison, WI, USA
e-mail: cannon@urology.wisc.edu; nakada@urology.wisc.edu

H.-Y. Wu et al. (eds.), *Pediatric Urology for the Adult Urologist*,
https://doi.org/10.1007/978-3-032-10306-2_9

A study of Olmstead County, Minnesota, interpolated national incidence rates among children, with similar findings of a 4% average annual increase in nephrolithiasis in a 25-year period between 1984 and 2008 [2]. Incidence was estimated at 14.5 per 100,000 person-years in 2003–2008, with higher rates among adolescents (23.9 per 100,000 person-years in ages 12–17) but no significant differences in incidence by gender [2]. A large administrative claims database study reported a stone incidence of 59.5 per 100,000 person-years from 2005 to 2016, with a peak in incidence of 65.2 cases per 100,000 person-years in 2011 [7]. Future studies may show stabilization or further increase in stone incidence among children.

Increases in incidence are attributed to changes in dietary habits (increased intake of salt, sugar, animal protein, carbonated beverages, and vitamin C) and decreased fluid intake [6, 8, 9]. While childhood obesity has been proposed as a contributor to increased incidence of pediatric nephrolithiasis, comparative studies of obesity trends and stone incidence rates suggest a more complex relationship between body weight, diet, lithogenic solute concentrations, and urinary pH [4]. The underlying etiology of gender-based differences in stone incidence are less clear. Regional or geographic differences in stone incidence are not well studied in children.

Stone compositions differ between pediatric and adult stone formers, likely due to a greater disposition to underlying metabolic risks in children with stone disease. Like adults, calcium-based calculi are most common in children, found in 60–90% of cases [2, 4, 10–12]. Calcium phosphate stones are more common and uric acid stones are less common in children, related to slightly higher urinary pH and higher excretion of uric acid when compared to adults [4, 11]. Struvite has been observed as the major component in 13–17% of cases [4, 11]. A higher incidence of struvite stones is attributed to patterns of urinary tract infection (UTI) among younger children and lower citrate excretion due to degradation by bacterial enzymes [4, 11]. Prompt and effective UTI treatment may be responsible for decreases in struvite incidence over time.

While pediatric nephrolithiasis may be increasing, trends in hospitalizations for management of nephrolithiasis are less clear. Shoag et al. studied the National Inpatient Sample (NIS) and identified that pediatric hospitalizations for upper tract urinary stones decreased from 0.16% of all pediatric hospitalizations in 2001 to 0.12% in 2014, and surgical interventions during the hospitalization increased from 38.6% to 52.4% [13]. However, other studies have identified an increase [3], decrease [14], or no trend in hospitalization rate [15].

Metabolic Risk Factors and Genetic Causes

In children, contributors to stone formation include metabolic risk factors (95%), anatomic factors (32%), and UTIs (24%), alone or in combination [16]. Genetic conditions often lead to increased metabolic and/or anatomic risk. Hypercalciuria is the most common metabolic risk for stone disease in children; while hypocitraturia was thought to be rare among children, it may be nearly as common [17] as hypercalciuria. Frequency and etiology of metabolic risk factors are shown in Table 9.1. Because metabolic causes are common in pediatric nephrolithiasis, it is critical to obtain a 24-hour urine study to assess metabolic risk in all children.

Genetic evaluation may also be important to identify patients with monogenic causes of nephrolithiasis. There are 46 genes associated with monogenic causes of nephrolithiasis; 14 genes are responsible for 15% of pediatric nephrolithiasis or nephrocalcinosis cases [18–20]. Common monogenic stone conditions include cystinuria (SLC3A1, SLC7A9), Renal Tubular Acidosis (SCL4A1 and SCL4A4), Primary Hyperoxaluria Type 1 (AGXT), Type 2 (GRHPR), and Type 3 (HOGA1) [21]. Monogenic causes of hypercalciuria have been discovered in those with previously presumed idiopathic causes (Infantile idiopathic hypercalcemia [CYP24A1,

Table 9.1 Metabolic causes of pediatric nephrolithiasis

Metabolic risk	Definition	Percentage (%)	Causes
Hypercalciuria	Urine calcium >4 mg/kg on 24-hour test	50–97	Idiopathic; inherited: polygenic (renal, absorptive, resorptive), monogenic (Dent and Bartter diseases); hypercalcemia: vitamin D excess, hyperparathyroidism, sarcoidosis, malignancy, Williams syndrome; primary distal renal tubular acidosis; metabolic acidosis; loop diuretics, glucocorticoids, ketogenic diet; immobilization; excessive sodium intake; medullary sponge kidney
Hyperoxaluria	Urinary oxalate >45 mg/1.73 m^2 on 24-hour test	10–20	Idiopathic; primary hyperoxaluria types I–III; secondary hyperoxaluria: excessive oxalate ingestion (ethylene glycol, ascorbic acid, and methoxyflurane); fat malabsorption (cystic fibrosis, celiac disease, inflammatory bowel disease, short bowel syndrome, pancreatitis); medication: orlistat
Hypocitraturia	Urine Citrate <365 mg/1.73 m^2 in males or <310 mg/1.73 m^2 in females on 24-hour test	20–60	Idiopathic; chronic metabolic acidosis (chronic diarrhea, distal tubular acidosis, medication: topiramate, acetazolamide); hypokalemia; ketogenic diet
Hyperuricosuria	Uric acid >815 mg/1.73 m^2 (< 484 mmol) on 24-hour test	2–8	Idiopathic; dietary: excessive purine intake, ketogenic diet; metabolic syndrome; overproduction of uric acid: tumor lysis syndrome, malignant proliferative disorders; genetic disorders: Lesch–Nyhan syndrome, glycogen storage disease
Cystinuria	–	5	Cystinuria: types I, II, and III

Adapted from Pecoraro et al. [12] and Kovacevic [16]

SLC34A1, and SLC34A3]) [21]. Additional monogenic causes may be identified in the future, as the study of patients with idiopathic metabolic risk continues.

Next-generation sequencing (NGS) has allowed for more cost-effective testing of multiple genes in a short time frame, paving the way for gene panels and whole-exome sequencing. Gene panels are less expensive than whole-exome sequencing or genome-wide association studies and are more commonly used in a clinical setting [22]. Diagnostic yield of genetic testing for stones in children is between 12% and 21%, depending on the stringency of the criteria for a diagnostic result [20]. The relatively high yield lowers the threshold to recommend genetic testing for hereditary stone disease in children, and some advocate for targeted nephrolithiasis gene panels for all stone-formers ≤25 years old [12, 16, 20]. Early identification of underlying genetic risk for stone disease may aid with improved preventive care and reduced long-term costs associated with care [12]. Research on appropriate selection of pediatric patients for genetic testing is currently limited, but it may balance the costs and ethical concerns of indiscriminate testing with the costs of care for underdiagnosed hereditary stone disease.

Clinical Management

Acute Presentation

Pain is the primary presenting symptom of obstructing kidney stones in children, but atypical symptoms are also more common. In prior studies of presenting symptoms in children, the most common symptoms are pain (47–81%) and gross hematuria (32–55%) [4]. Children with complex medical conditions may present with atypical or more severe symptoms. A study of 27 nonverbal, nonambulatory children seen in a kidney stone clinic at a tertiary children's hospital reported that 22% of those with an obstructing stone presented with sepsis, and another 22% presented with an afebrile UTI [23]. Medically complex children often have one or more additional risk factors for stone formation, including enteral feeding, anticonvulsant medications, and bladder management requiring diapers or catheterization, lowering the threshold to evaluate for nephrolithiasis as a cause for sepsis or UTI [23].

The most important decision during the initial presentation is whether a patient requires urgent urinary decompression. Indications for urinary decompression mirror those in the adult population: patients with evidence of an obstructing stone with concern for pyelonephritis, solitary kidney, signs of renal function decline, uncontrolled pain, or oral intake intolerance [9, 24]. Surgical decompression with a ureteral stent or percutaneous nephrostomy (PCN) are both options. Ureteral stent placement can be limited by access to equipment and stents appropriately sized for a younger, smaller patient. PCN may be associated with higher risk of tube dislodgement requiring replacement. PCN is likely more appropriate for larger obstructing stones, with a prior randomized trial showing higher failure and mucosal complications using ureteral stent for ureteral stones >2 cm [24, 25] .

Emergency room protocols for initial evaluation and management of pediatric nephrolithiasis have proven benefits for the patient and urologist. Such protocols ensure appropriate assessment prior to urologic consultation and can reduce unnecessary testing and imaging. Large tertiary children's centers most often employ these protocols, citing improvements in recommending medical expulsive therapy, increased spontaneous stone passage rates, reduced frequency of stone surgery, and reduced use of CT imaging as the first imaging modality [24, 26–28]. Emergency room protocols can increase the involvement of urologists in decision-making; urologic consultation has been previously demonstrated to increase the rate of recommending medical expulsive therapy, resulting in reduced surgical intervention [27].

Imaging

While computed tomography (CT) is considered the gold standard for imaging of nephrolithiasis, renal–bladder ultrasound (US) is the first-line modality for the initial diagnostic imaging for children with suspected nephrolithiasis. Ionizing radiation exposure is a significant concern for all patients with nephrolithiasis, as repeated imaging is often required for longitudinal stone management. Pediatric patients may be more susceptible to radiation-induced injury due to rapidly dividing tissue and longer lifespan [29].

The US is radiation-free and holds sufficient capability in accurately identifying kidney stones in general, and those that will require surgical management [30]. Prior studies of the US report 70% sensitivity and 100% specificity, and positive and negative predictive values of 96% and 62%, respectively [30, 31]. While US is less sensitive and specific than CT, the As Low As Reasonably Achievable (ALARA) principle and Image Gently campaign support the use of US rather than CT as the initial imaging choice [32, 33]. Guidelines from the American Urological Association (AUA) and the European Association of Urology also recommend US over CT for initial imaging in most children [34, 35].

Ziemba et al. performed a cross-sectional, single-institutional study of CT use in pediatric nephrolithiasis and found that older age and smaller stone size were associated with CT utilization [28]. Nearly three-quarters (71%) of the patients underwent CT as the first imaging study, despite wide and continuous access to ultrasound, and similarly high rates of CT utilization have been identified in studies of nationwide administrative data [28, 36–38]. A study of ED imaging practices using Healthcare Utilization Project (HCUP) data from 2006 to 2010 demonstrated that while 87% of patients underwent CT alone to image for suspected nephrolithiasis, ultrasound utilization increased over the study period, possibly correlating with the introduction of the Image Gently Campaign [36]. More recent epidemiologic studies of pediatric stone disease have noted similar trends in increasing ultrasound utilization over time [7]. Patient characteristics (age, insurance status) and institutional characteristics (teaching hospital, region) both contribute to CT utilization [28, 36].

Noncontrast, low-dose CT is highly sensitive and specific for the identification of stones and serves as an important tool when used judiciously for diagnostic and surgical planning purposes. CT can be helpful when US cannot clearly identify the presence of a stone, and low-dose radiation protocols minimize radiation exposure while maintaining high sensitivity and specificity for stone detection (95% and 97%, respectively) [39]. CT is critical for surgical planning for pediatric patients with a large stone burden and for whom surgery is being considered. AUA guidelines recommend CT prior to proceeding with percutaneous nephrolithotomy (PCNL) in pediatric patients [29].

Follow-up imaging is recommended for pediatric nephrolithiasis in the setting of active surveillance of nonobstructing stones as outlined by AUA guidelines, after stone treatment, or to ensure spontaneous passage of an obstructing ureteral stone [29, 37]. A Marketscan claims database study identified that among children with ED presentations for nephrolithiasis, 44% received ultrasound and plain film (KUB), 24% underwent CT, and 32% had no follow-up imaging at all [37]. Among children presenting with a ureteral stone, 28% did not receive any follow-up imaging [37]. Many children do not receive guideline-based kidney stone care, particularly related to imaging.

Medical Management

Acute

Immediate management of an acute kidney stone episode often entails a nonoperative trial of stone passage or watchful waiting. In children, spontaneous passage of a stone is not directly correlated to age or patient size, but rather to stone size. Stones that are ≤5 mm in size are more likely to pass spontaneously, and a trial of passage can be reasonably offered in the otherwise healthy patient for stones ≤1 cm in size [24, 29]. Prior studies in children have reported spontaneous passage rates of 32–50% and 41–63% of renal and ureteral stones, respectively [9].

Medical expulsive therapy with alpha-adrenergic receptor blockers (alpha blockers) or calcium channel blockers is a well-established approach to stone passage in the adult patient, but the utility of alpha-blockers in pediatric patients is less clear. Alpha-blockers and calcium channel blockers promote relaxation of ureteral smooth muscle, aiding in stone passage time and analgesia [9]. A recent systematic review of the use of alpha-blockers for pediatric nephrolithiasis suggests increased stone expulsion rates and decreased analgesic requirements when using alpha-blockers, though noted heterogeneity of existing studies [40]. Importantly, alpha-blockers appear to be safe for off-label use in a pediatric population; low rates of nasal congestion have been reported in randomized controlled trials of medical expulsive therapy [24, 41, 42]. AUA guidelines encourage a trial of passage for stones ≤1 cm, with or without alpha-blockers [29].

Alpha-blockers are also a useful adjunct in the surgical management of pediatric nephrolithiasis. A multi-institutional study reported tamsulosin use one week before ureteroscopy was associated with higher likelihood of ureteral access, although patient age and size may have been confounders [43]. Single institution studies suggest improved rates ureteral access with preoperative tamsulosin, mirroring studies of preoperative alpha-blocker use in adults [43–45].

Prevention

A thorough evaluation of the pediatric patient with stone disease is valuable in identifying metabolic, anatomic, or genetic risk for recurrent stone episodes. A complete history includes medical, dietary, and family history. Medical conditions, such as history of UTIs, congenital anomalies of the kidney and urinary tract (CAKUT), malabsorption concerns like Crohn's disease or short gut syndrome can help guide treatment plans for stone prevention. Ongoing use of medications such as anticonvulsants, diuretics, corticosteroids, or chemotherapeutics can persistently elevate stone formation risk, and working closely with specialists who prescribe these medications can help balance stone risk with medical management for other conditions. While an extensive and complete dietary history is optimal, an abbreviated dietary history focusing on fluid, sodium, protein, and oxalate intake is effective in identifying common dietary risk factors. Use of supplements or special diets (such as ketogenic diets for patients with severe forms of epilepsy) is important to note as well. Family history of stone disease may increase suspicion for genetic stone disease. While the physical exam may be unremarkable in most children, concerns such as obesity, growth failure, dysmorphic features, or rickets can alert to syndromic conditions that predispose to stone formation [16].

Because metabolic risks of stone formation are common among children, a complete metabolic evaluation is recommended, including serum studies and 24-hour urine testing for metabolic risks after their first stone episode. AUA guidelines recommend 24-hour urine testing for high-risk patients, and children are considered metabolically active and therefore high-risk [30, 46, 47]. A urine calcium-to-creatinine ratio can be calculated from a "spot" urine test to identify hypercalciuria and can be obtained in a non–toilet-trained child [30]. Typical serum studies include a basic metabolic panel, calcium, vitamin D, magnesium, phosphorus, and uric acid. Stone analysis should be performed if stone material was obtained after passage or during surgical treatment.

Patient size is an important consideration for interpreting 24-hour urine testing in a pediatric cohort. Values are indexed to weight, body surface area, and creatinine, and an appropriate collection is determined by urine creatinine, with normal values of 15–25 mg/kg/24 hours [30].

There are several limitations to 24-hour urine testing in children. First, 24-hour urine studies can be challenging to perform, with low compliance and high lab rejection rates [46]. Children most often complete a 24-hour urine collection on the weekend, when dietary habits may differ from weekday intake [46]. Finally, collections can be costly, and a repeat test due to inappropriate collection further adds to the high cost. Prior retrospective studies present a conflicting picture of whether management is affected by 24-hour urine test results [46, 48]. These studies propose that urologists may be less likely than nephrologists to initiate medical management in response to a 24-hour urine test, and center-specific 24-hour ordering practices may influence the overall management impact of 24-hour urine testing [46]. The ideal frequency of follow-up 24-hour urine testing for patients with metabolic risk is also unclear [30].

Medical management of recurrent stone disease in children should take into consideration a higher risk of metabolic or genetic etiology of stone disease, but it should also emphasize the importance of dietary modification strategies. Low fluid intake is a common cause of nephrolithiasis in both children and adults. Fructose consumption is highest among children and increases urinary excretion of calcium and oxalate [30]. It is recommended that fructose or sugary fluids are limited. Similar to adults, adolescents should aim for fluid intake that supports 2 L of urine output daily [30]. Sodium intake should be limited, particularly in patients with hypercalciuria (2–3 mEq/kg/day in children, 2.4 g in adolescents) [30]. While calcium, animal protein, and oxalate intake are not typically limited in children, some advocate for counseling patients on avoiding excessive animal protein, oxalate-rich, or purine-rich foods [18]. However, calcium and animal protein intake are vital to appropriate growth in childhood and should meet the recommended dietary allowance recommendations [30].

Long-term medical management may be required for patients with metabolic abnormalities on 24-hour urine studies, such as hypercalciuria, hypocitraturia, hyperoxaluria, or hyperuricosuria. For children with hypercalciuria and calcium stones, thiazide diuretics such as hydrochlorothiazide (1–2 mg/kg per day, older children 25–100 mg/day) are first-line therapy [16, 30]. Primary hyperoxaluria is treated with pyridoxine (5–10 mg/kg/day), but secondary hyperoxaluria requires targeted treatment based on the underlying cause [16]. Treatment of hyperuricosuria with allopurinol (4–10 mg/kg/day, older children 300 mg/day) requires close monitoring of liver function tests [16]. Urine alkalinization with agents such as potassium citrate can also be helpful to address metabolic abnormalities in the setting of high urine pH. Dietary supplementation with "lemonade" has also been used to alkalinize the urine. Compared to adults, fewer studies have focused on the efficacy of citrate agents or dietary supplementation with citrate-rich liquids in a pediatric cohort [16, 30]. A robust study of the efficacy and treatment adherence in adults has yet to be replicated in children. Because the side effects and practical considerations of medications used for preventive management may present significant barriers to treatment adherence, further characterization of real-world outcomes for long-term medical management of pediatric recurrent stone disease is needed.

Surgical Management

Open surgery is rarely needed or used for the surgical management of stone disease in pediatric patients. Minimally invasive techniques include extracorporeal shockwave lithotripsy (ESWL), ureteroscopy with laser lithotripsy and/or stone basket extraction (URS), and percutaneous nephrolithotomy (PCNL). Patient and stone characteristics, as well as hospital and surgeon factors, determine the appropriate surgical technique for stone treatment. AUA guidelines provide specific recommendations for surgical treatment choice based on stone size and location; for stones ≤20 mm, URS or ESWL are considered first-line treatment, and for stones ≥20 mm, PCNL is considered first line [29].

ESWL

ESWL is the most minimally invasive treatment option for smaller stones in children. Several studies have demonstrated its safety and efficacy in children [49]. ESWL utilizes a lithotripter that delivers high-energy shockwaves to a focused target zone. In children, positioning and technical considerations are important to maximize the success of ESWL. Patients should be securely positioned on the lithotripter table to avoid movement, and the focus of the shockwave generator and acoustic gel bridge should be appropriate to the size of the child [49]. Fluoroscopic guidance is typically used to target stones and confirm fragmentation, but ultrasound guidance has been shown to be safe and effective [50].

Stone-free rates in children range from 57% to 97% with retreatment rates ranging between 14% and 54% [51]. Sedation or general anesthesia is required to reduce discomfort. Factors such as stone size, stone durability, collecting system anatomy, and number of stones impact the success of ESWL [51]. Stone-free rates decrease with increasing stone size, and harder stones like calcium oxalate monohydrate reduce the likelihood of successful stone treatment. While stone fragments tend to transit the collecting system more quickly in children, lower pole stone location or anomalous collecting system anatomy can decrease the passage of stone fragments [49, 51].

Long-term effects on renal function have not been reported in children undergoing ESWL, but risks of transient kidney injury and intra- and perirenal hematoma are well described [52]. A reduction in energy and shocks is recommended for children. Energy should start at the lowest level (14 kV) and increase only to the level needed for fragmentation, at a maximum of 20 kV [53]. A maximum of 1000–1500 shocks for very young children (under 5 years old) and 2500 shocks in children older than 5 is recommended [53].

URS

URS, or retrograde intrarenal surgery (RIRS) is widely utilized for stone treatment in adults and children. A ureteroscope is advanced retrograde through the collecting system, and laser lithotripsy and/or stone basket extraction is used to treat stones. A ureteral access sheath can be used to aid with stone fragment removal, especially for stones >1 cm [54]. While ureteral access sheaths reduce postoperative sepsis by decreasing intrarenal pressure, they increase the risk of ureteral injury, particularly in a pediatric ureter [54]. Use of smaller inner diameter sheaths (8 Fr or 10 Fr) in older children and limited use of sheaths in children under 5 years may be advisable [54]. Fluoroscopic guidance is necessary for safe passage of instruments and stent placement, although fluoroscopy-free techniques have been described [55, 56].

Stone-free rates in children are reported between 58% and 100%, though a systematic review of published studies in pediatric cohorts supports a high stone-free rate of around 90% [57]. Complication rates are around 11%, with the most common complications including ureteral or mucosal injuries, postoperative fever, and hematuria [57]. Risk factors for complications include increased stone burden and Hounsfield Units (HU) [58]. For stone burden >2 cm, PCNL or ESWL is recommended over URS, and PCNL is ideal for large lower pole stones [29].

Advances in technology may further increase the utility of URS in children. Continued miniaturization of both URS and PCNL offers an opportunity for reduced tissue trauma with the possibility of similar stone-free rates. Mini-URS utilizes a 4.85 Fr ureteroscope and 200 μm or 270 μm holmium:yttrium–aluminum–garnet (Ho:YAG) laser fiber. In older children and adolescents, mini-URS may reduce the risk of ureteral complications and decrease the need for postoperative ureteral stent; for younger children, it may allow for retrograde stone treatment where larger ureteroscopes cannot be used. In preschool-aged children, miniURS has demonstrated minimal complications with similar stone-free rates, and reasonable accessibility for commonly used components of URS, such as retrograde pyelography, stone baskets, and safety wires [59, 60]. Newer laser technologies adopted for adult stone treatment are now being explored for their utility in pediatric URS. The thulium fiber laser (TFL) is more efficient at stone ablation and can be delivered at a wider range of energy and frequency settings than Ho:YAG lasers. A single-center retrospective study of pediatric patients found that TFL was associated with increased stone-free rates, increased laser time, and similar complication rates and overall operative times when compared with Ho:YAG laser URS [61]. The authors also cited several arguments for increased ease-of-use with TFL, including availability of a more maneuverable 150 μm fiber, 110 V compatible generator, and minimal stone retropulsion during treatment [61]. Simulations of thermal effects of Ho:YAG laser lithotripsy in a pediatric patient suggest increased risk of tissue heating, but intermittent laser activity and continuous irrigation can mitigate risk [62]. As TFL use in children increases, technique modifications in the pediatric population such as pressure irrigation and increased off-laser time, can reduce thermal injury [61, 63].

PCNL

PCNL is the gold-standard approach for large and complex stone burden in both children and adults. After obtaining percutaneous access to the kidney through an upper or lower pole calyx, the tract is dilated to allow for sheath placement and passage of tools for stone removal. Traditional PCNL tract size 24–32 Fr poses an increased risk of bleeding and renal injury in a pediatric patient. Advances in mini- and micro-PCNL have improved safety outcomes with minimal reduction in efficacy. Mini-PCNL utilizes sheath sizes 14–20Fr, although it was originally described using an 11 Fr peel-away vascular access sheath [64, 65]. Mini-PCNL has reported low rates of blood transfusion or urosepsis, and a high stone-free rate of 85–85% [64]. Mini-PCNL typically utilizes a nephroscope and laser or lithotripter, and it is ideal for stone burden <2.5 cm [65]. Ultra-mini-PCNL (11–13 Fr sheath size) and micro-PCNL (16 G angiocath needle) require the use of a laser fiber and are recommended for even smaller stone burdens <1.5 cm [65]. A survey of European urology societies suggests mini-PCNL is the prevailing approach over traditional PCNL, although traditional PCNL may still be the optimal choice for a large staghorn calculus [66].

PCNL can be performed in the prone or supine position. Prone positioning reduces respiratory compliance and increases the potential for airway-related complications [65]. A systematic review and meta-analysis of studies comparing prone to supine positioning demonstrated decreased operative time in the supine position with equivalent stone-free and complication rates [67]. Similar results have been reported in children, with the suggestion of improved complication rates [68, 69]. Disadvantages of the supine position include a limited puncture area and increased kidney movement [65].

Postoperative urinary drainage is typically ensured with a PCN, but tubeless variations of PCNL are increasingly being studied in the pediatric population. In a comparison study of tubeless mini-PCNL to mini-PCNL with postoperative PCN, the tubeless approach was associated with reduced anesthesia and fluoroscopy time, and similar stone-free rates [70]. A systematic review and meta-analysis of tubeless PCNL in children identified advantages, including shorter hospital stay, reduced postoperative fever or urinary leakage, and increased stone-free rates [71]. Authors of this review noted that many studies include cases where surgeon preference determines who receives a PCN, suggesting that surgeon experience, patient characteristics, and stone factors may limit these findings [71].

Surgical Decision-Making

The optimal surgical treatment for an individual patient is multifactorial. In addition to stone characteristics such as size, location, hardness, and probable stone composition, patient characteristics like size, age, medical conditions, and family/patient preferences must also be considered.

Nomograms can help aid decision-making for the surgical treatment of stones. A systematic review of existing nomograms identified seven nomograms for stone treatment, two of which were externally validated in a pediatric cohort and were used to predict the success of ESWL [72]. Further research and validation of pediatric stone nomograms will likely decrease re-treatment rates and improve the efficacy of treatments through appropriate patient selection.

Patient-reported outcomes can be helpful to counsel patients and families on optimal medical and surgical plans to balance effective treatment with a patient-centered approach. Comparative effectiveness research for stone disease is beneficial for shared decision-making, in that it provides information about the benefits and tradeoffs between multiple options for treatments or interventions [73]. Within stone disease research, few studies utilize patient-reported outcomes or engage stakeholders during the research design and development process [73]. A recent multicenter comparative effectiveness study of ESWL, URS, and PCNL in children utilized a patient-centered, pragmatic approach and includes patient-reported measures related to physical, emotional, and social health; early data from this study may shape decision-making for both surgeons and patients as they consider surgical approaches for stone treatment [74].

Transition to Adulthood

Transition to adult care for patients with a history of stone disease can be relatively straightforward, as the treatment approach for preventive and surgical management is likely familiar to the adult urologist and nephrologist. Many conditions contribute to recurrent nephrolithiasis, such as Dent disease, cystinuria, primary hyperoxaluria, and familial hypomagnesemia with hypercalciuria and nephrocalcinosis [75]. Through adulthood, stone preventive care and metabolic risk should be optimized to reduce stone recurrence. However, more complex diseases, such as myelomeningocele and/or surgically complex patients, such as those with intestinal segment diversions, may require a urologist with knowledge of the intricacies of care in these patients [75].

Conclusion

Although stone disease is less common in children than adults, stone incidence has risen over the last two decades and may continue to rise in the future. While calcium-based stones are most common among children, they are less likely to have uric acid stones. Metabolic and genetic causes of stone disease should be strongly considered, so a thorough history is critical in the initial evaluation and can help determine if genetic testing is helpful. Children and adolescents are considered high risk for stone recurrence; testing for metabolic causes should include 24-hour urine testing, despite known challenges to reliable completion of the test among pediatric patients. Dietary modifications and targeted medical therapy may be useful in stone prevention, although further research is required on the effects of treatment nonadherence on prevention outcomes.

Imaging is fundamental in the management of stone disease, and choosing the optimal imaging modality for the pediatric patient is especially critical. Although ultrasound is often ideal for the pediatric patient, CT is sometimes necessary to diagnose and localize stones or to facilitate surgical planning. Overutilization of CT in the acute setting can be curtailed by involvement of a urologist in the initial diagnostic decision-making. Surgical management of stones in children is also nuanced; stone and patient factors will determine the optimal surgical approach. Advances in surgical technology, such as miniaturization of instrumentation and increased laser fiber power, have the potential to improve outcomes for minimally invasive stone surgery in children. Patient-reported outcomes should also be considered in surgical decision-making. While relatively rare, pediatric stone disease may impact patients in a general urology practice; knowledge of the specific considerations for management of stones in children and adolescents remains valuable.

Summary

- The incidence of pediatric stone disease has risen in the last 2 decades, likely due to changes in diet and fluid intake.
- Compared to adults, pediatric patients are more likely to have recurrent stone disease, due to increased risk of metabolic, anatomic, and/or genetic causes.
- Ultrasound is the first-line imaging modality for children with nephrolithiasis and is recommended by AUA guidelines. Many children do not receive guideline-based imaging, and CT is overutilized in the acute management of stones.
- Medical management in acute and preventive care for pediatric stone formers aligns with principles of management in adult patients, but more robust research on treatment adherence and outcomes in children is needed.
- ESWL, URS/RIRS, and PCNL are all options for stone surgery in children. Stone and patient characteristics should be considered to determine the optimal surgical approach in each case.

References

1. Wang H-HS, Wiener JS, Lipkin ME, Scales CD, Ross SS, Routh JC. Estimating the nationwide, hospital based economic impact of pediatric urolithiasis. J Urol. 2015;193:1855–9.
2. Dwyer ME, Krambeck AE, Bergstralh EJ, Milliner DS, Lieske JC, Rule AD. Temporal trends in incidence of kidney stones among children: a 25-year population based study. J Urol. 2012;188:247–52.
3. Routh JC, Graham DA, Nelson CP. Epidemiological trends in pediatric urolithiasis at United States freestanding pediatric hospitals. J Urol. 2010;184:1100–5.
4. Sas DJ. An update on the changing epidemiology and metabolic risk factors in pediatric kidney stone disease. Clin J Am Soc Nephrol. 2011;6:2062–8.
5. Tasian GE, Ross ME, Song L, Sas DJ, Keren R, Denburg MR, Chu DI, Copelovitch L, Saigal CS, Furth SL. Annual incidence of nephrolithiasis among children and adults in South Carolina from 1997 to 2012. Clin J Am Soc Nephrol. 2016;11:488–96.
6. VanDervoort K, Wiesen J, Frank R, Vento S, Crosby V, Chandra M, Trachtman H. Urolithiasis in pediatric patients: a single center study of incidence, clinical presentation and outcome. J Urol. 2007;177:2300–5.
7. Ward JB, Feinstein L, Pierce C, Lim J, Abbott KC, Bavendam T, Kirkali Z, Matlaga BR. Pediatric urinary stone disease in the United States: the urologic diseases in America project. Urology. 2019;129:180–7.
8. Shoag J, Tasian GE, Goldfarb DS, Eisner BH. The new epidemiology of nephrolithiasis. Adv Chronic Kidney Dis. 2015;22:273–8.

9. Hernandez JD, Ellison JS, Lendvay TS. Current trends, evaluation, and management of pediatric nephrolithiasis. JAMA Pediatr. 2015;169:964–70.
10. Kalorin CM, Zabinski A, Okpareke I, White M, Kogan BA. Pediatric urinary stone disease--does age matter? J Urol. 2009;181:2267–71.
11. Kirejczyk JK, Porowski T, Filonowicz R, Kazberuk A, Stefanowicz M, Wasilewska A, Debek W. An association between kidney stone composition and urinary metabolic disturbances in children. J Pediatr Urol. 2014;10:130–5.
12. Pecoraro L, Zuccato A, Vitella R, Pietrobelli A, Piacentini G, Brugnara M. Pediatric nephrolithiasis: a changing landscape through time and space. Medicina (Kaunas). 2024; https://doi.org/10.3390/medicina60121993.
13. Modi PK, Kwon YS, Davis RB, Elsamra SE, Dombrovskiy V, Olweny EO. Pediatric hospitalizations for upper urinary tract calculi: epidemiological and treatment trends in the United States, 2001-2014. J Pediatr Urol. 2018;14:13.e1–6.
14. Kusumi K, Becknell B, Schwaderer A. Trends in pediatric urolithiasis: patient characteristics, associated diagnoses, and financial burden. Pediatr Nephrol. 2015;30:805–10.
15. Bush NC, Xu L, Brown BJ, Holzer MS, Gingrich A, Schuler B, Tong L, Baker LA. Hospitalizations for pediatric stone disease in United States, 2002–2007. J Urol. 2010;183:1151–6.
16. Kovacevic L. Diagnosis and management of nephrolithiasis in children. Pediatr Clin N Am. 2022;69:1149–64.
17. Kovacevic L, Wolfe-Christensen C, Edwards L, Sadaps M, Lakshmanan Y. From hypercalciuria to hypocitraturia—a shifting trend in pediatric urolithiasis? J Urol. 2012;188:1623–7.
18. Scoffone CM, Cracco CM. Pediatric calculi: cause, prevention and medical management. Curr Opin Urol. 2018;28:428–32.
19. Halbritter J, Baum M, Hynes AM, et al. Fourteen monogenic genes account for 15% of nephrolithiasis/nephrocalcinosis. J Am Soc Nephrol. 2015;26:543–51.
20. Geraghty R, Lovegrove C, Howles S, Sayer JA. Role of genetic testing in kidney stone disease: a narrative review. Curr Urol Rep. 2024;25:311.
21. Hoppe B, Martin-Higueras C. Inherited conditions resulting in nephrolithiasis. Curr Opin Pediatr. 2020;32:273–83.
22. Arora V, Anand K, Chander Verma I. Genetic testing in pediatric kidney disease. Indian J Pediatr. 2020;87:706–15.
23. Fernandez N, Silverii H, Dangle P, Yonekawa K. Atypical clinical presentation and management of urinary stone disease in non-verbal non-ambulatory children. J Pediatr Urol. 2023;19:560.e1–6.
24. Van Batavia JP, Tasian GE. Clinical effectiveness in the diagnosis and acute management of pediatric nephrolithiasis. Int J Surg. 2016;36:698–704.
25. Elsheemy MS, Shouman AM, Shoukry AI, Elshenoufy A, Aboulela W, Daw K, Hussein AA, Morsi HA, Badawy H. Ureteric stents vs percutaneous nephrostomy for initial urinary drainage in children with obstructive anuria and acute renal failure due to ureteric calculi: a prospective, randomised study. BJU Int. 2015;115:473–9.
26. Ellison JS, Crowell CS, Clifton H, Whitlock K, Haaland W, Chen T, Merguerian P, Migita R, Vora SB. A clinical pathway to minimize computed tomography for suspected nephrolithiasis in children. J Pediatr Urol. 2019;15:518.e1–7.
27. Salevitz D, Lin CY, Alcanzo B, Namjoshi A, Lee P, Monteilh C, Grimsby G. Standardization of the management of pediatric urolithiasis in the emergency department. J Pediatr Urol. 2024;20:89.e1–6.
28. Ziemba JB, Canning DA, Lavelle J, Kalmus A, Tasian GE. Patient and institutional characteristics associated with initial computerized tomography in children presenting to the emergency department with kidney stones. J Urol. 2015;193:1848–54.
29. Kidney Stones: Surgical Management Guideline - American Urological Association. https://www.auanet.org/guidelines-and-quality/guidelines/kidney-stones-surgical-management-guideline. Accessed 26 May 2025.

30. Tasian GE, Copelovitch L. Evaluation and medical management of kidney stones in children. J Urol. 2014;192:1329–36.
31. Passerotti C, Chow JS, Silva A, et al. Ultrasound versus computerized tomography for evaluating urolithiasis. J Urol. 2009;182:1829–34.
32. Strauss KJ, Kaste SC. The ALARA (as low as reasonably achievable) concept in pediatric interventional and fluoroscopic imaging: striving to keep radiation doses as low as possible during fluoroscopy of pediatric patients - a white paper executive summary. Pediatr Radiol. 2006;36:110–2.
33. Goske MJ, Applegate KE, Boylan J, et al. The "Image Gently" campaign: increasing CT radiation dose awareness through a national education and awareness program. Pediatr Radiol. 2008;38:265–9.
34. Fulgham PF, Assimos DG, Pearle MS, Preminger GM. Clinical effectiveness protocols for imaging in the management of ureteral calculous disease: AUA technology assessment. J Urol. 2013;189:1203–13.
35. EAU Guidelines on Urolithiasis - UROweb. https://uroweb.org/guidelines/urolithiasis Accessed 10/24/2025.
36. Johnson EK, Graham DA, Chow JS, Nelson CP. Nationwide emergency department imaging practices for pediatric urolithiasis: room for improvement. J Urol. 2014;192:200–6.
37. Ellison JS, Merguerian PA, Fu BC, Holt SK, Lendvay TS, Gore JL, Shnorhavorian M. Follow-up imaging after acute evaluations for pediatric nephrolithiasis: trends from a national database. J Pediatr Urol. 2018;14:525–31.
38. Raghavan VR, Porter JJ, Monuteaux MC, Neuman MI, Nelson KA. Imaging trends and surgical outcomes for nephrolithiasis in the pediatric emergency department. Am J Emerg Med. 2025;92:104–8.
39. Poletti PA, Platon A, Rutschmann OT, Schmidlin FR, Iselin CE, Becker CD. Low-dose versus standard-dose CT protocol in patients with clinically suspected renal colic. AJR Am J Roentgenol. 2007;188:927–33.
40. Haddad F, Farhat WA, Cannon S. The use of alpha-adrenergic antagonists in pediatric nephrolithiasis: a systematic review. Front Pediatr. 2024;12:1396659.
41. Tasian GE, Cost NG, Granberg CF, Pulido JE, Rivera M, Schwen Z, Schulte M, Fox JA. Tamsulosin and spontaneous passage of ureteral stones in children: a multi-institutional cohort study. J Urol. 2014;192:506–11.
42. Aldaqadossi HA, Shaker H, Saifelnasr M, Gaber M. Efficacy and safety of tamsulosin as a medical expulsive therapy for stones in children. Arab J Urol. 2015;13:107–11.
43. Meyer KM, Asantey K, Ellison JS, et al. The effect of preoperative tamsulosin on pediatric ureteroscopic access: a multi-institutional experience. Urol Pract. 2025; https://doi.org/10.1097/UPJ.0000000000000793.
44. Morley C, Hajiran A, Elbakry AA, Al-Qudah HS, Al-Omar O. Evaluation of preoperative tamsulosin role in facilitating ureteral orifice navigation for school-age pediatric ureteroscopy. Res Rep Urol. 2020;12:563.
45. McGee LM, Sack BS, Wan J, Kraft KH. The effect of preoperative tamsulosin on ureteroscopic access in school-aged children. J Pediatr Urol. 2021;17:795.e1–6.
46. Carnes K, Howe A, Feustel PJ, Listman JA, White M, Kogan BA. 24-hour urine collection for first time pediatric stone formers: is it worth it? J Pediatr Urol. 2021;17:387.e1–7.
47. Pearle MS, Goldfarb DS, Assimos DG, Curhan G, Denu-Ciocca CJ, Matlaga BR, Monga M, Penniston KL, Preminger GM, Turk TM, White JR; American Urological Assocation. Medical management of kidney stones: AUA guideline. J Urol. 2014 Aug;192(2):316-24. https://doi.org/10.1016/j.juro.2014.05.006. Epub 2014 May 20. PMID: 24857648.
48. Tasian GE, Kabarriti AE, Kalmus A, Furth SL. Kidney stone recurrence among children and adolescents. J Urol. 2017;197:246–52.
49. Lahme S. Shockwave lithotripsy and endourological stone treatment in children. Urol Res. 2006;34:112–7.
50. Grabsky A, Tsaturyan A, Musheghyan L, Minasyan G, Khachatryan Y, Shadyan G, Qocharyan A, Mosoyan M, Kallidonis P. Effectiveness of ultrasound-guided shockwave lithotripsy and

predictors of its success rate in pediatric population: a report from a national reference center. J Pediatr Urol. 2021;17:78.e1–7.
51. Güzel R, Yildirim Ü, Sarica K. Contemporary minimal invasive surgical management of stones in children. Asian J Urol. 2023;10:239–45.
52. Goel MC, Baserge NS, Babu RVR, Sinha S, Kapoor R. Pediatric kidney: functional outcome after extracorporeal shock wave lithotripsy. J Urol. 1996;155:2044–6.
53. Akin Y, Yucel S. Long-term effects of pediatric extracorporeal shockwave lithotripsy on renal function. Res Rep Urol. 2014;6:21.
54. Tanidir Y, Sekerci CA, Bujons A, et al. The utility and safety of ureteral access sheath during retrograde Intrarenal surgery in children. Urology. 2024;187:71–7.
55. Ozan T, Karakeci A, Yilmaz K, Pirincci N, Osmanlioglu F, Yuvanc E, Yilmaz E, Orhan I. Is there a safe no radiation option for endoscopic kidney stone treatment in children? multicenter results of modified retrograde intrarenal surgery without fluoroscopy in pediatric patients. Urolithiasis. 2025;53:46.
56. Reda A, Mahmoud Abdelsalam Y, Shehata ML, Shaker SED, Faragallah MA. Ultrasound versus fluoroscopy-guided ureteroscopy for distal ureteric stones in adults. Arab J Urol. 2022;20:197–203.
57. Rob S, Jones P, Pietropaolo A, Griffin S, Somani BK. Ureteroscopy for stone disease in paediatric population is safe and effective in medium-volume and high-volume centres: evidence from a systematic review. Curr Urol Rep. 2017;18:92.
58. Lim EJ, Traxer O, Madarriaga YQ, et al. Outcomes and lessons learnt from practice of retrograde intrarenal surgery (RIRS) in a paediatric setting of various age groups: a global study across 8 centres. World J Urol. 2022;40:1223–9.
59. Utangaç MM, Sancaktutar AA, Tepeler A. Micro-ureteroscopy for the treatment of distal ureteral calculi in children. J Pediatr Surg. 2017;52:512–6.
60. Hernández RP, Caballero Romeu JP, Galiano Baena JF, Montoya Lirola MD, García Tabar PJ, Galán Llopis JA, Gonzálvez Piñera J, Mira Marcelí NA, Budía Alba A. Technical considerations about micro-ureteroscopy in children. J Pediatr Surg. 2017;52:1216.
61. Jaeger CD, Nelson CP, Cilento BG, Logvinenko T, Kurtz MP. Comparing pediatric ureteroscopy outcomes with SuperPulsed thulium fiber laser and low-power holmium:YAG laser. J Urol. 2022;208:426–33.
62. Ellison JS, MacConaghy B, Hall TL, Roberts WW, Maxwell AD. A simulated model for fluid and tissue heating during pediatric laser lithotripsy. J Pediatr Urol. 2020;16:626.e1–8.
63. Ellison JS. Editorial comment. J Urol. 2022;208:432.
64. Jackman SV, Hedican SP, Peters CA, Docimo SG. Percutaneous nephrolithotomy in infants and preschool age children: experience with a new technique. Urology. 1998;52:697–701.
65. Softness KA, Kurtz MP. Pediatric stone surgery: what is hot and what is not. Curr Urol Rep. 2022;23:57–65.
66. Pietropaolo A, Geraghty R, Griffin S, et al. Worldwide trends of practice and intervention in paediatric endourology: comparison of European versus non-European responses. Cent European J Urol. 2023;76:245.
67. Liu L, Zheng S, Xu Y, Wei Q. Systematic review and meta-analysis of percutaneous nephrolithotomy for patients in the supine versus prone position. J Endourol. 2010;24:1941–6. https://home-liebertpub-com.ezproxy.library.wisc.edu/end.
68. Fang H, Zhu F, Cui K, Liu X, Wu S, Hua Y, Lin T, He D, Wei G, Zhang D. An updated systematic review and meta-analysis on the efficacy of supine versus prone position for pediatric PCNL. Int Urol Nephrol. 2025:1–14.
69. Ramez M, Desoky EAE, EL-Nahas AR. Supine versus prone pediatric percutaneous nephrolithotomy: a systematic review and meta-analysis. Arab J Urol. 2024;22:253.
70. Bilen CY, Gunay M, Ozden E, Inci K, Sarikaya S, Tekgul S. Tubeless mini percutaneous nephrolithotomy in infants and preschool children: a preliminary report. J Urol. 2010;184:2498–503.
71. Fang H, Wang Z, Wei K, Liu X, Wu S, Hua Y, Lin T, He D, Wei G, Zhang D. Safety and efficacy of standard vs. tubeless percutaneous nephrolithotomy in pediatric populations: an updated systematic review and meta-analysis. BMC Urol. 2025;25:110.

72. Brown G, Juliebø-Jones P, Keller EX, De Coninck V, Beisland C, Somani BK. Current status of nomograms and scoring systems in paediatric endourology: a systematic review of literature. J Pediatr Urol. 2022;18:572–84.
73. Dangle P, Tasian GE, Chu DI, Shannon R, Spiardi R, Xiang AH, Jadcherla A, Arenas J, Ellison JS. A systematic scoping review of comparative effectiveness studies in kidney stone disease. Urology. 2024;183:3–10.
74. Ellison JS, Lorenzo M, Beck H, et al. Comparative effectiveness of paediatric kidney stone surgery (the PKIDS trial): study protocol for a patient-centred pragmatic clinical trial. BMJ Open. 2022; https://doi.org/10.1136/BMJOPEN-2021-056789.
75. Lambert SM. Transitional care in pediatric urology. Semin Pediatr Surg. 2015;24:73–8.

Pediatric Genitourinary Trauma 10

Marie-Therese Valovska, Matthew P. Kirschenbaum, George E. Koch, and Judith C. Hagedorn

Renal Trauma

Epidemiology

Trauma is the leading cause of death in children in the United States, primarily due to firearm injuries, motor vehicle accidents, or falls [16, 41, 64]. Pediatric anatomy renders children much more susceptible to significant renal trauma than their adult counterparts [3]. The relatively larger proportion of the pediatric kidneys, reduced perirenal fat, and weaker ribs and abdominal musculature are all contributing factors. One study found that of all the renal injuries registered in the National Trauma Database (NTDB), 25% occurred in pediatric patients [23]. The vast majority (85–90%) of pediatric renal trauma is blunt in nature and more commonly occurs after age 5. In fact, approximately 5–20% of pediatric patients with blunt abdominal trauma will have renal trauma, and renal trauma is rarely an isolated injury [20, 23, 47, 54]. An additional consideration in the pediatric population is that up to 23% may have a renal injury concomitant with a pre-existing congenital renal anomaly or pediatric renal tumor [21, 55]. As in adults, renal preservation is critical and remains the primary goal when managing pediatric patients with renal trauma. Familiarity with management by the adult urologist is crucial, as most of these

M.-T. Valovska · J. C. Hagedorn (✉)
University of Washington, Department of Urology, Seattle, WA, USA
e-mail: mvalosk@uw.edu; judithch@uw.edu

M. P. Kirschenbaum
University of Washington, School of Medicine, Seattle, WA, USA
e-mail: mattk93@uw.edu

G. E. Koch
The Ohio State University, Department of Urology, Columbus, OH, USA
e-mail: george.koch@osumc.edu

H.-Y. Wu et al. (eds.), *Pediatric Urology for the Adult Urologist*, https://doi.org/10.1007/978-3-032-10306-2_10

children are treated at adult hospitals, where, unfortunately, the rate of nephrectomy has been cited as up to three times higher than in pediatric hospitals [23]. Nevertheless, the overall rate of nephrectomy in pediatric renal trauma has been reported to be in the range of 0–3.2%, which is nearly half the rate reported in the adult renal trauma population [28].

Diagnosis/Imaging

Renal injuries are graded according to the revised American Association for the Surgery of Trauma (AAST) Organ Injury Scale (Table 10.1) [5]. Rapid acceleration or deceleration, or direct impact to the flank, should raise the suspicion for a potential blunt renal injury (Fig. 10.1). Penetrating injury may involve the kidneys if entry or exit wounds are in the proximity of the flank. When assessing the child with a potential renal injury, it is important to remember that hypotension manifests much later in the pediatric population as compared to adults due to their significant physiological reserve [47]. It is, therefore, important to have a much higher index of suspicion in this population. Similarly, the degree of hematuria does not always correlate with the severity of an injury. For example, one study found that 17% of pediatric patients with Grade IV renal trauma had normal urinalyses [28]. Accordingly, any child with blunt renal trauma and any degree of microscopic or gross hematuria, or suspicion of renal injury despite normal urinalysis, should be evaluated for renal injury [20]. Any clinical history or presentation concerning potential high-grade renal injury warrants full evaluation with CT imaging, including delayed-phase imaging to evaluate the collecting system. The adult Urotrauma Guidelines recommend repeat imaging for Grades IV and V renal injury or those with clinical signs of complications [42]. Some argue that due to the low rate of operative intervention and complications, routine repeat imaging may be avoidable in children with high-grade renal injury [35, 56].

Table 10.1 AAST renal injury grading and management [4]

Grade	Description	Intervention[a]
I	Subcapsular hematoma or contusion	O
II	≤1.0 cm cortical laceration	O
III	>1.0 cm cortical laceration without extravasation	O
IV	Segmental vessel laceration, collecting system injury	A, UD
V	Complete avulsion, hilum disruption, or shattered kidney	A (if stable) N (if unstable)

[a]*O* Observation, *A* Angioembolization, *UD* Urinary Diversion (Stent/Catheter), *N* Nephrectomy
Vascular injury includes pseudoaneurysms and AV fistulas. Grading is based on the most severe injury seen on imaging, surgery, or pathology. If multiple injuries are present, the highest grade is assigned, advancing one grade for each subsequent injury up to Grade III

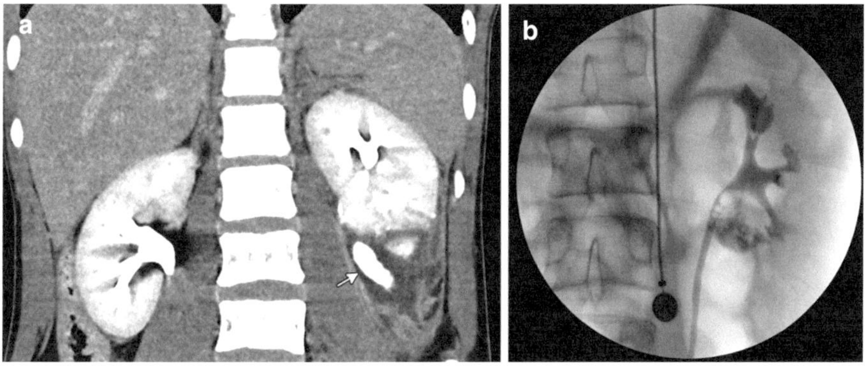

Fig. 10.1 (**a**) CT urogram (excretory phase) showing a left Grade 4 renal laceration in a 15-year-old boy with lower pole urine leak in a 15-year-old patient after a pedestrian versus motor vehicle collision. (**b**) Shows the same injury on retrograde pyelography at the time of ureteral stent placement

Management

As in the adult world, management of renal trauma has trended away from early operative intervention in an effort to maximize renal preservation and minimize morbidity. One recent study performed a systematic review and meta-analysis of 51 articles on pediatric renal trauma. Based on the meta-analysis and Grading of Recommendations Assessment, Development, and Evaluation profile, they formulated several recommendations regarding pediatric renal trauma. First, initial management of any blunt renal trauma should be managed conservatively so long as the patient is clinically stable. Stable patients with high-grade renal trauma and ongoing or delayed bleeding should undergo angioembolization versus surgical intervention. Early operative management is generally reserved for hemodynamically unstable patients, severe penetrating injuries, and patients with other concomitant injuries that necessitate exploration [25].

Studies have proven that conservative management of even high-grade renal injuries is often successful, though the protocol for conservative management varies between institutions [22, 37]. At our institution, conservative management entails PICU admission for Grades III–V injuries, mandatory Urology consult, consideration of Interventional Radiology consult if concern for ongoing bleeding, monitoring of hemoglobin and hematocrit (with liberalization once stable for 24 hours), holding DVT prophylaxis, and possible repeat imaging after 48–72 hours if concern for a persistent urine leak or continuous bleeding. Bed rest is not mandated for any degree of injury at our institution. One systematic review of 32 studies found that short and long-term outcomes of conservative management for high-grade renal injury are favorable [37]. Importantly, even the failure of conservative management still results in improved renal salvage rates when compared to upfront surgical exploration (12.1% vs. 57.1%) [47]. Suggested factors that may be predictive of a higher likelihood for urological intervention of any type include higher Injury

Severity Score, higher grade injuries (e.g., vascular pedicle avulsion, etc.), penetrating injuries, anemia, transfusion requirement, size of perinephric hematoma >2.2–3.5 cm, and persistent urinary contrast extravasation [34, 36, 47].

In accordance with the aforementioned risk factors, renal exploration rate for blunt pediatric renal trauma varies vastly in contemporary series from that of penetrating pediatric renal trauma. In one study, almost 90% of cases were managed conservatively after blunt trauma, as opposed to only half of the cases after penetrating trauma [23]. One retrospective study of 374 pediatric renal injuries found that the renal exploration rate for blunt pediatric renal trauma was less than 2%, as opposed to penetrating trauma, which had an exploration rate of 76%. Nevertheless, their overall renal salvage rate was greater than 99% [6]. Possible explanations for the increased failure of conservative management in cases of penetrating renal trauma include increased likelihood of higher-grade injuries and increased likelihood of concomitant injuries to other organs [47].

Failure of conservative management can present as either hemodynamic instability, persistent bleeding with clinical stability, or delayed bleeding. While hemodynamic instability unresponsive to resuscitation warrants surgical exploration, it has been otherwise established that minimally invasive endovascular procedures such as angioembolization are safe and effective even in the management of high-grade renal trauma so long as the patient is hemodynamically stable [33]. While involvement of Interventional Radiology has been widely adopted in the adult world, it is underutilized in the pediatric population. One NTDB study found that angioembolization comprised 3.5% of all interventions for those patients undergoing immediate intervention, and only 3.1% of all procedures after failure of conservative management. However, it is important to note that they defined failure of conservative management as the need for intervention 4 hours after presenting to the Emergency Department [47]. As such, it is important to emphasize that angioembolization has been shown to be safe and effective in the management of pediatric renal trauma [25, 33].

Failure can also present in the form of persistent urinary contrast extravasation, or symptomatic urinary extravasation with fevers and infection, or uncontrolled flank pain. Typically, this is managed in a minimally invasive fashion with ureteral stent placement and a period of Foley catheter drainage for maximal decompression [47]. If a ureteral stent fails, additional drainage can be achieved with a percutaneous drain. Follow-up thereafter includes repeat assessment of the leak prior to definitive stent or drain removal. For younger patients in our practice, this typically involves a return to the operating room for a repeat retrograde pyelogram. This spares radiation exposure in comparison to evaluation with a CT scan, and also allows for stent removal under anesthesia rather than in the clinic.

Follow-Up

Pediatric patients with renal trauma should have routine blood pressure checks on follow-up to diagnose hypertension [25]. In a review of 15 years of literature on pediatric renal trauma, LeeVan et al. reported that conservative management did not increase the likelihood of secondary hypertension. In their review, the incidence of pediatric hypertension after conservative management was typically between 0% and 15%, and self-limited in nature, or in severe instances cured by subsequent operation [37].

Ureteral Trauma

Epidemiology

Ureteral trauma is rare, accounting for less than 1% of all cases of pediatric urological trauma, and is seen more commonly in polytrauma [27, 48, 58]. Ureteral injuries are more common in penetrating trauma, but blunt injuries such as ureteral contusion, laceration, or ureteropelvic junction (UPJ) avulsion can also occur due to the hyperextensible vertebral column in children [27].

Diagnosis/Imaging

A high-grade ureteral injury, such as a ureteral transection or UPJ avulsion (Fig. 10.2), may occur with the absence of hematuria; therefore, index of suspicion should remain high based on clinical history, such as penetrating trauma to the flank or deep abdomen, or significant deceleration injury, respectively [13, 51]. While some recommend diagnosis of ureteral injuries by retrograde pyelogram, the reality is that these patients typically have polytrauma that warrants CT imaging. CT findings of perirenal hematoma, low-density fluid around the urinary tract, or hydronephrosis raise concern for a ureteral injury [10, 27]. Additionally, concomitant injury

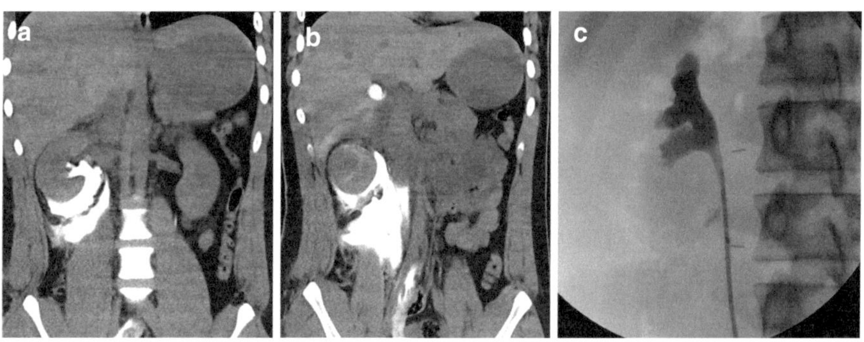

Fig. 10.2 (**a**) and (**b**) Delayed phase imaging showing right ureteropelvic junction avulsion after an unrestrained motor vehicle accident in a 16-year-old boy with large volume contrast extravasation into the retroperitoneum. This was immediately surgically repaired with pyeloplasty over a ureteral stent. (**c**) 1-month postoperative retrograde pyelography at the time of ureteral stent removal, showing a well-healed ureter with smooth contour and no leak or stricture

to the lumbar vertebral transverse processes should raise suspicion for a UPJ avulsion [51].

If a renal injury or ureteral injury is suspected, patients should have delayed excretory phase imaging to complete stage the injury and detect a collecting system or ureteral injury [10, 53, 58]. If a patient is taken directly to the operating room for exploratory laparotomy and a ureteral injury is suspected, direct inspection of the ureter should be performed if possible, or a retrograde pyelogram can be considered [10]. The Ureter Organ Injury Scale was proposed in 1992 by Moore et al. and aimed to provide an injury classification scale based on anatomic description, and can be used to describe injury severity after direct inspection (Table 10.2) [40].

Management

Low-grade ureteral lesions (i.e., contusion, partial laceration) may be managed by ureteral stenting [58]. Ureteral stenting may also be employed in cases of delayed diagnosis of partial ureteral injury; if this fails then a percutaneous nephrostomy followed by delayed repair is indicated [10, 69].

In cases where conservative management with stenting has failed, or where high-grade ureteral injury is diagnosed expeditiously or on exploratory laparotomy, then surgical repair should be performed so long as the patient is hemodynamically stable. A diagnosis of ureteropelvic junction avulsion necessitates expeditious exploration and repair if not already indicated secondary to polytrauma injury burden [20].

Method of repair for ureteral injuries depends on both location as well as etiology of injury. Principles for repair in pediatric patients follow those of adult patients. When performing primary repair, the mechanism of injury should be considered. For example, blast effect from gunshot wounds can impart nearby microvascular tissue damage up to a radius of approximately 2 cm and require debridement or resection of potentially compromised tissue [1]. Generally, proximal injuries above the level of the iliac vessels can be repaired primarily, whereas distal ureteral injuries can be repaired primarily or with ureteral reimplantation with or without elaboration with a psoas hitch or Boari flap. Repairs should be performed over a ureteral

Table 10.2 AAST ureteral injury grading and management [4]

Grade	Key injury features	Intervention[a]
I	Hematoma without devascularization	O
II	Laceration <50% transection	US
III	Laceration ≥50% transection	US, DR
IV	Complete transection with <2.0 cm devascularization	DR
V	Complete transection with ≥2.0 cm devascularization	DR

[a]*O* Observation, *US* Ureteral Stent, *DR* Delayed Repair or Reconstruction

stent [10, 69]. A drain can be placed to help diagnose an early leak. Duration of stenting may vary based on surgical factors and level of concern, but typically, in our practice, it ranges between 3 and 4 weeks after surgical ureteral repair. Whether imaging is necessary prior to stent removal is up to the surgeon's discretion [68]. If a highly complex repair (i.e., buccal ureteroplasty, trans-ureteroureterostomy, ileal ureter, appendiceal interposition) is indicated, such as in rare scenarios involving significant loss of viable ureter, then temporizing measures can be considered (e.g., ureteral ligation with nephrostomy tube placement or cutaneous ureterostomy) until a detailed conversation can be had about risks and benefits of these approaches.

Follow-Up

Whether managed with ureteral stenting alone or with primary repair and ureteral stent placement, most patients will have a ureteral stent for approximately 3–4 weeks. In the pediatric population, stent removal is most often done under anesthesia rather than in the clinic. If there is concern for a leak or other complication, retrograde urography can be performed at this time, and a stent can be replaced if needed. This approach minimizes potential additional radiation exposure with CT scans. Following stent removal, patients should be monitored with renal ultrasound for the development of silent hydronephrosis in the near-term, and for the development of ureteral stricture long term. The interval and duration of monitoring can be influenced by both the degree of clinical concern and the level of patient or family concern.

Bladder Trauma

Epidemiology

Pediatric bladder injuries account for less than 2% of abdominal injuries in children requiring surgery, and are mostly caused by blunt trauma from motor vehicle collisions, falls, or impact from a heavy object [59, 65]. The pediatric bladder is more vulnerable to blunt trauma than the adult bladder due to its higher abdominal position above the pelvic ring, limited muscular and adipose protection, incompletely ossified pelvic bones, and developing rectus muscles, especially when distended [58]. Pediatric bladder injuries are frequently linked with pelvic fractures, as up to 29% of children with pelvic fractures have bladder injuries, and 55–57% of those with bladder ruptures have associated pelvic fractures—a lower incidence than in adults, where up to 90% of bladder injuries are associated with pelvic fractures [2, 10, 11, 59, 62, 65].

Diagnosis/Imaging

Bladder imaging is indicated in pediatric trauma patients with (1) gross hematuria and pelvic fracture, or (2) inability to void [62, 65]. Retrograde cystography, via CT or radiography, is highly reliable (sensitivity >90%, specificity ~100%) [29, 52, 59, 65]. CT is preferred for its ability to detect associated renal, ureteral, or urethral injuries, with adjusted pediatric radiation levels when possible (Fig. 10.3) [17]. Proper bladder distension with contrast [(age+2) x 30 mL] is critical for accuracy [24]. Pediatric bladder trauma is classified using the AAST scale (Table 10.3) [4, 17]. Intraperitoneal ruptures (~17%), more common in children than adults due to the bladder positioning, involve contrast extravasation into the peritoneal cavity [11, 29, 59, 65]. Extraperitoneal ruptures (~83%), often with pelvic fractures, show a flame/starburst pattern confined to the pelvis [11, 38, 59]. Imaging with both distended and post-drainage views ensures thorough evaluation [29, 59].

Treatment

Uncomplicated extraperitoneal ruptures are typically managed conservatively with 2–3 weeks of transurethral catheter drainage, followed by cystography to confirm healing, as recommended by the AUA [11, 42, 58]. Intraperitoneal ruptures generally require double-layer surgical repair with monofilament absorbable sutures and urethral catheter drainage for ~2 weeks [4, 10, 11, 59]. Proper assessment and tailored management are essential to optimize outcomes, as surgical repair significantly reduces in-hospital mortality, with evidence suggesting an 82% reduction [11].

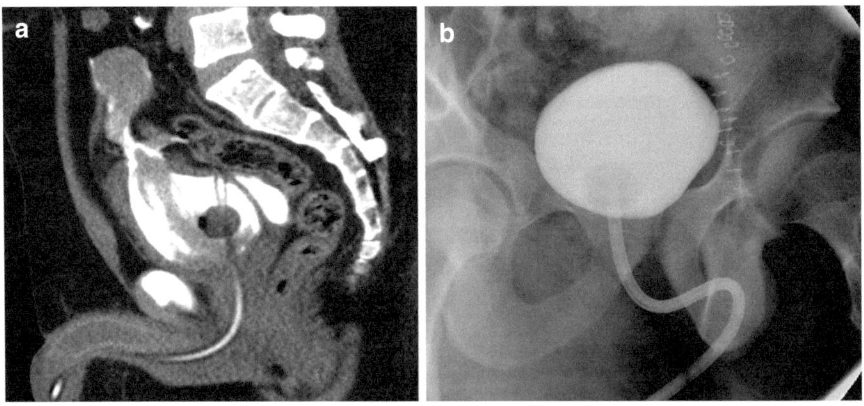

Fig. 10.3 (**a**) Sagittal view of a CT cystogram showing an intraperitoneal bladder rupture in a 19-year-old boy after a motor vehicle accident. (**b**) 2-week postoperative cystogram prior to Foley catheter removal, confirming no leak

Table 10.3 AAST bladder injury grading and management [4]

Grade	Key injury features	Intervention[a]
I	Hematoma with partial thickness laceration	O
II	Extraperitoneal laceration (<2.0 cm)	CD
III	Extraperitoneal laceration (≥2.0 cm) or Intraperitoneal laceration (<2.0 cm)	CD (extraperitoneal) SR (intraperitoneal)
IV	Intraperitoneal laceration (≥2.0 cm)	SR
V	Laceration extending into neck or trigone	SR

[a]*O* Observation, *CD* Catheter Drainage, *SR* Surgical Repair

Follow-Up

Follow-up care in pediatric bladder trauma is crucial for detecting complications such as peritonitis, urine absorption leading to elevated serum creatinine, wound sepsis, and renal dysfunction [58, 65]. For nonoperative management of uncomplicated extraperitoneal injuries, a cystogram can be done at 2–4 weeks, depending on the size of the injury, to evaluate persistent leakage or other complications before catheter removal. If the leak persists, cystogram can be repeated again in 2 weeks or longer if needed [4, 58]. Cystogram is similarly done approximately 2–4 weeks after surgical repair depending on complexity of repair to evaluate for persistent leakage. As with extraperitoneal injuries, if there is a leak then the catheter can be continued, and cystogram can be repeated in another 2 weeks or longer if needed [10, 67].

Urethral Trauma

Epidemiology

Pediatric urethral injuries are uncommon and often occur at the proximal urethra in the setting of severe blunt trauma, usually associated with pelvic fracture-associated urethral injury (PFUI) [26, 32, 63]. Pelvic fractures in children are more likely to be unstable, leading to more severe injuries, including complete separation of the prostatic urethra and bladder neck [43, 49, 57]. Posterior male urethral disruption is particularly challenging due to the immaturity of the prostate and puboprostatic ligaments, increasing the risk of avulsion or transection [26, 43, 49]. For prepubertal females, pelvic fractures, especially with vaginal lacerations or sacral spine injuries, present a high risk of bladder neck and urethral involvement [11, 12, 46, 49]. Anterior urethral injuries typically result from direct straddle trauma or iatrogenic injury [14, 32, 49]. Pediatric PFUI are present in 0.6% to 13.5% of anterior pelvic fractures, with the risk increasing by 10% for every 1 mm increase in pubic symphysis diastasis [10, 49, 57, 61].

Diagnosis/Imaging

Pediatric urethral imaging is indicated by a triad of (1) blood at the meatus or vaginal introitus, (2) perineal or genital hematoma, and (3) difficulty or significant pain with urination [4, 26, 49]. Retrograde urethrography (RUG) is the gold standard for diagnosing male urethral trauma, with high sensitivity when a catheter or small feeding tube is used to inject contrast and obtain oblique radiographs after stabilization [14, 26, 32, 46, 49]. For females, endoscopic evaluation under anesthesia is preferred due to the shorter and less rigid urethra [12, 26, 49]. Blunt trauma with pubic rami fractures and pubic symphysis diastasis should prompt evaluation due to the high risk of urethral injury (Fig. 10.4) [26, 32, 43, 57]. CT scans can identify associated injuries but are less specific for urethral trauma [14, 26, 46, 49]. MRI may aid in surgical planning by providing detailed anatomical views without ionizing radiation. Recognition of concurrent rectal injuries is crucial to avoid complications such as abscesses and infections [26, 32, 43].

Treatment

The treatment of pediatric urethral trauma starts with ensuring urinary drainage, monitoring urine output, and administering prophylactic antibiotics, especially in unstable patients [10, 26, 42, 46]. If the patient has voided after the trauma and urethral rupture is not suspected on physical examination, a transurethral catheter may be placed [10, 46, 49]. If the catheter does not pass easily, RUG should be performed [14, 26, 42, 46]. A suprapubic tube is typically placed percutaneously or in the operating room if immediate exploration is necessary for life-threatening injuries [42, 43, 46, 58]. For isolated bulbous urethral or straddle injuries, a transurethral catheter is often sufficient for managing bleeding and voiding discomfort

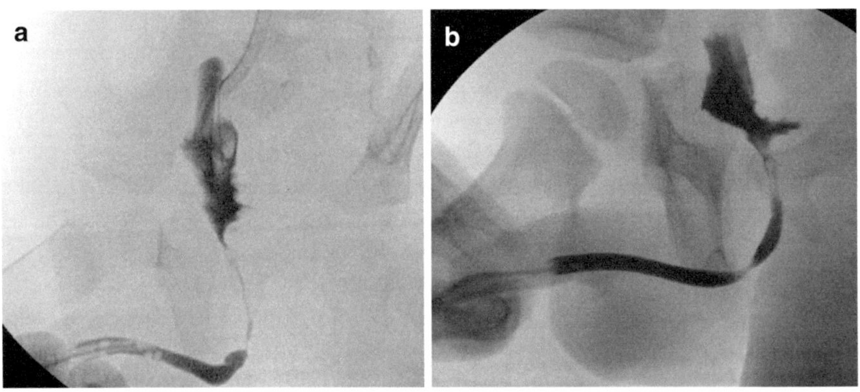

Fig. 10.4 (**a**) Retrograde urethrogram in a 3-year-old boy after pelvic fracture urethral injury. (**b**) Repeat retrograde urethrogram approximately 4 weeks postoperatively at the time of catheter removal shows contrast going into the bladder and no urine extravasation

[14, 26, 31, 32]. The management of posterior urethral injuries remains controversial, with some advocating for primary realignment, while others suggest suprapubic drainage followed by delayed reconstruction [31, 46]. Delayed urethroplasty has shown success in pediatric cases, with high rates of stricture-free urethras and good continence outcomes [26, 46, 61]. Primary realignment via catheter can also be used, though it carries a higher risk of strictures and incontinence [31, 46, 49].

Follow-Up

For patients with urinary drainage via transurethral or suprapubic catheter, regular monitoring of urine output and signs of infections is necessary [26, 42, 46]. Follow-up imaging is recommended after 2–3 weeks to confirm urethral healing before catheter removal [14, 42, 49]. Imaging can entail either pericatheter RUG or voiding cystourethrogram (VCUG) based on clinical judgment. Stricture formation can occur with high rates after trauma despite efforts such as realignment or primary repair; therefore, clinicians may choose to keep the suprapubic tube if present until urethral patency is confirmed at follow-up [9]. After urethroplasty, we monitor patients at 3- and 12-month postoperatively with uroflowmetry and ultrasound residual volumes, and cystoscopy when indicated.

Trauma to External Genitalia

Epidemiology

Traumatic genital injuries in the pediatric population are often minor and do not require procedural intervention. These genital injuries encompass about 0.5–0.8% of all pediatric traumatic injuries, not including sexual abuse, which is outside the scope of this chapter. This represents about 0.35 genital injuries/1000 children/year [8].

Two large studies of the National Electronic Injury Surveillance System, spanning 1991–2020 demonstrated that injuries to girls (54.2–56.6%) were slightly more common than boys (39.7–43.4%) [8, 45]. Patients tend to be younger, with an average age of less than 10 years in most studies [15, 18, 39]. Given that isolated genital injuries are typically soft-tissue injuries, patients most often present with visible signs of injury, making the physical examination essential for management. A large retrospective review of female pediatric genital injuries demonstrated that bleeding ($N = 182$, 90.1%), pain ($N = 126$, 62.3%), dysuria ($N = 54$, 26.7%), urinary retention ($N = 19$, 9.4%), and hematuria ($N = 7$, 3.5%) were the most common presenting symptoms [15].

Diagnosis/Imaging

Diagnosing traumatic genital injuries in children relies heavily on the physical examination, which can be difficult due to patient cooperation and pain in this population [15, 60]. Small, blunt mechanism lacerations to the scrotum, vulva, and vagina are a common scenario. These injuries will occur secondary to falls from standing in younger children or secondary to accidents with toys or playground equipment, with straddle injuries being common. More severe injuries are often associated with high injury severity scores and polytrauma and should be evaluated in a multidisciplinary approach. A review of female pediatric injuries from the National Trauma Data Bank reported that almost half of these patients presented after being struck by a motor vehicle [18]. Onen et al. classified genital injury severity in a retrospective analysis of 116 children [15, 44]. While not used in clinical practice, this classification supports the assertion that isolated injuries are often minor and appropriate for conservative management, while polytraumatic injuries often occur secondary to high-energy mechanisms.

The physical examination should be thorough but focused on areas of high concern to ensure the least amount of distress for the child. Parents should be recruited to help soothe and distract whenever possible. If a thorough exam is not possible, given patient distress, light sedation in the Emergency Room can often be achieved with intranasal or intravenous opiates, benzodiazepines, or ketamine. However, given the goal of minimizing these medications, the urologist evaluating injuries under sedation should have all the implements needed to treat small injuries ready and in hand during these sensitive examinations.

For girls, vulvar and vaginal lacerations secondary to straddle injuries should be examined closely to ensure no involvement of the urethra [60]. Urethral involvement is rare but may require a formal exam under anesthesia and cystoscopy [15]. Invasive imaging is rarely necessary for isolated female pediatric genital injuries, although a post-void residual may be helpful when the urethra is close to or involved with a vaginal laceration [15, 60].

Boys may be more likely to have injuries that require operative intervention, given the exposure of the gonads outside of the pelvis. Physical examinations should focus on ruling out urethral injury and ensuring testicular integrity. For urethral injuries, the perineum should be closely evaluated for ecchymosis and hematomas. Either of these injury patterns or blood at the urethral meatus should prompt retrograde urethrography or cystoscopy. For older boys, urethrography may be possible with either coaching or light sedation. For more anxious boys and younger boys, this may need to be done in the operating room. Further, for very mild cases associated with low-impact injuries, imaging may be deferred. However, this decision should only be made in close consultation between the urologist and parents, and only for patients who can demonstrate a low post-void residual, absence of pain with voiding, and who can follow-up closely as outpatients.

For concerns for testicular injury, including ecchymosis or hematomas of the scrotum, soft, tender testicles, or inability to delineate testicular structures on physical examination, providers should obtain a scrotal ultrasound in the emergency department [19]. These exams are generally low-cost and can be done with little discomfort for even pediatric patients. Ultrasounds with testicular ruptures, significant testicular heterogeneity, or large hematoceles should prompt operative intervention by the urologist [19]. Sensitivity and specificity for ultrasound in diagnosing testicular rupture have been reported to be as high as 95%, respectively [7].

Treatment

The treatment for genital injuries in the pediatric population is variable and injury-dependent. Small and superficial lacerations of the external genitalia can often be treated with local wound care alone. Deeper lacerations may require primary closure with absorbable sutures, but this can often be done safely at the time of a sedated examination in the emergency department. One study of pediatric vaginal injuries at a pediatric referral center found that <20% of patients require operative intervention [60]. The decision point about whether to repair lacerations should be made in consultation with the patient's parents. A good rule of thumb is to evaluate the patient's tolerance of the physical examination as a proxy for their ability to tolerate wound care at home. If patients are unable to tolerate an exam or application of dressings, then they likely require repair. Laceration repairs should include copious irrigation of the wound, judicious debridement of devitalized tissue, and primary closure with absorbable suture. It is paramount that wounds remain both aesthetic and functional, given the sensitive nature of the area. If this is not possible, then reconstructive urology, plastic surgery, or gynecology should be engaged for assistance [18].

For urethral injuries, urinary drainage is the mainstay of treatment. Female urethral injuries should be given the opportunity to heal over a catheter in most cases, as long as they do not extend to the bladder neck. Male urethral injuries should also be given the opportunity to heal over a catheter, although a suprapubic tube may be necessary if the urethra is obliterated.

Testicular injuries should be managed using the same algorithm as adult injuries [41]. A midline raphe incision will allow access to the bilateral testicles as necessary. For salvageable testicles, devitalized tissue should be debrided, and the tunica albuginea should be closed primarily. A tunica vaginalis flap can be created to help complete a closure if there is not enough available tunica albuginea [30]. For a non-salvageable testis, urologists should proceed with orchiectomy. However, given the age of the patient and the sensitive nature of these injuries, it may be beneficial to salvage viable gonadal tissue, even if it is a minority of the affected testicle. For blunt injuries, the rate of testicular salvage is 80–90% with prompt management [50].

Follow-Up

Follow-up for external genital wounds is dependent on the nature of the injury and the repair. For lacerations, urologists should consider close interval follow-up for a wound check. If wounds are healing well, follow-up can be discontinued.

For urethral injuries managed with a urethral catheter, the catheter can be discontinued after 2–4 weeks in most cases. The patient should pass a trial of void prior to leaving the office, and then should follow-up again to ensure safe, durable, unobstructed bladder emptying. The patient should then be followed up for a year to monitor for urethral strictures [66]. Patients with a urethral injury requiring a suprapubic tube should be referred to a reconstructive urologist before their first suprapubic tube exchange, as they will likely require reconstruction [66].

Finally, boys who undergo scrotal exploration should be seen for a wound check following surgery. Follow-up can then be determined on a case-by-case basis. For those who underwent an orchiectomy, either the urologist or the patient's primary care doctor should ensure appropriate developmental milestones and puberty progression, with consideration of endocrinological evaluation or referral if there is concern.

Conclusion

Management of pediatric GU trauma requires a multidisciplinary approach that prioritizes conservative, nonoperative strategies whenever feasible. Pediatric physiology shifts our framework for clinical concern, as children's robust physiological reserve can mask early instability, while pediatric anatomy increases susceptibility to specific injuries. Renal injuries, most commonly from blunt trauma, are typically managed conservatively unless severe or life-threatening. Less common injuries to the bladder, ureters, urethra, and external genitalia may occur in polytraumatized children, requiring tailored management based on severity and location. By maintaining a high suspicion, following pediatric-focused guidelines, and collaborating across specialties, adult urologists can improve outcomes for pediatric patients with GU trauma.

Summary

- Genitourinary trauma in children is a relatively uncommon, but the adult urologist should be familiar with the presentation, workup, and management of these injuries.
- If there is a high index of suspicion based on the mechanism of injury, physicians should rule out urologic trauma even if patients are hemodynamically stable and without hematuria, as these are not always reliable markers in children.

- Any clinical history or presentation concerning potential high-grade renal injury warrants full evaluation with CT imaging, including delayed-phase imaging to evaluate the collecting system.
- Pediatric patients have anatomic differences that render them more susceptible to certain blunt traumatic urologic injuries, e.g., ureteropelvic junction avulsion and bladder ruptures.
- Pelvic fractures in children are more likely to be unstable, leading to more severe injuries, including complete separation of the prostatic urethra and bladder neck.

Bibliography

1. Amato JJ, Billy LJ, Gruber RP, Lawson NS, Rich NM. Vascular injuries. An experimental study of high and low velocity missile wounds. Arch Surg. 1970;101:167–74.
2. Becker A, Yaslowitz O, Dubose J, Peleg K, Daskal Y, Givon A, Israel Trauma Group, Kessel B. Is computed tomography cystography indicated in children with pelvic fractures? Chin J Traumatol. 2020;23:181–4.
3. Brown SL, Elder JS, Spirnak JP. Are pediatric patients more susceptible to major renal injury from blunt trauma? A comparative study. J Urol. 1998;160:138–40.
4. Bryk DJ, Zhao LC. Guideline of guidelines: a review of urological trauma guidelines. BJU Int. 2016;117:226–34.
5. Buckley JC, McAninch JW. Revision of current American Association for the Surgery of Trauma Renal Injury grading system. J Trauma. 2011;70:35–7.
6. Buckley JC, McAninch JW. Pediatric renal injuries: management guidelines from a 25-year experience. J Urol. 2004;172:687–90; discussion 690.
7. Buckley JC, McAninch JW. Use of ultrasonography for the diagnosis of testicular injuries in blunt scrotal trauma. J Urol. 2006;175:175–8.
8. Casey JT, Bjurlin MA, Cheng EY. Pediatric genital injury: an analysis of the National Electronic Injury Surveillance System. Urology. 2013;82:1125–30.
9. Chen Y-T, Wang T-M, Cheng C-T, Tee Y-S, Liao C-H, Hsieh C-H, Fu C-Y. Timing of male urethral injury treatment in patients with polytrauma: a retrospective study. Injury. 2024;55:111339.
10. Coccolini F, Moore EE, Kluger Y, Biffl W, Leppaniemi A, Matsumura Y, Kim F, Peitzman AB, Fraga GP, Sartelli M, Ansaloni L, Augustin G, Kirkpatrick A, Abu-Zidan F, Wani I, Weber D, Pikoulis E, Larrea M, Arvieux C, Manchev V, Reva V, Coimbra R, Khokha V, Mefire AC, Ordonez C, Chiarugi M, Machado F, Sakakushev B, Matsumoto J, Maier R, di Carlo I, Catena F, WSES-AAST Expert Panel. Kidney and uro-trauma: WSES-AAST guidelines. World J Emerg Surg. 2019;14:54.
11. Deibert CM, Glassberg KI, Spencer BA. Repair of pediatric bladder rupture improves survival: results from the National Trauma Data Bank. J Pediatr Surg. 2012;47:1677–81.
12. Delaney KM, Reddy SH, Dayama A, Stone ME Jr, Meltzer JA. Risk factors associated with bladder and urethral injuries in female children with pelvic fractures: an analysis of the National Trauma Data Bank. J Trauma Acute Care Surg. 2016;80:472–6.
13. Elliott SP, McAninch JW. Ureteral injuries: external and iatrogenic. Urol Clin North Am. 2006;33:55–66, vi.
14. Elsingergy MM, Bellah RD, Back SJ, Weiss DA, Darge K. Retrograde urethrography in children: a decade of experience at a children's hospital. Pediatr Radiol. 2023;53:862–74.
15. Encisco EM, Sundaram K, McNinch NL, Wulkan ML, Huntington JT, Heinzerling NP, Iocono JA. The management of accidental perineal injuries in pediatric females: retrospective review at a single institution. J Pediatr Surg Open. 2023;2:100021.

16. Evans M, Rajasekaran K, Murala A, Moreira A. Development and validation of a pediatric model predicting trauma-related mortality. BMC Pediatr. 2023;23:637.
17. Expert Panel on Urological Imaging, Heller MT, Oto A, Allen BC, Akin O, Alexander LF, Chong J, Froemming AT, Fulgham PF, Mackenzie DC, Maranchie JK, Mody RN, Patel BN, Schieda N, Turkbey IB, Venkatesan AM, Wang CL, Lockhart ME. ACR appropriateness criteria® penetrating trauma-lower abdomen and pelvis. J Am Coll Radiol. 2019;16:S392–8.
18. Fan SM, Grigorian A, Chaudhry HH, Allen A, Sun B, Jasperse N, Albertson S, Nahmias J. Female pediatric and adolescent genitalia trauma: a retrospective analysis of the National Trauma Data Bank. Pediatr Surg Int. 2020;36:1235–41.
19. Fenton LZ, Karakas SP, Baskin L, Campbell JB. Sonography of pediatric blunt scrotal trauma: what the pediatric urologist wants to know. Pediatr Radiol. 2016;46:1049–58.
20. Fernández-Ibieta M. Renal trauma in pediatrics: a current review. Urology. 2018;113:171–8.
21. Fraser JD, Aguayo P, Ostlie DJ, St Peter SD. Review of the evidence on the management of blunt renal trauma in pediatric patients. Pediatr Surg Int. 2009;25:125–32.
22. Graziano KD, Juang D, Notrica D, Grandsoult VL, Acosta J, Sharp SW, Murphy JP, St Peter SD. Prospective observational study with an abbreviated protocol in the management of blunt renal injury in children. J Pediatr Surg. 2014;49:198–200; discussion 200–1.
23. Grimsby GM, Voelzke B, Hotaling J, Sorensen MD, Koyle M, Jacobs MA. Demographics of pediatric renal trauma. J Urol. 2014;192:1498–502.
24. Guerra LA, Keays MA, Purser MJ, Wang SY, Leonard MP. Pediatric cystogram: are we considering age-adjusted bladder capacity? Can Urol Assoc J. 2018;12:378–81.
25. Hagedorn JC, Fox N, Ellison JS, Russell R, Witt CE, Zeller K, Ferrada P, Draus JM Jr. Pediatric blunt renal trauma practice management guidelines: collaboration between the Eastern Association for the Surgery of Trauma and the Pediatric Trauma Society. J Trauma Acute Care Surg. 2019;86:916–25.
26. Hagedorn JC, Voelzke BB. Pelvic-fracture urethral injury in children. Arab J Urol. 2015;13:37–42.
27. Hirsch K, Heinz M, Wullich B. Diagnosis and therapeutic management in kidney, ureter and bladder trauma. Aktuelle Urol. 2017;48:64–71.
28. Ishida Y, Tyroch AH, Emami N, McLean SF. Characteristics and management of blunt renal injury in children. J Emerg Trauma Shock. 2017;10:140–5.
29. Iverson AJ, Morey AF. Radiographic evaluation of suspected bladder rupture following blunt trauma: critical review. World J Surg. 2001;25:1588–91.
30. Jian PY, Nelson ED, Roth DR. Use of a vascularized tunica vaginalis flap for repair of testicular rupture in a pediatric patient. Urology. 2012;79:1363–4.
31. Joe W, Owen K, Ivander A, Jaya AP, Palgunadi IN, Adhyatma KP, Soebhali B, Nasution R. A systematic review and meta-analysis of surgical approaches in pelvic fracture-associated urethral injury in children: primary endoscopic realignment versus delayed urethroplasty. Injury. 2024;55:111728.
32. Kaba M, Kılıç S, Gecit İ. Evaluation of urethral traumas in children: a retrospective analysis. Turk Assoc Pediatr Surg. 2024; https://doi.org/10.62114/jtaps.2024.3.
33. Kiankhooy A, Sartorelli KH, Vane DW, Bhave AD. Angiographic embolization is safe and effective therapy for blunt abdominal solid organ injury in children. J Trauma. 2010;68:526–31.
34. Latabi AF, Aitzirri K, Moudouni SM, Lakmichi MA, Dahami Z, Sarf I. Facteurs prédictifs d'échec du traitement conservateur du traumatisme rénal grade III–V. Prog Urol. 2019;29:416–22.
35. Lee AS, Broadwell NH, Tong CMC, Lucas JW, Bhatia VP, Abelson B, Ellis JL, Weiss DA, Ho C, Mecca D, Balthazar A, Kitchens DM, Russell RT, Rana MS, Wang M-H, Clayton D. Presentation, hospital course and outcomes of children with high grade renal trauma-results from the traumatic renal injury collaborative in kids multi-center consortium. Urology. 2025; https://doi.org/10.1016/j.urology.2025.01.072.
36. Lee JN, Lim JK, Woo MJ, Kwon SY, Kim BS, Kim HT, Kim T-H, Yoo ES, Chung SK. Predictive factors for conservative treatment failure in grade IV pediatric blunt renal trauma. J Pediatr Urol. 2016;12:93.e1–7.

37. LeeVan E, Zmora O, Cazzulino F, Burke RV, Zagory J, Upperman JS. Management of pediatric blunt renal trauma: a systematic review: a systematic review. J Trauma Acute Care Surg. 2016;80:519–28.
38. Mathew JE, Chaudhary K, Devana SK, Sharma AP. High rising flames: a sign of complex extraperitoneal bladder rupture. Ann R Coll Surg Engl. 2022;104:e35–6.
39. McLaughlin CJ, Martin KL. Mechanism of injury and age predict operative intervention in pediatric perineal injury. Pediatr Emerg Care. 2023;39:230–5.
40. Moore EE, Cogbill TH, Jurkovich GJ, McAninch JW, Champion HR, Gennarelli TA, Malangoni MA, Shackford SR, Trafton PG. Organ injury scaling iii: chest wall, abdominal vascular, ureter, bladder, and urethra. J Trauma Acute Care Surg. 1992;33:337.
41. Morey AF, Brandes S, Dugi DD, Armstrong JH, Breyer BN, Broghammer JA, Erickson BA, Holzbeierlein J, Hudak SJ, Pruitt JH, Reston JT, Santucci RA, Smith TG, Wessells H. Urotrauma: AUA guideline. J Urol. 2014; https://doi.org/10.1016/j.juro.2014.05.004.
42. Morey AF, Broghammer JA, Hollowell CMP, McKibben MJ, Souter L. Urotrauma Guideline 2020: AUA Guideline. J Urol. 2021;205:30–5.
43. Nerli RB, Koura AC, Ravish IR, Amarkhed SS, Prabha V, Alur SB. Posterior urethral injury in male children: long-term follow up. J Pediatr Urol. 2008;4:154–9.
44. Onen A, Oztürk H, Yayla M, Basuguy E, Gedik S. Genital trauma in children: classification and management. Urology. 2005;65:986–90.
45. Pandher M, Song A, Mahajan J, Srinivasan N, Berg C, Fernandez G, Chang C, Medina C, Alwaal A, Weiss R. Characterization of pediatric genital injuries due to consumer products from 2011 to 2020. Urology. 2022;167:201–6.
46. Patel AB, Osterberg EC, Satarasinghe PN, Wenzel JL, Akbani ST, Sahi SL, Emigh BJ, Wolf JS Jr, Brown CVR. Urethral injuries: diagnostic and management strategies for critical care and trauma clinicians. J Clin Med. 2023;12:1495. https://doi.org/10.3390/jcm12041495.
47. Patel M, Glassman T, Burjonrappa S. Predictors of conservative management failure in pediatric renal trauma: National Trauma Database insights. J Pediatr Surg. 2024;60:162024.
48. Pereira BMT, Ogilvie MP, Gomez-Rodriguez JC, Ryan ML, Peña D, Marttos AC, Pizano LR, McKenney MG. A review of ureteral injuries after external trauma. Scand J Trauma Resusc Emerg Med. 2010;18:6.
49. Pichler R, Fritsch H, Skradski V, Horninger W, Schlenck B, Rehder P, Oswald J. Diagnosis and management of pediatric urethral injuries. Urol Int. 2012;89:136–42.
50. Pogorelić Z, Jurić I, Biočić M, Furlan D, Budimir D, Todorić J, Milunović KP. Management of testicular rupture after blunt trauma in children. Pediatr Surg Int. 2011;27:885–9.
51. Pumberger W, Stoll E, Metz S. Ureteropelvic junction disruption following blunt abdominal trauma. Pediatr Emerg Care. 2002;18:364–6.
52. Quagliano PV, Delair SM, Malhotra AK. Diagnosis of blunt bladder injury: a prospective comparative study of computed tomography cystography and conventional retrograde cystography. J Trauma. 2006;61:410–21; discussion 421–2.
53. Radmayr C, Bogaert G, Bujons A, Burgu B, Castagnetti MS, O'Kelly F, Pakkasjärvi NA, Quaedackers J, Rawashdeh YFH, Silay MS, Gnech M, Skott M, van Uitert A. EAU guidelines on paediatric urology. https://tashpmi.uz/wp-content/uploads/2024/07/eau-pocket-on-paediatric-urology-2024.pdf. Accessed 22 Feb 2025
54. Rogers CG, Knight V, MacUra KJ, Ziegfeld S, Paidas CN, Mathews RI. High-grade renal injuries in children—is conservative management possible? Urology. 2004;64:574–9.
55. Schmidlin FR, Iselin CE, Naimi A, Rohner S, Borst F, Farshad M, Niederer P, Graber P. The higher injury risk of abnormal kidneys in blunt renal trauma. Scand J Urol Nephrol. 1998;32:388–92.
56. Schmidt J, Loftus CJ, Skokan A, Hagedorn JC. Routine repeat imaging may be avoidable for asymptomatic pediatric patients with renal trauma. J Pediatr Urol. 2022;18:76.e1–8.
57. Silber JS, Flynn JM, Koffler KM, Dormans JP, Drummond DS. Analysis of the cause, classification, and associated injuries of 166 consecutive pediatric pelvic fractures. J Pediatr Orthop. 2001;21:446–50.

58. Singer G, Arneitz C, Tschauner S, Castellani C, Till H. Trauma in pediatric urology. Semin Pediatr Surg. 2021;30:151085.
59. Sivit CJ, Cutting JP, Eichelberger MR. CT diagnosis and localization of rupture of the bladder in children with blunt abdominal trauma: significance of contrast material extravasation in the pelvis. AJR Am J Roentgenol. 1995;164:1243–6.
60. Spitzer RF, Kives S, Caccia N, Ornstein M, Goia C, Allen LM. Retrospective review of unintentional female genital trauma at a pediatric referral center. Pediatr Emerg Care. 2008;24:831–5.
61. Sreeranga YL, Joshi PM, Bandini M, Kulkarni SB. Comprehensive analysis of paediatric pelvic fracture urethral injury: a reconstructive centre experience. BJU Int. 2022;130:114–25.
62. Tarman GJ, Kaplan GW, Lerman SL, McAleer IM, Losasso BE. Lower genitourinary injury and pelvic fractures in pediatric patients. Urology. 2002;59:123–6; discussion 126.
63. Tasian GE, Bagga HS, Fisher PB, McCulloch CE, Cinman NM, McAninch JW, Breyer BN. Pediatric genitourinary injuries in the United States from 2002 to 2010. J Urol. 2013;189:288–93.
64. Theodorou CM, Galganski LA, Jurkovich GJ, Farmer DL, Hirose S, Stephenson JT, Trappey AF. Causes of early mortality in pediatric trauma patients. J Trauma Acute Care Surg. 2021;90:574–81.
65. Tyroch AH, Matlock K. Pediatric and adult blunt traumatic bladder rupture: a comparative review. Panam J Trauma Crit Care Emerg Surg. 2015;4:11–5.
66. Wessells H, Morey A, Souter L, Rahimi L, Vanni A. Urethral stricture disease guideline amendment. J Urol. 2023;210:64–71.
67. Yeung LL, McDonald AA, Como JJ, Robinson B, Knight J, Person MA, Lee JK, Dahm P. Management of blunt force bladder injuries: a practice management guideline from the Eastern Association for the Surgery of Trauma. J Trauma Acute Care Surg. 2019;86:326–36.
68. Zebib L, Skupin P, Barboglio-Romo P, Blair Y, Malaeb BS, Stoffel JT, Ambani SN. Surveillance after ureteroneocystostomy: is it necessary? Urology. 2022;167:224–8.
69. Urotrauma Guideline - American Urological Association. https://www.auanet.org/guidelines-and-quality/guidelines/urotrauma-guideline. Accessed 28 Feb 2025

Part II

Long-Term Follow-Up

Persistent Hydronephrosis After Pyeloplasty

11

Madeline Cancian

Incidence and Pathophysiology of Persistent Hydronephrosis After Pyeloplasty

By definition, kidneys that undergo pyeloplasty are hydronephrotic; this imaging finding is perhaps the only unifying trait among the diverse set of patients who present with ureteropelvic junction (UPJ) obstruction. Interestingly, not all hydronephrosis resolves after surgery. For some patients, persistent hydronephrosis is a sign of a failed surgery, with the swelling being a marker of continued obstruction. However, a subset of patients will have a successful pyeloplasty, defined by resolution of symptoms and good flow of urine from the kidney, but will have hydronephrosis on postoperative imaging. The incidence of persistent hydronephrosis is not well understood, in part because there is no standard definition of hydronephrosis in this setting (Fig. 11.1). Värelä et al. found that 10% of their successful postpyeloplasty children had persistent hydronephrosis, as defined by an anterior-pelvic diameter (APD) of ≥10 mm or an APD that was greater than 50% of the preoperative APD at 12 months of ultrasound [1]. In contrast, Carpenter et al. used a more stringent definition of APD = 0 cm and found that only 13.8% reached this milestone in long-term follow-up (107–2707 days) [2]. There are no patient-specific characteristics that have been identified that predict persistent hydronephrosis, and there is no consensus that the size of the renal pelvis preoperatively is correlated to the presence of persistent hydronephrosis postoperatively [1, 2].

The rate at which hydronephrosis resolves postoperatively is not well understood. While some authors note up to 10% of their patients show complete resolution on initial 3-month ultrasounds, others report complete resolution occurring between 2 and 4 years postoperatively, and even up to 8 years [2, 3]. Oktar et al.

M. Cancian (✉)
Warren Alpert School of Medicine, Brown University, Providence, RI, USA

H.-Y. Wu et al. (eds.), *Pediatric Urology for the Adult Urologist*,
https://doi.org/10.1007/978-3-032-10306-2_11

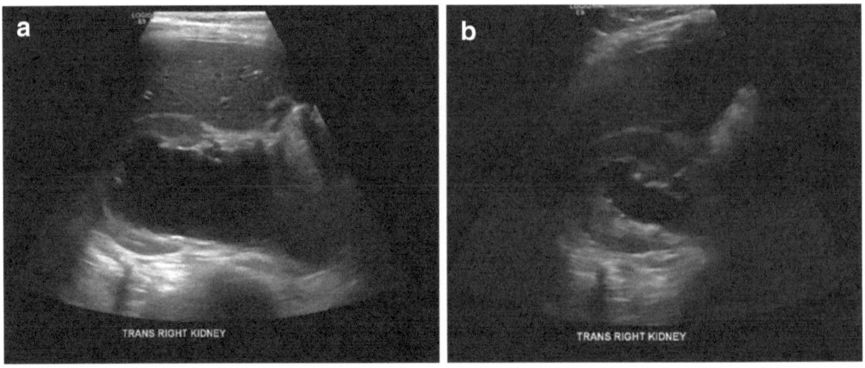

Fig. 11.1 (**a**) Preoperative renal ultrasound of the right kidney with UPJ obstruction. (**b**) 6 months post successful pyeloplasty, ultrasound of right kidney with improved, but persistent, hydronephrosis

found improvement in hydronephrosis on ultrasounds plateaued at 60 months postoperatively, with minimal improvement noted beyond that time point [4].

Reduction of the renal pelvis at the time of pyeloplasty is a technique that was part of the original Anderson–Hynes pyeloplasty description in 1949. Potential benefits include reducing stasis of urine in the postoperative period and decreasing kinking at the UPJ. Additionally, reducing the renal pelvis size has been shown to produce a very modest improvement in renal pelvis size at 6 months postoperative ultrasound as compared to patients who did not have renal pelvis reductions [5, 6]. This technique has not translated into better postoperative drainage parameters, nor does it affect pyeloplasty success either positively or negatively. While it may decrease, although not eradicate, early postoperative hydronephrosis, it has not been found to serve any functional purpose and is done at the discretion of the surgeon.

Despite commonly finding some degree of renal dilation after successful pyeloplasty, it is not clear what causes persistent hydronephrosis. Renal pressure-flow studies from the 1980s have shown that not all renal pelvises react the same to obstruction; the degree of hydronephrosis and impaired compliance varies even when the same obstructive force is applied [7–9]. Similarly, it makes intuitive sense that not all renal pelvises would react the same when the obstructive force is removed. Perhaps pelvises that have lost compliance are unable to return to their normal size.

Presentation and Workup

Since persistent hydronephrosis after pyeloplasty can be a common finding, it is critically important to identify the subset of patients who require repeat intervention to preserve renal function. Unfortunately, there is no standard definition of a "failed" pyeloplasty; this is invariably defined in studies by the need for reintervention. The decision to reintervene is based on many factors, typically taking into account worsening hydronephrosis, decreasing renal function, increasing flank pain, developing urinary tract infections, or growing new kidney stones [10–12]. Pediatric patients are usually followed closely for 6–12 months after surgery with renal US and office visits, so a change in condition can be picked up quickly and further investigated. Diagnosing failed pyeloplasty in patients who present as adults with a history of pyeloplasty as a child can be a more difficult task. Often, there is no readily available previous imaging to compare degrees of hydronephrosis. Pain alone can be multifactorial and unreliable in diagnosing a UPJ obstruction.

Renal scintigraphy is a useful adjunct to help determine obstructive parameters in a hydronephrotic kidney, although it must be interpreted in the context of the patient. False positive studies for obstruction can occur with dehydration, underlying renal disease, or a full bladder [13]. Equivocal or nonobstructive studies can be misleading, as patients may be having renal colic from an underlying UPJ abnormality even in the setting of a normal scintigraphy. Additionally, an obstructive result with preserved ipsilateral renal function in an asymptomatic patient does not necessarily portend future renal decline. A small series of ten patients with obstructive scintigraphy and no additional symptoms were followed conservatively, with none requiring surgery and no decline in ipsilateral renal function [14].

Additional invasive diagnostics can be employed if the above imaging is not adequate to determine if the patient requires further surgical intervention to fix an underlying obstruction. Retrograde pyelography can further elucidate renal anatomy to show if there is a true narrowing in the proximal ureter, kinking at the UPJ, or a nondependent ureteral insertion (Fig. 11.2). Having ureteroscopy available at

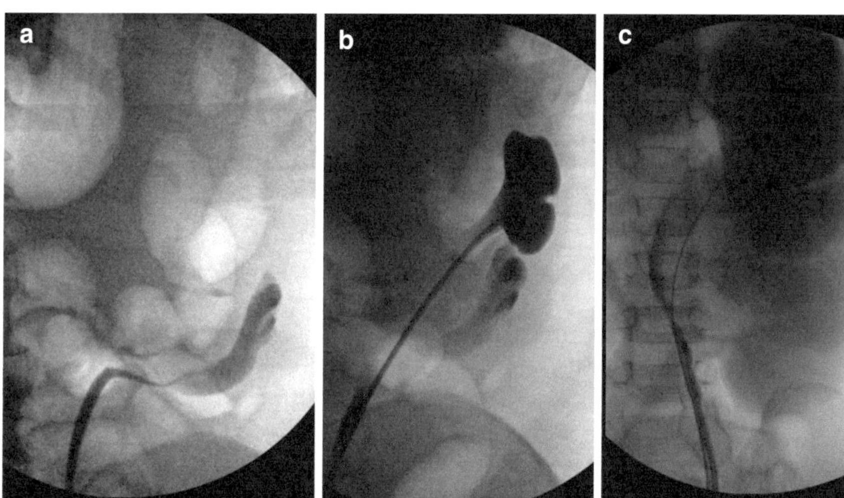

Fig. 11.2 Retrograde pyelogram in patients with previous pyeloplasties. (**a**) Contrast flowing smoothly through UPJ into dilated bifid lower pole renal pelvis; (**b**) Same patient, 5 Fr open-ended catheter in the upper pole calyces, with dilation of the calyces without stricture, kinking, or other signs of obstruction; (**c**) Different patient with open UPJ; however, massively dilated renal calyces causing nondependent drainage through the reconstructed UPJ

that time can be helpful to directly visualize the UPJ. If pain is the presenting symptom, a percutaneous nephrostomy (PCN) or ureteral stent can be inserted; if the pain resolves, it is reasonable to proceed to surgical intervention. Unfortunately, PCNs and stents can bring additional discomfort, and so their diagnostic value is often not as high as one might think. If a PCN is being considered, a Whitaker test can be done at the time of placement, or even if the PCN is foregone. This test measures the renal pelvis and bladder pressures to identify an obstruction at the level of the ureter. While a somewhat antiquated test, it has a potential role for patients with poor renal function, persistent pain with negative scintigraphy, or suspected intermittent obstruction [15].

Treatment

Endoscopic Management

Treatment options for recurrent UPJ obstruction are similar to primary treatments for the condition. Endoscopic treatment, a mainstay in every urologist's arsenal, encompasses either balloon dilation or endopyelotomy for the area of recurrent obstruction. Small series consistently show a 50% success rate for endopyelotomy in recurrent UPJ obstruction and slightly lower success, 30%, for balloon dilation [11, 12, 16]. A longer stenosed segment may be associated with a lower success rate of endoscopic management [16, 17], a principle which is mirrored in data for endoscopic management of both ureteral and urethral stricture disease.

Another consideration in the use of endoscopic management is the possible presence of a "missed" crossing vessel. The crossing vessel could have been missed at the time of initial pyeloplasty; thus, recurrence is due to persistent extrinsic compression of the UPJ. It is also possible that in recurrent UPJ obstruction patients who re-present as adults, the crossing vessel was not there at the time of initial pyeloplasty, or has newly become obstructive. The incidence of missed crossing vessels varies widely in the literature; Aresenio et al. found that 3/5 (60%) of redo pyeloplasties had a missed crossing vessel [10], while other studies have shown it to be a rarer occurrence (0–22%) [11, 12, 18] (Fig. 11.3). Small series suggested a retroperitoneal approach to pyeloplasty led to a higher rate of missed crossing vessels [19], however, meta-analysis of retroperitoneal versus transperitoneal approaches shows no difference in success rates and no increase in missed crossing vessels [20].

It is generally thought that endopyelotomy is less successful in the setting of a crossing vessel, as this vessel is not directly addressed endoscopically, although there is little data to support this conjecture. Corbett and Mullassery found through a systematic review that 31% of failed endopyelotomies who went on to have a pyeloplasty were found to have a crossing vessel; however, it is unknown how many of the successful endopyelotomies had a crossing vessel [21]. Van Cangh et al. looked at endopyelotomies, mostly in the primary UPJ setting, and found patients with high-grade hydronephrosis and a crossing vessel had a significantly lower rate of success compared to patients with neither of these characteristics (39% vs 95%)

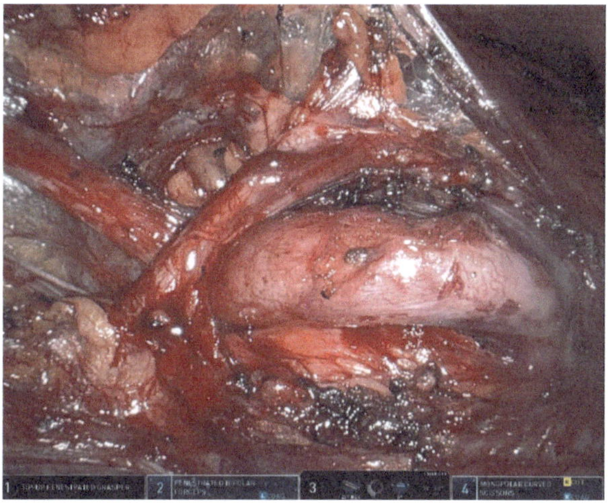

Fig. 11.3 Crossing vessel seen indenting right UPJ, causing upstream renal pelvic dilation

[22]. There is also a possibility of incising the vessel endoscopically, causing significant bleeding that may necessitate open exploration [23]. To minimize this risk, the incision should always be made in a posterolateral position.

There are many techniques described for completing an endopyelotomy. It can be performed antegrade or retrograde and involves a full-thickness incision of the ureter through the stenotic segment. This can be accomplished with a cold knife, electrocautery, laser, or cutting balloon, and may be followed by a balloon dilation. There is no consensus that any difference in technique significantly affects the success rates of the procedure [21].

Redo Pyeloplasty

A redo pyeloplasty carries a higher success rate in recurrent UPJ obstruction than endoscopic management, with rates of success between 83% and 92% [10–12]. Mittal et al. compared primary and redo robotic pyeloplasties and noted that, while operative times for redos were higher, complications and outcomes were equivalent in the two groups [24]. However, careful preoperative evaluation can reveal that the narrowed proximal ureter in redo cases can be longer than expected, and not all cases can be accomplished with a repeat Anderson–Hynes dismembered pyeloplasty. For longer strictures or in patients with altered anatomy, a local flap using the renal pelvis can be utilized. This may involve either a Foley Y-V plasty, in which a "V" of pelvic tissue is pulled down to the apex of a long spatulation on the ureter, or a spiral flap can be taken from the redundant pelvis and used to augment a strictured ureter.

If there is not an adequate pelvis for reconstruction, right-sided procedures can be performed using the appendix, either as an inlay or onlay flap. The inlay technique is ideal for a completely obliterated ureteral segment where the intact tubular appendix can be anastomosed to the healthy proximal and distal ends of the ureter with wide spatulations at both ends. In contrast, for a strictured but patent lumen, the appendix can be detubularized on the anti-mesenteric aspect and used to augment the intact ureter. For the onlay technique, the appendiceal flap is sewn to either the dorsal or ventral ureterotomy [25]. The appendix is harvested in the same technique as would be used for a Mitrofanoff channel, taking care to keep the appendiceal mesentery intact. Often, the right colon needs to be mobilized to allow the appendix to reach the proximal ureter. In the setting of ureteral strictures, success rates for this technique at >1 year are above 90% [26, 27].

If there are no flaps available, grafting can be accomplished with a buccal graft. Buccal grafts can be placed either ventrally or dorsally after the ureter is opened longitudinally. If a dorsal graft is used, the omentum can be secured to the graft to provide a stable blood supply, whereas a ventral graft can be quilted to the psoas muscle (Fig. 11.4). While the perinephric fat is readily available for UPJ strictures, our experience suggests it does not supply a suitable blood supply to guarantee graft take. We are not aware of any direct comparisons between dorsal and ventral graft placement, but we feel both techniques offer similar results. A small series of buccal graft augmentations for pyeloplasty failure has shown between 80% and 100% success rates at 10 months [28, 29].

Most of the flap or graft techniques utilize a nontransecting approach, which is potentially advantageous in redo surgery. By leaving the ureter intact, the surgeon is preserving the antegrade and retrograde collateral blood supply, thus theoretically minimizing scarring with healing. There have been no comparative studies of transecting versus nontransecting approaches to redo pyeloplasties, and with the overall paucity of patients undergoing this surgery, there are unlikely to be any such comparisons in the future. However, it is especially important when embarking on repeat

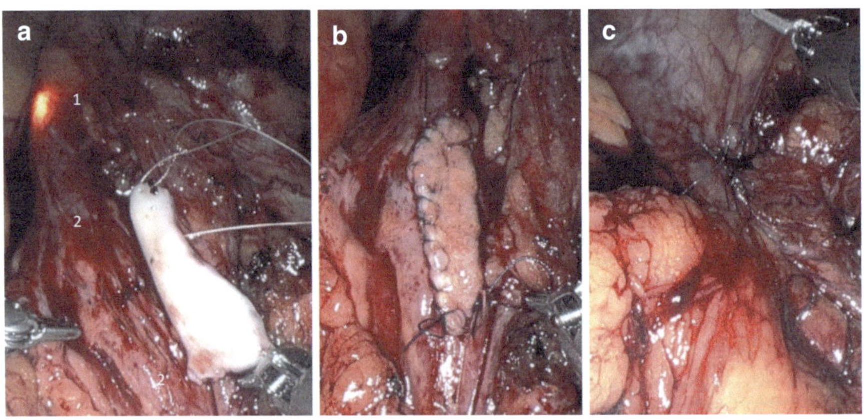

Fig. 11.4 (**a**) Ureteroscope in the ureter (1, light visible) with ureterostomy through a strictured ureteral segment (2). Buccal graft with mucosa exposed alongside ureterostomy; (**b**) Buccal mucosa sewn into dorsal ureterotomy; (**c**) Omentum sutured over graft and quilted to exposed underside of graft to provide blood supply

surgery to keep in mind the fundamental tenets of reconstructive surgery: preserve vasculature and create a watertight and tension-free anastomosis. The technique that is most likely to accomplish these goals should be chosen and varies based on the patient, surgeon comfort, and anatomy.

Ureterocalycostomy

A final option to salvage a failed pyeloplasty is a ureterocalycostomy. This procedure is traditionally reserved for patients with insufficient extra-renal pelvis dilation or massively dilated calyces such that the renal pelvis is no longer the most dependently-draining portion of the hydronephrotic kidney (Fig. 11.5). It can also be utilized for patients with a long proximal ureteral stricture where it is not feasible to place a graft or flap to bridge the scarred segment. Robotic-assisted procedures have been shown to be safe and effective, with a success rate of 75–92% [30, 31]. Whether done open or robotically, it is important to make a generous incision into the renal parenchyma, often requiring excising a saucer of the lower pole of the kidney to allow for a wide-open anastomosis and minimize the risk of stenosis. The renal

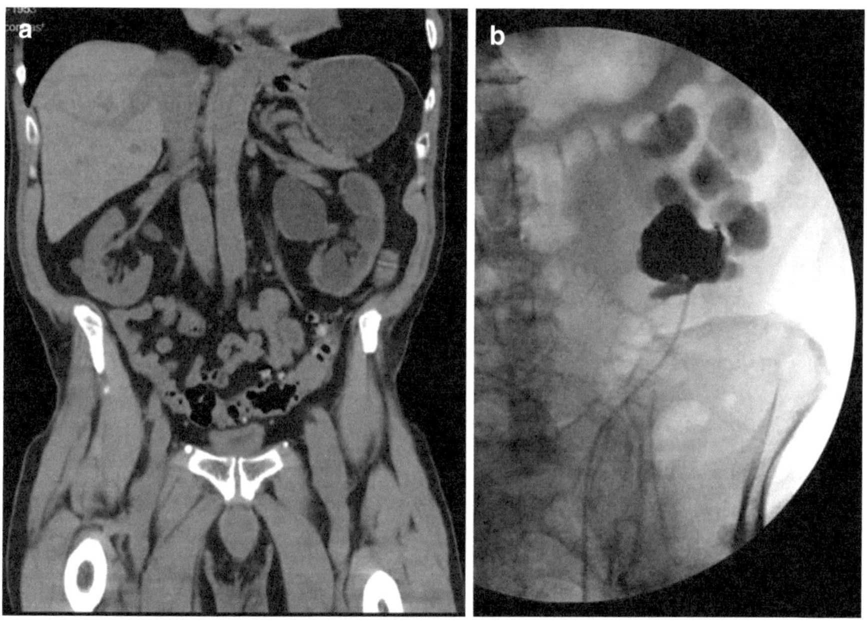

Fig. 11.5 (**a**) Preoperative CT scan showing a hydronephrotic left kidney with dilated calyces and thinning of the lower pole renal parenchyma; (**b**) Postoperative retrograde pyelogram after ureterocalycostomy showing a 5 Fr catheter extending directly into the lower pole, contrast opacifying the dilated calyceal system

pelvis is ligated, and the healthy proximal ureter is then transposed to the opened lower pole calyx. A downward nephropexy can be utilized to minimize tension on the uretero-calyx anastomosis.

Summary

- Persistent hydronephrosis following pyeloplasty is common and often does not indicate persistent renal obstruction.
- Identifying recurrent or persistent obstruction can be difficult and requires assimilating patient symptoms with renal imaging, renal scintigraphy, uretero-pelvic fluoroscopy, and/or ureteroscopy.
- Endoscopic management of recurrent UPJ obstruction is moderately successful and ideally utilized in the setting of short strictures with no crossing vessels.
- Redo pyeloplasty is highly successful; however, adjunctive surgical maneuvers may be necessary in the setting of longer strictures or altered anatomy, including renal pelvis flaps, appendiceal flaps, or buccal mucosa grafts.

References

1. Värelä S, Omling E, Börjesson A, Salö M. Resolution of hydronephrosis after pyeloplasty in children. J Pediatr Urol. 2021;17(1):102.e1–7. https://doi.org/10.1016/j.jpurol.2020.10.031. Epub 2020 Nov 4
2. Carpenter CP, Tolley E, Tourville E, Sharadin C, Giel DW, Gleason JM. Hydronephrosis after pyeloplasty: "will it go away?". Urology. 2018;121:158–63.
3. Fernández-Ibieta M, Nortes-Cano L, Guirao-Piñera MJ, et al. Radiation-free monitoring in the long-term follow-up of pyeloplasty: are ultrasound new parameters good enough to evaluate a successful procedure? J Pediatr Urol. 2016;12(4):230e1–7. https://doi.org/10.1016/j.jpurol.2016.04.026.
4. Oktar T, Selvi I, Ifran Donmez M, et al. What to expect on the Long-term follow-up of pediatric Pyeloplasty: critical time intervals and risk factors. J Pediatr Surg. 2024;59(6):1170–6.
5. Burgu B, Suer E, Aydogdu O, Soygur T. Pelvic reduction during pyeloplasty for antenatal hydronephrosis: does it affect outcome in ultrasound and nuclear scan postoperatively? Urology. 2010;76:169e74.
6. Morsi HA, Mursi K, Abdelaziz AY, ElSheemy MS, Salah M, Eissa MA. Renal pelvis reduction during dismembered pyeloplasty: is it necessary? J Pediatr Urol. 2013;9(3):303–6. https://doi.org/10.1016/j.jpurol.2012.03.002.
7. Jones DA, Lupton EW, George NJR, et al. Compliance studies, pressure flow measurements and renal function assessment in patients with upper urinary tract dilatation. J Urol. 1987;138:571–3.
8. Koff SA. Determinants of progression and equilibrium in hydro-nephrosis. Urology. 1983;21:496–500.
9. BullockKN WRH. Upper urinary tract compliance: its importance in obstructive hydronephrosis. Ann Acad Med Singap. 1984;13:585–9.
10. Asensio M, Gander R, Royo GF, Lloret J. Failed pyeloplasty in children: is robot-assisted laparoscopic reoperative repair feasible? J Pediatr Urol. 2015;11(2):69.e1–6. https://doi.org/10.1016/j.jpurol.2014.10.009. Epub 2015 Feb 24

11. Ceyhan E, Dogan HS, Tekgul S. Our experience on management of failed pediatric pyeloplasty. Pediatr Surg Int. 2020;36(8):971–6. https://doi.org/10.1007/s00383-020-04699-9. Epub 2020 Jun 15
12. Romao RL, Koyle MA, Pippi Salle JL, Alotay A, Figueroa VH, Lorenzo AJ, Bagli DJ, Farhat WA. Failed pyeloplasty in children: revisiting the unknown. Urology. 2013;82(5):1145–7. https://doi.org/10.1016/j.urology.2013.06.049. Epub 2013 Sep 12
13. Volkan-Salanci B, Erbaş B. Diuretic renal scintigraphy in adults: practical aspects and reporting. Semin Nucl Med. 2022;52(4):445–52., ISSN 0001-2998. https://doi.org/10.1053/j.semnuclmed.2021.12.006.
14. Kinn AC. Ureteroplevic junction obstruction: Long-term follow up of adults with and without surgical treatment. J Urol. 164:652–6.
15. Lupton EW, George NJR. The Whitaker test: 35 years on. BJUI. 2010;105(1):94–100.
16. Braga LH, Lorenzo AJ, Skeldon S, Dave S, Bagli DJ, Khoury AE, Pippi Salle JL, Farhat WA. Failed pyeloplasty in children: comparative analysis of retrograde endopyelotomy versus redo pyeloplasty. J Urol. 2007;178(6):2571–5; discussion 2575. https://doi.org/10.1016/j.juro.2007.08.050. Epub 2007 Oct 22.
17. Abdrabuh AM, Salih EM, Aboelnasr M, Galal H, El-Emam A, El-Zayat T. Endopyelotomy versus redo pyeoloplasty for management of failed pyeloplasty in children: a single center experience. J Pediatr Surg. 2018;53(11):2250–5. https://doi.org/10.1016/j.jpedsurg.2018.06.002. Epub 2018 Jun 7
18. Abdulfattah S, Zirel L, Mittal S, Srinivasan A, Shukla AR. The missed crossing vessel during open pyeloplasty: a potential advantage of the robot-assisted approach in children. J Robot Surg. 2024;18(1):285. https://doi.org/10.1007/s11701-024-02006-5.
19. Rehman J, Landman J, Sundaram C, Clayman RV. Missed anterior crossing vessels during open retroperitoneal pyeloplasty: laparoscopic transperitoneal discovery and repair. J Urol. 2001;166(2):593–6. https://doi.org/10.1016/S0022-5347(05)65990-3.
20. Chua ME, Ming JM, Kim JK, et al. Meta-analysis of retroperitoneal vs transperitoneal laparoscopic and robot-assisted pyeloplasty for the management of pelvi-ureteric junction obstruction. BJUI Int. 2021;127(6):687–702.
21. Corbett HJ, Mullassery D. Outcomes of endopyelotomy for pelviureteric junction obstruction in the paediatric population: a systematic review. J Pediatr Urol. 2015;11(6):328–36. https://doi.org/10.1016/j.jpurol.2015.08.014.
22. Van Cangh PJ, Wilmart JF, Opsomer RJ, Abi-Aad A, Wese FX, Lorge F. Long-term results and late recurrence after endoureteropyelotomy: a critical analysis of prognostic factors. J Urol. 1994;151(4):934–7. https://doi.org/10.1016/s0022-5347(17)35126-1.
23. Tállai B, Salah MA, Flaskó T, Tóth C, Varga A. Endopyelotomy in childhood: our experience with 37 patients. J Endourol. 2004;18:952–8.
24. Mittal S, Aghababian A, Eftekharzadeh S, et al. Primary vs redo robotic pyeloplasty: a comparison of outcomes. J Pediatr Urol. 2021;17(4):528.e1–7. https://doi.org/10.1016/j.jpurol.2021.02.016.
25. O'Rourke T, Gn M, Patel H, et al. The urologist and the appendix: a review of appendiceal use in genitourinary reconstructive surgery. Urology. 2022;159:10–5. https://doi.org/10.1016/j.urology.2021.10.007.
26. Wang J, Xiong S, Fan S, et al. Appendiceal onlay flap ureteroplasty for the treatment of complex ureteral strictures: initial experience of nine patients. J Endourol. 2020;34(8):874.
27. Jun MS, Stair S, Xu A, et al. A multi-institutional experience with robotic appendiceal ureteroplasty. Urology. 2020;145:287–91. https://doi.org/10.1016/j.urology.2020.06.062.
28. Ahn JJ, Shapiro ME, Ellison JS, Lendvay TS. Pediatric robot-assisted redo pyeloplasty with buccal mucosa graft: a novel technique. Urology. 2017;101:56–9. https://doi.org/10.1016/j.urology.2016.12.036. Epub 2016 Dec 27
29. Lee M, Nagoda E, Strauss D, et al. Role of buccal mucosa graft ureteroplasty in the surgical management of pyeloplasty failure. Asian J Urol. 2024;11(3):373–6. https://doi.org/10.1016/j.ajur.2023.09.001.

30. Adamic BL, Lombardo A, Andolfi C, Hatcher D, Gundeti MS. Pediatric robotic-assisted laparoscopic ureterocalycostomy: salient tips and technical modifications for optimal repair. BJUI Compass. 2020;2(1):53–7. https://doi.org/10.1002/bco2.53.
31. Mittal S, Aghababian A, Eftekharzadeh S, Saxena S, Janssen K, Lombardo A, Adamic B, Dinardo L, Weaver J, Fischer K, Andolfi C, Long C, Weiss D, Kirsch A, Srinivasan A, Gundeti M, Shukla AR. Robot-assisted laparoscopic ureterocalicostomy in the setting of ureteropelvic junction obstruction: a multi-institutional cohort. J Urol. 2022;208(1):180–5. https://doi.org/10.1097/JU.0000000000002484. Epub 2022 Feb 21

Management of Patients with a History of Posterior Urethral Valves

12

Venkat M. Ramakrishnan, Dicken S. C. Ko, and Rena Xu

Key Points

- Posterior urethral valves represent a major cause of pediatric urologic disease and can have significant ramifications in adults who were treated with valve ablation as children.
- Valve bladder syndrome can persist despite successful valve ablation. Advanced forms of the syndrome can necessitate renal replacement therapy or renal transplantation.
- Urodynamic studies are required for pretransplant evaluation.
- Aggressive bladder management optimizes transplant outcomes.
- Preemptive transplantation with a well-managed bladder can yield excellent outcomes.

Introduction

Posterior urethral valves (PUV) constitute abnormal membranous structures within the male posterior urethra that create varying degrees of bladder outlet obstruction. These congenital anomalies can develop during early fetal life and lead to profound consequences for the developing urinary system [1, 2]. The obstruction can result in elevated bladder pressures that transmit retrograde to the kidneys, resulting in

V. M. Ramakrishnan · R. Xu (✉)
Department of Urology, Boston Children's Hospital, Harvard Medical School, Boston, MA, USA
e-mail: Venkat.Ramakrishnan@childrens.harvard.edu; rena.xu@childrens.harvard.edu

D. S. C. Ko
Division of Urology, The Warren Alpert Medical School, Brown University, Providence, RI, USA
e-mail: dicken_ko@brown.edu

H.-Y. Wu et al. (eds.), *Pediatric Urology for the Adult Urologist*,
https://doi.org/10.1007/978-3-032-10306-2_12

hydronephrosis, parenchymal damage, and potential renal dysplasia. In severe cases, reduced fetal urine output leads to oligohydramnios with subsequent pulmonary hypoplasia.

The clinical spectrum of PUV extends from life-threatening neonatal presentations to subtle voiding symptoms that may not manifest until later childhood or adolescence [3, 4]. Recent data indicate that despite improvements in prenatal detection and postnatal management, PUV represents the most common cause of congenital bladder outlet obstruction in males and a leading urological cause of pediatric kidney transplantation, accounting for approximately 15% of all pediatric renal transplant recipients [5]. Despite advances in prenatal detection and early valve ablation, PUV remains responsible for 22–30% of chronic kidney disease (CKD) cases by late adolescence, with 8–21% progressing to end-stage renal disease (ESRD) requiring renal replacement therapy [6, 7]. The clinical challenge, then, extends well beyond initial valve management to encompass decades of evolving bladder dysfunction.

Valve bladder syndrome, characterized by persistent storage and voiding dysfunction despite successful ablation, affects 50–60% of PUV patients and represents a major determinant of long-term graft survival [5]. For adult urologists managing these complex patients, understanding the nuances of bladder optimization before transplantation is essential for achieving successful long-term outcomes. This chapter seeks to provide evidence-based guidance on preparing the bladder for renal transplantation in PUV patients, focusing on evaluation protocols, timing of interventions, and strategies to optimize graft survival.

Epidemiology

Population-based studies report PUV incidence between 1 in 3800 and 1 in 10,000 male live births. Recent epidemiological data from Australia documented an incidence of 1.28 per 10,000 live births, while an audit in the UK found similar rates of approximately 1 in 7800 [8, 9] . These variations likely reflect methodological differences in case identification, as less severe forms may escape early detection [10].

Prenatal ultrasound screening has substantially altered detection patterns, with current antenatal diagnosis rates reaching 46–53% of cases. However, significant numbers continue to present postnatally, with approximately 45% during the neonatal period and the remainder throughout childhood, highlighting persistent diagnostic challenges [8].

Embryology and Pathologic Classification

Hugh Hampton Young's 1919 classification describes Type I valves (over 95% of cases) as membranous folds extending distally from the verumontanum, representing persistent Wolffian structures [11]. Type III valves (5%) appear as circumferential diaphragm-like membranes. The existence of Type II valves—described as membranous folds from the verumontanum to the bladder neck—is now questioned.

Pathophysiology

The pathophysiology of PUV in adults reflects decades of progressive urinary tract changes that initiated during fetal development. While the primary obstruction is addressed through valve ablation in infancy, cascading effects persist and evolve throughout life, creating unique challenges for adult management. The initial posterior urethral obstruction induces compensatory bladder changes, including detrusor hypertrophy, increased collagen deposition (types I and III), trabeculations, and reduced compliance due to fibrotic remodeling [12]. These changes define "valve bladder syndrome"—persistent dysfunction despite successful valve ablation, affecting 50–60% of adult patients [13]. First described by Mitchell in the 1980s, this syndrome encompasses upper tract dilation, bladder wall thickening, reduced compliance, and incomplete emptying. It arises from a vicious cycle of poor compliance leading to elevated storage pressures, while concurrent polyuria from renal tubular dysfunction further stresses the bladder [14, 15].

Upper tract damage occurs through pressure transmission via the ureterovesical junctions, causing hydronephrosis, disrupted nephrogenesis, and progressive nephron loss. Vesicoureteral reflux, present in 50–61% of cases, compounds injury through exposure to infected urine [16, 17]. When obstruction occurs early in fetal development, renal dysplasia with primitive ducts and reduced nephron number can create irreversible functional limitations, including lung hypoplasia [18].

For adult urologists, understanding this developmental context is essential. Bladder dysfunction is not static but evolves from childhood overactivity to adult myogenic failure [19, 20]. The transition from adolescence to adulthood often coincides with deteriorating function, making this a critical intervention period. Polyuria associated with CKD—often exceeding 3–4 liters daily—can place extraordinary demands on the already compromised bladder, accelerating progression to decompensation [21]. This dynamic pathophysiology underscores the complexity of preparing these bladders for renal transplantation.

Clinical Presentation and Diagnostic Evaluation: A Pediatric Context

Severe cases with early-onset oligohydramnios carry grave prognoses due to associated pulmonary hypoplasia [22]. The "multicentre validation of a fetal urine peptidome-based classifier to predict postnatal renal function in posterior urethral valves" (ANTENATAL) consortium has developed standardized protocols for fetal assessment and prognostication [6].

Affected newborns typically demonstrate palpably distended bladders, weak or dribbling urinary streams, respiratory compromise in severe cases, laboratory abnormalities including azotemia, hyperkalemia, and metabolic acidosis, and signs of urinary infection [23, 24]. Therefore, the immediate postnatal period represents a critical window in which prompt diagnosis and intervention can preserve renal function. Later childhood presentations are characterized by recurrent febrile urinary tract infections, persistent daytime wetting, straining to void with poor stream, secondary enuresis, growth failure from CKD, and, more rarely, serious consequences such as acute urinary retention or spontaneous bladder perforation [3, 25–27]. Of importance to the general urologic audience, studies demonstrate that despite widespread prenatal screening programs, a substantial number of PUV cases present throughout childhood, necessitating continued clinical awareness [8].

Urodynamics (UDS): The Cornerstone of Pretransplant Evaluation

A comprehensive UDS evaluation is generally performed for PUV patients 3–6 months after valve ablation [28, 29]. The frequency with which UDS should be repeated throughout childhood and adolescence is debated. UDS facilitates early detection of bladder dysfunction and can inform pharmacologic therapy. It is mandatory for those being considered for renal transplantation and should be performed early in the transplant evaluation process, as abnormal findings may necessitate months of bladder rehabilitation before transplantation can proceed safely. Notably, normal upper tract imaging does not exclude significant bladder dysfunction, and clinical symptoms correlate poorly with urodynamic findings in this population [20]. This underscores the importance of obtaining UDS as part of pretransplant evaluation, even in patients with normal imaging and minimal or no symptoms.

Key UDS parameters requiring assessment include bladder capacity, compliance, detrusor pressure at capacity, presence of detrusor overactivity, voiding pressures and patterns, and postvoid residual. Poor compliance, defined as less than 10 mL/cm H_2O, occurs in approximately 35% of adult PUV patients and represents a significant risk factor for graft dysfunction [30]. End-filling pressures exceeding 40 cm H_2O indicate unsafe storage conditions that will transmit damaging pressures to the transplanted kidney.

UDS patterns in adult PUV patients typically fall into three categories [31]. The first is the overactive bladder with reduced compliance, characterized by detrusor overactivity, reduced functional capacity, and elevated storage pressures. The second pattern is myogenic failure, featuring a large capacity bladder with poor contractility, incomplete emptying, and overflow incontinence. The third pattern combines elements of both, with poor compliance during filling but inadequate contractility during voiding. Each pattern requires different management strategies, emphasizing the importance of accurate UDS characterization.

Video UDS can provide additional valuable information by demonstrating bladder neck hypertrophy (present in over 50% of patients) [32], bladder diverticula that may require surgical management, and vesicoureteral reflux patterns during filling and voiding [33]. The presence of high-grade reflux into the native kidneys raises concerns about reflux into the transplanted ureter and may influence surgical planning [34].

Transplantation Versus Hemodialysis

The strongest predictor of progression to CKD is the nadir creatinine after initial valve ablation [35]. Values exceeding 0.85 mg/dL (75 μmol/L) uniformly predict CKD at puberty, while levels below 0.4 mg/dL (35 μmol/L) indicate a favorable prognosis [36]. Therefore, the decision between continuing renal replacement therapy versus proceeding with transplantation requires careful consideration of multiple factors specific to PUV patients. Current guidelines support preemptive listing for transplant when the estimated glomerular filtration rate (eGFR) falls below 15 mL/min/1.73 m^2 with confirmed irreversibility [37]. Multiple studies have demonstrated superior outcomes with preemptive transplantation as compared to transplantation after hemodialysis initiation. The mortality risk is significantly reduced, with a relative risk of 0.74 (95% CI 0.60–0.91) for living donor transplants [38]. Graft survival improves by 25% for both living and deceased donor transplants when performed preemptively [39]. These clinical benefits translate to substantial economic advantages, with annual Medicare costs of $35,000 for transplant recipients versus $89,000 for dialysis patients [40]. Additionally, preemptive transplantation offers a superior quality of life through the avoidance of dialysis-related morbidity and dietary restrictions.

Importantly, a brief hemodialysis exposure of less than 6 months does not significantly impact long-term outcomes if transplantation occurs within this window [41]. However, transplantation should be deferred in patients with uncontrolled bladder pressures despite maximal medical therapy, active urinary tract infections, need for bladder augmentation with uncertain outcomes, or inadequate family support for complex posttransplant care. For children with small-capacity bladders, clean intermittent catheterization (CIC) is critical yet depends on parental adherence to catheterization regimens, which can vary widely [42] Social services involvement and Mitrofanoff creation may help to alleviate compliance challenges, but delayed transplantation may be necessary until adequate family support is established.

Early peritoneal dialysis (PD) also presents timing challenges for bladder augmentation in PUV patients. Bladder augmentation requires opening the peritoneal cavity and manipulating bowel segments, which can compromise the peritoneal membrane's function for dialysis [43]. PD complications include peritoneal scarring, adhesion formation, and increased infection risk, with peritonitis being the most common dialysis-related complication in pediatric patients [43]. The surgical manipulation required for enterocystoplasty may create peritoneal adhesions that interfere with PD catheter placement and function, potentially necessitating conversion to hemodialysis [44]. This creates a clinical dilemma: bladder augmentation may preclude PD as a dialysis modality, yet delaying bladder augmentation risks progressive bladder and renal deterioration.

Initial and Pretransplantation Bladder Management Strategies

Early management priorities in pediatric protocols include establishing reliable bladder drainage, correcting fluid and electrolyte imbalances, treating metabolic acidosis, instituting antibiotic prophylaxis, managing postobstructive diuresis, and supporting respiratory function when pulmonary hypoplasia exists, with structured protocols for catheter management facilitating subsequent definitive intervention [45]. Pretransplantation bladder management builds upon these same themes. The primary goal of pretransplant bladder optimization is to achieve safe storage pressures below 40 cm H_2O and complete bladder emptying. This is essential to protect the future allograft.

Primary endoscopic ablation of valves, the standard definitive therapy, employs cold knife incisions at the 5 and 7 o'clock positions to minimize thermal injury and bleeding while preserving continence mechanisms compared to electrocautery [46]. Success rates exceed 90% in experienced centers, despite complications including urethral stricture (5–10%), incomplete ablation (10–15%), and bladder neck obstruction. Early ablation before 6 months is associated with superior functional outcomes [47]. Additional interventions include bladder neck incision for demonstrated obstruction [48] and circumcision to reduce infection risk. Temporary vesicostomy is reserved for technical failures or medical instability, as upper tract diversion shows no long-term advantage over primary ablation [49].

Pharmacological management addresses specific dysfunction patterns following valve ablation, with treatment decisions guided by UDS findings and clinical presentations [50, 51]. Anticholinergic therapy is initiated for patients demonstrating elevated detrusor pressures during the storage phase (>20 cm H_2O), detrusor overactivity or instability, reduced bladder compliance, or persistent vesicoureteral reflux. Early anticholinergic use has been associated with improved bladder function in infants with high voiding pressures and low storage volumes, with first-line agents including oxybutynin [52]. Oxybutynin is initiated to inhibit stretch-induced bladder smooth muscle proliferation, thereby retaining normal intravesical pressure and reducing collagen infiltration in the detrusor. Beta-3 agonists such as mirabegron are useful for patients who experience intolerable anticholinergic side effects (particularly dry mouth, constipation, or cognitive effects) or demonstrate insufficient symptomatic improvement with anticholinergic therapy. Mirabegron, which received Food and Drug Administration (FDA) approval in March 2021 for neurogenic detrusor overactivity in pediatric patients aged ≥3 years, relaxes the detrusor muscle without affecting micturition pressure or postvoid residual [53].

Intravesical botulinum toxin injections are reserved for patients with refractory detrusor overactivity and/or poor bladder compliance who have failed to respond adequately to oral pharmacological therapy [54]. Specific indications include persistent detrusor overactivity with elevated end-fill pressures, compromised bladder compliance despite anticholinergic therapy, and risk of upper tract damage due to elevated bladder pressures. Approximately one-third of patients require persistent pharmacological therapy following valve ablation, with severe bladder dysfunction requiring clean intermittent catheterization (CIC) being predictive of end-stage renal disease [51].

Interestingly, CIC is often necessary regardless of urodynamic pattern, with pretransplant CIC associated with better long-term graft outcomes [5]. CIC is indicated when postvoid residual volume exceeds 10% with myogenic failure on UDS, as well as pronounced bladder dysfunction with poor emptying, unsafe pressure levels, high-grade vesicoureteral reflux, and progressive renal impairment [55]. The probability of requiring CIC increases with serum nadir creatinine, with 26% progressing to CIC by age 10 [56].

Early CIC institution at a median age of 8 months counteracts renal function deterioration, while discontinuation results in a median GFR decline of 24% [55]. From a transplant perspective, pretransplant CIC is associated with better long-term graft outcomes [5], and CIC in children under 12 years does not negatively impact graft survival [57]. Benefits include decreased detrusor instability, improved compliance, and increased bladder capacity beyond age-expected norms [55], supporting aggressive bladder management as essential for optimizing both native renal preservation and posttransplant outcomes.

Patient education should emphasize the likely permanence of CIC, since bladder function rarely improves after transplantation. Families often have the misconception that renal transplantation will also fix the bladder dysfunction. PUV boys with sensate urethras may experience pain and discomfort with CIC. Only 65% achieve long-term compliance after 2 years despite 85% initial acceptance [58]. Patient comfort level is the best predictor of protocol success [59]. The compliance concern in these boys contributes to the rationale for catheterizable channels as originally described by Mitrofanoff [56]. The creation of a catheterizable channel should be considered for patients unable or unwilling to perform urethral catheterization, as evidence suggests such procedures may improve compliance with CIC and delay renal function deterioration [60].

Nocturnal bladder drainage deserves special attention due to the combination of polyuria and impaired sensation leading to massive nocturnal bladder overdistention that perpetuates bladder deterioration, with options including overnight indwelling catheterization, planned nocturnal CIC, or continuous drainage via Mitrofanoff. Studies by Koff and colleagues demonstrated marked improvement in hydronephrosis with nocturnal drainage alone [61].

When medical management fails to achieve safe storage parameters, surgical intervention becomes necessary. Bladder neck incision may improve voiding parameters in patients with demonstrated obstruction [48]. Vesicostomy should be considered when conservative medical management and CIC fail. The decision should be based on clinical indicators such as worsening hydronephrosis, vesicoureteral reflux, recurrent UTIs, and increasing renal insufficiency despite CIC. The procedure is effective, well-tolerated, and reversible [62]. Vesicostomy closure can be performed after a mean bladder rest period of 38.7 months, with the bladders of young infants regaining normal function after the vesicostomy is closed and normal bladder cycling is restored [63]. Moreover, approximately 75% of patients who underwent vesicostomy closure later in life achieved successful outcomes, with less than 5% of patients requiring later augmentation for bladder or renal deterioration [64].

An alternate diversion strategy, cutaneous ureterostomy, should be considered as a last-resort option and only when bladder-level drainage is insufficient. It is typically employed when the obstructive uropathy is unresponsive to lower urinary tract drainage [65]. It should not be considered a permanent method of urinary diversion and may be performed when the patient's chances of survival are limited or when the surgeon is not prepared to perform more definitive repair.

Augmentation cystoplasty represents the definitive surgical solution for refractory low compliance despite maximal medical therapy. Success is defined as achieving compliance greater than 20 mL/cm H_2O [66], storage pressures below 40 cm H_2O [67, 68], and a functional capacity exceeding 300 mL [69].

The optimal timing of augmentation cystoplasty in relation to transplantation remains controversial [70–72]. Arguments for pretransplant augmentation include establishing safe storage before immunosuppression, avoiding graft exposure to high pressures, improving technical ease without the transplant ureter present, and allowing complete healing before transplant. However, this approach may preclude peritoneal dialysis, and bladder dynamics may improve posttransplant, potentially making augmentation unnecessary [73].

Conversely, augmentation after transplantation allows for an assessment of bladder response to improved renal function, preserves the option of peritoneal dialysis, and may avoid unnecessary surgery if bladder function improves. The disadvantages include the risk of graft injury during augmentation, complicated healing under immunosuppression, and a period of graft exposure to a hostile bladder environment.

Current evidence from meta-analyses demonstrates no difference in graft survival between pretransplant, simultaneous, or posttransplant augmentation [71]. Therefore, individualized decision-making is essential. Pretransplant augmentation should be considered when compliance remains below 10 mL/cm H_2O despite maximal therapy and CIC. Augmentation may be deferred in patients with borderline parameters who may improve posttransplant.

Posttransplant Management

Successful transplantation requires continued vigilance regarding bladder function. The immediate posttransplant period necessitates bladder drainage for 3–5 days via urethral or suprapubic catheter, prophylactic antibiotics while catheterized, early institution of CIC if part of the pretransplant regimen, and monitoring for postobstructive diuresis [74–76]. Long-term surveillance includes repeat UDS at 6–12 months posttransplant to assess bladder response, then annually for the first 3 years if abnormal, and as indicated by clinical changes thereafter [30, 41].

Recurrent urinary tract infections occur more frequently in PUV patients (55% vs. 30% in controls) but do not necessarily impact graft survival if properly managed [5]. Management strategies include prophylactic antibiotics for patients on CIC, treatment of constipation, optimization of bladder emptying, and investigation for stones or vesicoureteral reflux. Progressive bladder dysfunction may require escalation of anticholinergic therapy, institution of CIC if not already performed, consideration of delayed augmentation, or, rarely, urinary diversion for refractory cases. Additionally, posttransplant patients with bladder augmentation face significantly increased malignancy risk. The incidence of bladder cancer is 15% in immunosuppressed transplant recipients as compared to 2.8% in augmented nontransplant patients. One series demonstrated that the cancer risk is increased by 7–8 fold for ileal/colonic augmentations and 14–15 fold for gastric augmentations, with cancer typically occurring 10–30 years postaugmentation [77]. However, annual screening for malignancy using cystoscopy and cytology is unlikely to be cost-effective at commonly accepted thresholds [78].

Outcomes and Future Directions

Contemporary series demonstrate that with appropriate bladder management, PUV patients achieve transplant outcomes comparable to nonurological causes of ESRD. Five-year graft survival reaches 85% with living donors and 75% with deceased donors, while 10-year graft survival approximates 70–75% with optimal bladder management, showing no significant difference from matched nonurological controls [41]. Favorable prognostic factors included living donor transplantation [hazard ratio (HR) 0.73 for graft loss], adequate bladder management with CIC, compliance exceeding 20 mL/cm H_2O, and absence of recurrent pyelonephritis. Conversely, risk factors for graft loss include persistent high-pressure bladder, recurrent febrile urinary tract infections (UTIs), noncompliance with CIC, and pretransplant dialysis exceeding 2 years.

Emerging strategies for optimizing transplant outcomes include biomarker development, with urinary neutrophil gelatinase-associated lipocalin (NGAL) and kidney injury molecule-1 (KIM-1) showing promise in predicting renal function decline and guiding intervention timing [79]. Noninvasive monitoring through contrast-enhanced ultrasound elastography may eventually replace invasive urodynamics [80, 81], while tissue engineering approaches offer hope for bladder regeneration as an alternative to enterocystoplasty [82].

Conclusion

Successful renal transplantation in PUV patients requires meticulous attention to bladder function from initial diagnosis through posttransplant care. The complex interplay between evolving bladder dysfunction and renal failure necessitates a multidisciplinary management approach involving pediatric and adult urologists, nephrologists, and transplant surgeons. Key principles for optimizing outcomes include early and regular urodynamic assessment beginning 6 months postvalve ablation, aggressive medical management to achieve safe storage parameters, timely institution of CIC when indicated, careful consideration of augmentation cystoplasty timing, preference for preemptive transplantation when possible, and lifelong surveillance of bladder function posttransplant. Through systematic evaluation, individualized management, and sustained follow-up, the majority of PUV patients can achieve excellent long-term transplant outcomes with preserved bladder function and continence.

References

1. Friedland GW, Fair WR, Govan DE, Filly R. Posterior urethral valves. Clin Radiol. 1977;28(4):367–80. https://doi.org/10.1016/s0009-9260(77)80142-6.
2. Krishnan A, de Souza A, Konijeti R, Baskin LS. The anatomy and embryology of posterior urethral valves. J Urol. 2006;175(4):1214–20. https://doi.org/10.1016/S0022-5347(05)00642-7.
3. Bomalaski MD, Anema JG, Coplen DE, Koo HP, Rozanski T, Bloom DA. Delayed presentation of posterior urethral valves: a not so benign condition. J Urol. 1999;162(6):2130–2. https://doi.org/10.1016/S0022-5347(05)68140-2.
4. Hendren WH. Posterior urethral valves in boys. A broad clinical spectrum. J Urol. 1971;106(2):298–307. https://doi.org/10.1016/s0022-5347(17)61278-3.
5. Amesty MV, Garcia-Vaz C, Espinosa L, Martinez-Urrutia MJ, Lopez-Pereira P. Long-term renal transplant outcome in patients with posterior urethral valves. Prognostic factors related to bladder dysfunction management. *Front Pediatr*. 2021;9:646923. https://doi.org/10.3389/fped.2021.646923.
6. Buffin-Meyer B, Klein J, van der Zanden LFM, Levtchenko E, Moulos P, Lounis N, et al. The ANTENATAL multicentre study to predict postnatal renal outcome in fetuses with posterior urethral valves: objectives and design. Clin Kidney J. 2020;13(3):371–9. https://doi.org/10.1093/ckj/sfz107.
7. Simforoosh N, Tabibi A, Basiri A, Noorbala MH, Danesh AD, Ijadi A. Is ureteral reimplantation necessary during augmentation cystoplasty in patients with neurogenic bladder and vesicoureteral reflux? J Urol. 2002;168(4 Pt 1):1439–41. https://doi.org/10.1016/S0022-5347(05)64469-2.

8. Brownlee E, Wragg R, Robb A, Chandran H, Knight M, McCarthy L, Baps C. Current epidemiology and antenatal presentation of posterior urethral valves: outcome of BAPS CASS National Audit. J Pediatr Surg. 2019;54(2):318–21. https://doi.org/10.1016/j.jpedsurg.2018.10.091.
9. Thakkar D, Deshpande AV, Kennedy SE. Epidemiology and demography of recently diagnosed cases of posterior urethral valves. Pediatr Res. 2014;76(6):560–3. https://doi.org/10.1038/pr.2014.134.
10. Ansari MS, Singh P, Mandhani A, Dubey D, Srivastava A, Kapoor R, Kumar A. Delayed presentation in posterior urethral valve: long-term implications and outcome. Urology. 2008;71(2):230–4. https://doi.org/10.1016/j.urology.2007.09.037.
11. Young HH, Frontz WA, Baldwin JC. Congenital obstruction of the posterior urethra. J Urol. 2002;3:289–365. J Urol. 1919; 167(1):265–7; discussion 268. Retrieved from https://www.ncbi.nlm.nih.gov/pubmed/11743334
12. Hodges SJ, Patel B, McLorie G, Atala A. Posterior urethral valves. ScientificWorldJournal. 2009;9:1119–26. https://doi.org/10.1100/tsw.2009.127.
13. Glassberg KI. The valve bladder syndrome. J Urol. 2002;167(1):298–9. Retrieved from https://www.ncbi.nlm.nih.gov/pubmed/11743344
14. Glassberg KI, Combs A. The valve bladder syndrome: 35+ years later. J Urol. 2016;196(1):16–7. https://doi.org/10.1016/j.juro.2016.04.049.
15. Mitchell ME. Persistent ureteral dilation following valve resection. Dial Pediatr Urol. 1982;5(8)
16. Heikkila J, Rintala R, Taskinen S. Vesicoureteral reflux in conjunction with posterior urethral valves. J Urol. 2009;182(4):1555–60. https://doi.org/10.1016/j.juro.2009.06.057.
17. Hoover DL, Duckett JW Jr. Posterior urethral valves, unilateral reflux and renal dysplasia: a syndrome. J Urol. 1982;128(5):994–7. https://doi.org/10.1016/s0022-5347(17)53313-3.
18. Sarhan OM. Posterior urethral valves: impact of low birth weight and preterm delivery on the final renal outcome. Arab J Urol. 2017;15(2):159–65. https://doi.org/10.1016/j.aju.2017.01.005.
19. De Gennaro M, Capitanucci ML, Mosiello G, Caione P, Silveri M. The changing urodynamic pattern from infancy to adolescence in boys with posterior urethral valves. BJU Int. 2000;85(9):1104–8. https://doi.org/10.1046/j.1464-410x.2000.00700.x.
20. Ghanem MA, Wolffenbuttel KP, De Vylder A, Nijman RJ. Long-term bladder dysfunction and renal function in boys with posterior urethral valves based on urodynamic findings. J Urol. 2004;171(6 Pt 1):2409–12. https://doi.org/10.1097/01.ju.0000127762.95045.93.
21. Taskinen S, Heikkila J, Rintala R. Effects of posterior urethral valves on long-term bladder and sexual function. Nat Rev Urol. 2012;9(12):699–706. https://doi.org/10.1038/nrurol.2012.196.
22. Holmes N, Harrison MR, Baskin LS. Fetal surgery for posterior urethral valves: long-term postnatal outcomes. Pediatrics. 2001;108(1):E7. https://doi.org/10.1542/peds.108.1.e7.
23. Greenfield SP, Hensle TW, Berdon WE, Geringer AM. Urinary extravasation in the newborn male with posterior urethral valves. J Pediatr Surg. 1982;17(6):751–6. https://doi.org/10.1016/s0022-3468(82)80441-7.
24. Merguerian PA, McLorie GA, Churchill BM, McKenna PH, Khoury AE. Radiographic and serologic correlates of azotemia in patients with posterior urethral valves. J Urol. 1992;148(5):1499–503. https://doi.org/10.1016/s0022-5347(17)36949-5.
25. Harper L, Botto N, Peycelon M, Michel JL, Leclair MD, Garnier S, et al. Risk factors for febrile urinary tract infection in boys with posterior urethral valves. Front Pediatr. 2022;10:971662. https://doi.org/10.3389/fped.2022.971662.
26. Hyuga T, Nakamura S, Kawai S, Kubo T, Furukawa R, Aihara T, et al. The changes of urethral morphology recognized in voiding cystourethrography after endoscopic transurethral incision for posterior urethral valve in boys with intractable daytime urinary incontinence and nocturnal enuresis. World J Urol. 2017;35(10):1611–6. https://doi.org/10.1007/s00345-017-2018-4.
27. Nishio H, Mizuno K, Kato T, Maruyama T, Yasui T, Hayashi Y. A case of posterior urethral valve identified in an older child by straining to void. Urol Case Rep. 2022;40:101886. https://doi.org/10.1016/j.eucr.2021.101886.

28. De Gennaro M, Mosiello G, Capitanucci ML, Silveri M, Capozza N, Caione P. Early detection of bladder dysfunction following posterior urethral valves ablation. Eur J Pediatr Surg. 1996;6(3):163–5. https://doi.org/10.1055/s-2008-1066497.
29. Mo Z, Li M, Xie X, Sun N, Zhang W, Tian J, Song H. Urodynamic changes before and after endoscopic valve ablation in boys diagnosed with the posterior urethral valve without chronic renal failure. BMC Urol. 2023;23(1):5. https://doi.org/10.1186/s12894-022-01170-w.
30. Salomon L, Fontaine E, Guest G, Gagnadoux MF, Broyer M, Beurton D. Role of the bladder in delayed failure of kidney transplants in boys with posterior urethral valves. J Urol. 2000;163(4):1282–5. Retrieved from https://www.ncbi.nlm.nih.gov/pubmed/10737529
31. Misseri R, Combs AJ, Horowitz M, Donohoe JM, Glassberg KI. Myogenic failure in posterior urethral valve disease: real or imagined? J Urol. 2002;168(4 Pt 2):1844–8; discussion 1848. https://doi.org/10.1097/01.ju.0000029633.06239.b7.
32. Sobhani S, Foroushani AR, Arshadi H, Hekmati P, Kajbafzadeh AM. Simultaneous primary posterior urethral valves ablation and bladder neck incision may decrease kidney and bladder failure in long-term follow-up in patients with bladder neck hypertrophy and poor bladder function at presentation: report of 301 cases. BMC Urol. 2024;24(1):154. https://doi.org/10.1186/s12894-024-01546-0.
33. Tourchi A, Kajbafzadeh AM, Aryan Z, Ebadi M. The management of vesicoureteral reflux in the setting of posterior urethral valve with emphasis on bladder function and renal outcome: a single center cohort study. Urology. 2014;83(1):199–205. https://doi.org/10.1016/j.urology.2013.07.033.
34. Concodora CW, Reddy PP, VanderBrink BA. The role of video urodynamics in the management of the valve bladder. Curr Urol Rep. 2017;18(3):24. https://doi.org/10.1007/s11934-017-0670-2.
35. DeFoor W, Clark C, Jackson E, Reddy P, Minevich E, Sheldon C. Risk factors for end stage renal disease in children with posterior urethral valves. J Urol. 2008;180(4 Suppl):1705–8; discussion 1708. https://doi.org/10.1016/j.juro.2008.03.090.
36. Coleman R, King T, Nicoara CD, Bader M, McCarthy L, Chandran H, Parashar K. Nadir creatinine in posterior urethral valves: how high is low enough? J Pediatr Urol. 2015;11(6):356 e351-355. https://doi.org/10.1016/j.jpurol.2015.06.008.
37. Rana Magar R, Knight S, Stojanovic J, Marks SD, Lafranca JA, Turner S, et al. Is preemptive kidney transplantation associated with improved outcomes when compared to non-preemptive kidney transplantation in children? A systematic review and meta-analysis. Transpl Int. 2022;35:10315. https://doi.org/10.3389/ti.2022.10315.
38. Rana Magar R, Knight SR, Maggiore U, Lafranca JA, Dor F, Pengel LHM. What are the benefits of preemptive versus non-preemptive kidney transplantation? A systematic review and meta-analysis. Transplant Rev (Orlando). 2023;37(4):100798. https://doi.org/10.1016/j.trre.2023.100798.
39. Kasiske BL, Snyder JJ, Matas AJ, Ellison MD, Gill JS, Kausz AT. Preemptive kidney transplantation: the advantage and the advantaged. J Am Soc Nephrol. 2002;13(5):1358–64. https://doi.org/10.1097/01.asn.0000013295.11876.c9.
40. Myers J. Preemptive kidney transplants: why aren't they more popular? 2019. Retrieved from https://www.kidney.org/news-stories/preemptive-kidney-transplants-why-aren-t-they-more-popular
41. Silverii H, Merguerian P, Fernandez N, Smith J, Shnorhavorian M, Ahn J. Posterior urethral valves and kidney transplantation: identifying opportunities for improvement. J Pediatr Urol. 2024;20(Suppl 1):S58–65. https://doi.org/10.1016/j.jpurol.2024.06.022.
42. Selekman RE, Sanford MT, Ko LN, Allen IE, Copp HL. Does perception of catheterization limit its use in pediatric UTI? J Pediatr Urol. 2017;13(1):48 e41–6. https://doi.org/10.1016/j.jpurol.2016.09.006.
43. Cho MH. Infectious and non-infectious complications of peritoneal dialysis in children. Child Kidney Dis. 2020;24(2):63–8. https://doi.org/10.3339/jkspn.2020.24.2.63.
44. Langer S, Radtke C, Gyori E, Springer A, Metzelder ML. Bladder augmentation in children: current problems and experimental strategies for reconstruction. Wien Med Wochenschr. 2019;169(3–4):61–70. https://doi.org/10.1007/s10354-018-0645-z.

45. Wu CQ, Blum ES, Patil D, Shin HS, Smith EA. Predicting childhood chronic kidney disease severity in infants with posterior urethral valve: a critical analysis of creatinine values in the first year of life. Pediatr Nephrol. 2022;37(6):1339–45. https://doi.org/10.1007/s00467-021-05271-w.
46. Pellegrino C, Capitanucci ML, Forlini V, Zaccara A, Lena F, Sollini ML, et al. Posterior urethral valves: role of prenatal diagnosis and long-term management of bladder function; a single center point of view and review of literature. Front Pediatr. 2022;10:1057092. https://doi.org/10.3389/fped.2022.1057092.
47. Kibar Y, Ashley RA, Roth CC, Frimberger D, Kropp BP. Timing of posterior urethral valve diagnosis and its impact on clinical outcome. J Pediatr Urol. 2011;7(5):538–42. https://doi.org/10.1016/j.jpurol.2010.08.002.
48. Kajbafzadeh AM, Payabvash S, Karimian G. The effects of bladder neck incision on urodynamic abnormalities of children with posterior urethral valves. J Urol. 2007;178(5):2142–7; discussion 2147–2149. https://doi.org/10.1016/j.juro.2007.07.046.
49. Khondker A, Chan JY, Malik S, Kim JK, Chua ME, Henderson B, et al. Primary ablation versus urinary diversion in posterior urethral valve: systematic review and meta-analysis. J Pediatr Urol. 2023;19(4):408–17. https://doi.org/10.1016/j.jpurol.2023.02.008.
50. Kim YH, Horowitz M, Combs AJ, Nitti VW, Borer J, Glassberg KI. Management of posterior urethral valves on the basis of urodynamic findings. J Urol. 1997;158(3 Pt 2):1011–6. https://doi.org/10.1097/00005392-199709000-00085.
51. Sharma S, Joshi M, Gupta DK, Abraham M, Mathur P, Mahajan JK, et al. Consensus on the management of posterior urethral valves from antenatal period to puberty. J Indian Assoc Pediatr Surg. 2019;24(1):4–14. https://doi.org/10.4103/jiaps.JIAPS_148_18.
52. Norris JJ, Raj JP, Thomas TT, Maleperambil TT, Shubha AM. Effects of oxybutynin in children with posterior urethral valves post fulguration: report in a select cohort of children. J Family Med Prim Care. 2021;10(10):3706–11. https://doi.org/10.4103/jfmpc.jfmpc_2554_20.
53. Keam SJ. Mirabegron: pediatric first approval. Paediatr Drugs. 2021;23(4):411–5. https://doi.org/10.1007/s40272-021-00452-4.
54. Naqvi S, Clothier J, Wright A, Garriboli M. Urodynamic outcomes in children after single and multiple injections for overactive and low compliance neurogenic bladder treated with abobotulinum toxin A. J Urol. 2020;203(2):413–9. https://doi.org/10.1097/JU.0000000000000540.
55. Holmdahl G, Sillen U, Hellstrom AL, Sixt R, Solsnes E. Does treatment with clean intermittent catheterization in boys with posterior urethral valves affect bladder and renal function? J Urol. 2003;170(4 Pt 2):1681–5; discussion 1685. https://doi.org/10.1097/01.ju.0000084142.71123.b5.
56. McLeod DJ, Szymanski KM, Gong E, Granberg C, Reddy P, Sebastiao Y, et al. Renal replacement therapy and intermittent catheterization risk in posterior urethral valves. Pediatrics. 2019;143(3) https://doi.org/10.1542/peds.2018-2656.
57. Marcou M, Galiano M, Tzschoppe A, Sauerstein K, Wach S, Taubert H, et al. Clean intermittent catheterization in children under 12 years does not have a negative impact on long-term graft survival following pediatric kidney transplantation. J Clin Med. 2023;13(1) https://doi.org/10.3390/jcm13010033.
58. Neel KF. Feasibility and outcome of clean intermittent catheterization for children with sensate urethra. Can Urol Assoc J. 2010;4(6):403–5. https://doi.org/10.5489/cuaj.955.
59. Van Savage JG, Sackett CK, Wilhelm CL, Sessions RP, Mesrobian HG. Indications for and outcomes of clean intermittent catheterization in children with normal genital sensation. J Urol. 1997;157(5):1866–8. https://doi.org/10.1097/00005392-199705000-00099.
60. Rickard M, Chua ME, Zu'bi F, Dos Santos J, Koyle MA, Lorenzo AJ, Farhat WA. Comparative outcome analysis of pediatric kidney transplant in posterior urethral valves children with or without pretransplant Mitrofanoff procedure. Pediatr Transplant. 2020;24(8):e13798. https://doi.org/10.1111/petr.13798.
61. Koff SA, Mutabagani KH, Jayanthi VR. The valve bladder syndrome: pathophysiology and treatment with nocturnal bladder emptying. J Urol. 2002;167(1):291–7. https://doi.org/10.1016/s0022-5347(05)65453-5.

62. Morrisroe SN, O'Connor RC, Nanigian DK, Kurzrock EA, Stone AR. Vesicostomy revisited: the best treatment for the hostile bladder in myelodysplastic children? BJU Int. 2005;96(3):397–400. https://doi.org/10.1111/j.1464-410X.2005.05638.x.
63. Podesta ML, Ruarte A, Herrera M, Medel R, Castera R. Bladder functional outcome after delayed vesicostomy closure and antireflux surgery in young infants with 'primary' vesico-ureteric reflux. BJU Int. 2001;87(6):473–9. https://doi.org/10.1046/j.1464-410x.2001.00095.x.
64. Jayanthi VR, McLorie GA, Khoury AE, Churchill BM. The effect of temporary cutaneous diversion on ultimate bladder function. J Urol. 1995;154(2 Pt 2):889–92. https://doi.org/10.1097/00005392-199508000-00155.
65. Rosen MA, Roth DR, Gonzales ET Jr. Current indications for cutaneous ureterostomy. Urology. 1994;43(1):92–6. https://doi.org/10.1016/s0090-4295(94)80274-2.
66. Husmann DA, Snodgrass WT, Koyle MA, Furness PD 3rd, Kropp BP, Cheng EY, et al. Ureterocystoplasty: indications for a successful augmentation. J Urol. 2004;171(1):376–80. https://doi.org/10.1097/01.ju.0000100800.69333.4d.
67. Grimsby GM, Menon V, Schlomer BJ, Baker LA, Adams R, Gargollo PC, Jacobs MA. Long-term outcomes of bladder neck reconstruction without augmentation cystoplasty in children. J Urol. 2016;195(1):155–61. https://doi.org/10.1016/j.juro.2015.06.103.
68. Veeratterapillay R, Thorpe AC, Harding C. Augmentation cystoplasty: contemporary indications, techniques and complications. Indian J Urol. 2013;29(4):322–7. https://doi.org/10.4103/0970-1591.120114.
69. Yang C, Chen X, Wang Y, Fang L, Sun W, Bi L, Yu D. Efficacy of complete laparoscopic ileal augmentation cystoplasty for the treatment of low bladder capacity and compliance: a case series. BMC Urol. 2022;22(1):58. https://doi.org/10.1186/s12894-022-01008-5.
70. Jesus LE, Pippi Salle JL. Pre-transplant management of valve bladder: a critical literature review. J Pediatr Urol. 2015;11(1):5–11. https://doi.org/10.1016/j.jpurol.2014.12.001.
71. Lopez Pereira P, Ortiz R, Espinosa L, Martinez Urrutia MJ, Lobato R, Alonso A, Jaureguizar E. Does bladder augmentation negatively affect renal transplant outcome in posterior urethral valve patients? J Pediatr Urol. 2014;10(5):892–7. https://doi.org/10.1016/j.jpurol.2014.01.011.
72. Nahas WC, Mazzucchi E, Arap MA, Antonopoulos IM, Neto ED, Ianhez LE, Arap S. Augmentation cystoplasty in renal transplantation: a good and safe option--experience with 25 cases. Urology. 2002;60(5):770–4. https://doi.org/10.1016/s0090-4295(02)01947-7.
73. Mizerski A, Ostrowska Clark K, Ostrowski M, Ciechanowski K, Kaminski M, Sulikowski J, et al. Postoperative adaptation of urinary bladder to variable volume of urine in the initial period following kidney transplantation. Transplant Proc. 2003;35(6):2174–5. https://doi.org/10.1016/s0041-1345(03)00778-4.
74. Gill IS, Hayes JM, Hodge EE, Novick AC. Clean intermittent catheterization and urinary diversion in the management of renal transplant recipients with lower urinary tract dysfunction. J Urol. 1992;148(5):1397–400. https://doi.org/10.1016/s0022-5347(17)36920-3.
75. Goodfellow M, Thompson ER, Tingle SJ, Wilson C. Early versus late removal of urinary catheter after kidney transplantation. Cochrane Database Syst Rev. 2023;7(7):CD013788. https://doi.org/10.1002/14651858.CD013788.pub2.
76. Green H, Rahamimov R, Gafter U, Leibovitci L, Paul M. Antibiotic prophylaxis for urinary tract infections in renal transplant recipients: a systematic review and meta-analysis. Transpl Infect Dis. 2011;13(5):441–7. https://doi.org/10.1111/j.1399-3062.2011.00644.x.
77. Husmann DA. Malignancy after gastrointestinal augmentation in childhood. Ther Adv Urol. 2009;1(1):5–11. https://doi.org/10.1177/1756287209104163.
78. Kokorowski PJ, Routh JC, Borer JG, Estrada CR, Bauer SB, Nelson CP. Screening for malignancy after augmentation cystoplasty in children with spina bifida: a decision analysis. J Urol. 2011;186(4):1437–43. https://doi.org/10.1016/j.juro.2011.05.065.
79. Bastos FM, Leal CRV, Vaz de Castro PAS, Vaz KKB, Oliveira KKR, Silva Filha RD, et al. Tubular and glomerular biomarkers of renal tissue function in the urine of fetuses with posterior urethral valves. J Pediatr Urol. 2022;18(3):368 e361–9. https://doi.org/10.1016/j.jpurol.2022.03.019.

80. Bosio M, Manzoni GA. Detection of posterior urethral valves with voiding cystourethrosonography with echo contrast. J Urol. 2002;168(4 Pt 2):1711–5; discussion 1715. https://doi.org/10.1097/01.ju.0000027283.78968.b5.
81. Chung PH, Leong JY, Machado P, Wessner CE, Trabulsi EJ, Halpern EJ, et al. Contrast-enhanced ultrasound and shear wave elastography: novel methods for the evaluation of urethral stricture disease. J Urol. 2022;207(1):152–60. https://doi.org/10.1097/JU.0000000000002146.
82. Ramakrishnan VM, Thaker H, Ocampo GL, Adam RM, Estrada CR Jr. Pediatric bladder tissue engineering: where have we been and where do we go next? J Pediatr Urol. 2025;21(3):550–7. https://doi.org/10.1016/j.jpurol.2025.01.001.

Hypospadias for the Adult Urologist

13

Annaliese Ionson and Hadley Wood

Acronyms

AUA	American Urological Association
DSD	Disorder of sexual differentiation
ED	Erectile dysfunction
EPA	Excision and primary anastomosis
IIEF-EF	International Index of Erectile Function—Erectile Function
LUTS	Lower urinary tract symptoms
RUG	Retrograde urethrogram
SAMHSA	Substance Abuse and Mental Health Administration
UTI	Urinary tract infection

1. *Long-term complications are common and often underreported including voiding and sexual dysfunction.* Lower urinary tract symptoms spraying dribbling and recurrent UTIs are frequent. These often stem from anatomic or functional sequelae like strictures sacculation or pelvic floor dysfunction. Sexual issues range from erectile to ejaculatory dysfunction sometimes with no identifiable organic cause.
2. *Testosterone deficiency and hypofertility are more prevalent.* Men should be counseled on these risks to identify problems in a timely fashion. Any testosterone supplementation should be weighed against the fertility goals of the patient.

A. Ionson · H. Wood (✉)
Cleveland Clinic Foundation, Cleveland, OH, USA
e-mail: ionsona@ccf.org; woodh@ccf.org

H.-Y. Wu et al. (eds.), *Pediatric Urology for the Adult Urologist*,
https://doi.org/10.1007/978-3-032-10306-2_13

3. *Adult repairs are often complex and require multistage approaches.* Reconstruction often requires grafts and staged urethroplasty, with perineal urethrostomy for severe cases.
4. *Psychosocial and psychosexual impact is understudied but likely significant.* A trauma-informed approach to care—emphasizing consent, communication, and patient comfort—can improve trust and outcomes.
5. *The paradigm of early surgery is shifting, particularly for distal hypospadias.* Shared decision-making, bodily autonomy, and respect for future patient agency are increasingly emphasized. This may lead to more adults seeking care for untreated hypospadias.

While the vast majority of primary repairs occur in childhood, many of these patients present to reconstructive urologists decades later with concerns regarding cosmesis, sexual function, voiding function, and fertility. In this chapter, we will review the classification, etiology, epidemiology, complications of hypospadias, and reoperation rates following primary repair, and the assessment and management of adult patients with a history of hypospadias repair. Lastly, we will discuss the evolving paradigm regarding surgical intervention in childhood and how it may impact subsequent medical intervention in adult life.

Classification, Epidemiology, and Etiology

Hypospadias is the most common congenital malformation of the penis, and the second most common congenital disorder in males after cryptorchidism [1]. The incidence varies by region and ranges from 2.1 to 39.1 per 10,000 live male births [2, 3]. Generally, hypospadias is characterized by [1]:

1. Ectopic location of the urethral meatus.
2. Incomplete development of the prepuce (dorsal hooded foreskin) and scrotum (penoscrotal transposition and bifid scrotum).
3. Ventral skin deficiency/penile curvature–chordee.

Hypospadias is a spectrum condition, and the postnatal phenotype can present with barely perceptible differences from a normal male phallus to a classic ambiguous genital presentation. Nearly 65–70% of hypospadias is distal, while approximately 10–25% is the more severe proximal phenotype [4]. The mega meatus intact prepuce is the mildest variant of hypospadias, without any foreskin defect or curvature, and characterized by a large "fish-mouth" urethral opening, deep fossa navicularis, and broad shovel-shaped glans [5]. Early classification systems evaluated the size of the glans, position of the urethra, and degree of curvature. More contemporary classification systems, such as the meatal, corpus spongiosum, glans, urethral plate (MCGU) from the International Hypospadias Society, also assess urethral plate quality, the degree of scrotal transposition, and the ano-scrotal distance [6].

Hypospadias is usually isolated on presentation, though 7–10% of patients have concomitant unilateral or bilateral cryptorchidism. These patients have a threefold higher risk of difference of sexual development (DSD) and are recommended to undergo a full DSD evaluation at presentation postnatally per American Urological Association (AUA) guidelines [7, 8]. Other associated conditions include inguinal hernia and/or hydrocele, and utricular cyst or dilation [4].

Primary Pediatric Surgical Repair and Complications

Surgical repair is elective, with the goal of achieving more normal urination, sexual function, and appearance. The American Academy of Pediatrics Section on Urology recommended timing for surgery between the ages of 6 and 12 months. The rationale for this is based on genital awareness, which is theorized to manifest around 18 months, procedural anxiety, and postoperative behavioral problems, which may be more severe in children >1 year [9, 10]. Typically, hypospadias repair includes urethroplasty and correction of chordee and associated scrotal transposition.

A survey of over 1200 patients post-hypospadias repair found 47% of complications manifested within the first year postoperatively. The median time to complication for all repair types was 69.2 months (interquartile range [IQR] 23–131.9) [11]. The complication rate varies by degree of severity of the initial presentation and ranges from 5% to 17.9% for distal repairs and 12% to 55.1% for proximal repairs [11–13]. Early complications of surgical repair include fistula, urethral stricture, wound dehiscence, and infection. Late complications include neourethral stricture or meatal stenosis, residual or recurrent ventral curvature, cosmetic dissatisfaction, and sexual dysfunction [14–16].

The reoperation rate following distal repair ranges from 3.3% to 12.6% [17, 18]. The reoperation rate following proximal repairs is much higher, up to 50–60% in published studies [19–21]. In a cohort of adults with complications from previous hypospadias surgery, 66% reported multiple surgeries [15]. Historically, primary hypospadias studies have had follow-up limited to childhood or young adulthood. While the rate of late complications is unknown, patients with a history of hypospadias often present with problems associated with their repairs in adult life to reconstructive urologists, so it is unlikely that existing literature truly captures late complications.

Assessment of Adults with a History of Hypospadias

The initial assessment of an adult patient presenting with a history of hypospadias should include a thorough history classifying the initial phenotype, the type of repair(s) they underwent, whether they required a graft or flap, any complications, and the number of reoperations. For late presentations, the patients often do not have this information, and relevant medical records have been destroyed or are inaccessible. It is imperative that a thorough physical exam examining prior scars, looking into the meatus, and evaluating the glans for morphology as well as the shaft for associated fistulae and chordee, is done initially (Fig. 13.1a). For this discussion, we will discuss complications in four not mutually exclusive categories: cosmesis, chordee, sexual function and fertility, and urinary function.

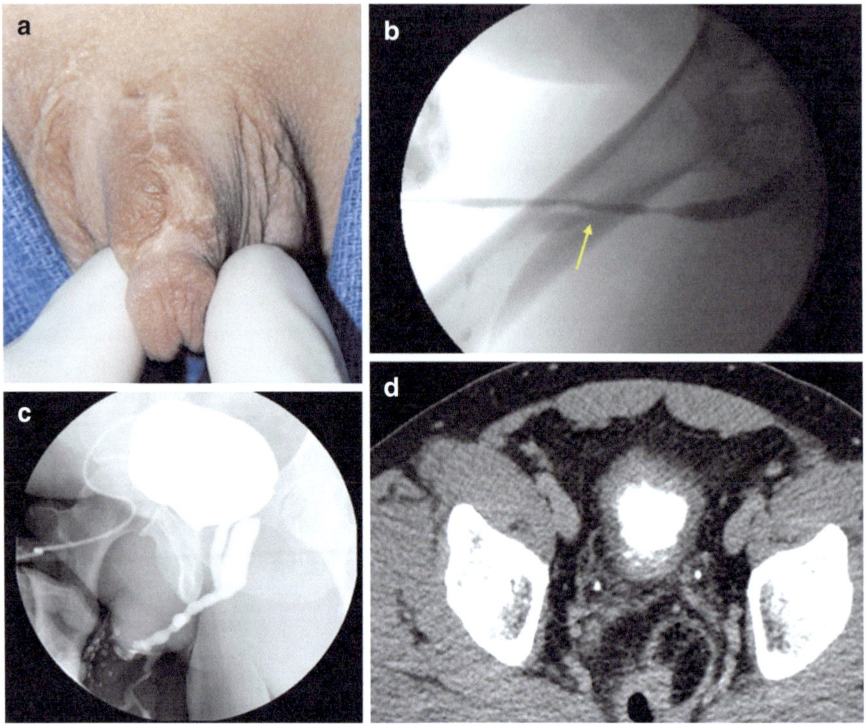

Fig. 13.1 Evaluation of any hypospadias patient should involve an assessment of penile length, glans size, and depth of glanular cleft, chordee, scarring from prior repairs, and scrotal anomalies (**a**). RUG before surgery will identify the length and caliber of strictures, associated fistulae (*yellow arrow*), as well as any concomitant strictures in the native urethra, which are common (**b**). Mostly seen in severe forms of proximal hypospadias, urogenital remnants can be a source of dribble and recurrent UTI (**c**). Co-existent bladder pathology may need to be assessed if patients have had long-standing obstruction or evidence on imaging of a thick-walled trabeculated bladder (**d**)

Cosmesis

The Penile Perception Score (PPS) was initially validated in children following hypospadias repair, but has since been expanded to the adult population [22, 23]. It is a survey to assess patient satisfaction with penile appearance, including length, skin, curvature, and urethral positioning. Generally, cosmetic satisfaction tends to be quite high in distal repairs, but as low as 11% in proximal repairs [24]. Objectively, patients with proximal hypospadias have shorter penile length and more curvature than matched controls, and PPS typically reflects this reality [25].

Chordee

Chordee must be objectively assessed in the erect state to accurately measure the maximal degree of curvature. Patients may provide photographs of their erect penis with both dorsal and lateral angles, or an erection can be induced in the office with intracavernosal injection with a vasodilatory medication, such as alprostadil. If the patient also has voiding dysfunction and is planned for surgery to address that, chordee can be assessed intraoperatively. Generally, curvature greater than 30 degrees is considered significant and more likely to impact sexual function [26]. In a study by Hoy and Rourke (2017) of adults presenting with hypospadias-related complications, 14% of adults with a history of repair report chordee, and 20% of those who underwent chordee release, suggesting that only a small percentage of patients post-repair have a significant degree of chordee that would benefit from intervention [27]. Even for chordee correction >30 degrees, it is critical to accept that straightening procedures may cause additional shortening of the phallus (and rarely surgery-associated neurological damage), so understanding the patient's bother and sexual interference is important for a shared decision-making approach to corrective surgery.

Sexual Function and Fertility

Rates of sexual dysfunction in this population range from 20.3% to 71.4% [14, 26]. Thus, these patients should be routinely screened and appropriately evaluated per guidelines. Complaints include erectile dysfunction (ED), ejaculatory dysfunction, and general sexual dissatisfaction. In a study by Gamidov et al. [14], patients with a history of hypospadias reporting an International Index of Erectile Function (IIEF) score < 16 underwent penile Doppler ultrasound, penile electromyography, and endocrine assessment. In nearly 47% of these patients, there was no organic cause for ED [14]. Higher rates of physiologic ED in this population may be due to greater corporal fibrosis and loss of elasticity, present both congenitally and inflicted from surgeries [28, 29].

Ejaculatory dysfunction includes prematurity, weak or anejaculation, pain, and postorgasmic milking of the urethra. The exact mechanism for weak ejaculation is not fully understood, but it possibly involves utricular obstruction, underdeveloped bulbospongiosus, meatal stenosis, urethral fistula, diverticulum, or sacculation [30]. In a study of men with chronic pelvic pain, painful ejaculations correlated most strongly with the inability to relax the pelvic floor [31]. Thus, patients who report painful ejaculation should be assessed for high-tone pelvic floor dysfunction. This can be done on a digital rectal exam, assessing for band-like tightness of the pelvic floor muscles and trigger points of tenderness.

As previously described, hypospadias associated with cryptorchidism is more likely associated with DSD and resulting hypofertility. However, even in isolated, nonsyndromic cases of hypospadias, oligo- or azoospermia was observed in 18.6% of young men [32]. Endocrine studies of this patient population demonstrated hypergonadotropic and hypogonadotropic hypogonadism in both mild and severe forms of hypospadias [33]. Mechanical factors, such as curvature, small phallus, and ejaculatory dysfunction, may also contribute to fertility challenges. In a population-based cohort of 1.2 million men in Sweden, hypospadias without cryptorchidism was associated with a lower paternity rate and higher use of assistive reproductive technologies [34]. Taken together, men with hypospadias should be counseled on potential challenges in conceiving and be offered timely referrals for infertility treatment if warranted.

Urinary Function

Voiding complaints and lower urinary tract symptoms (LUTS) are the chief complaint in more than half of adults with a history of hypospadias [27, 35]. Symptoms may include spraying, stranguria, or recurrent infections. There may be numerous causes, such as meatal stenosis, stricture (usually penile), urethrocutaneous fistula, urethral diverticulum, pelvic floor dysfunction, utricle enlargement/cyst, or hair/calcification in the urethra [15, 35]. Evaluation of voiding symptoms can include a patient survey such as the AUA Symptom Index, uroflowmetry, postvoid residual ultrasound, retrograde urethrogram (RUG), and selective urethroscopy (Fig. 13.1b and c). Care should be taken to use the smallest possible cystoscope, such as a 12 Fr flexible hysteroscope or a 7.5 Fr pediatric flexible cystoscope, due to the generally smaller lumen in these patients. In the event of a urethrocutaneous fistula, it is important to assess for a distal obstruction and address it concurrently with fistula repair. Spray is reported often and can be challenging to address. Spray is realized in both meatal stenosis and patulous or dehisced neo-meatus [36]. Addressing anatomic findings (stenosis or glans dehiscence) does not always improve spray and can often exacerbate the problem, so postoperative expectations should be very cautiously set. Postvoid dribbling stream, especially when more urine may be manually expressed, may be related to a urethral diverticulum, or just a lack of corpus spongiosal investment of the neourethra. Urodynamics and voiding cystourethrography studies may be indicated if there is concern for pelvic floor or bladder dysfunction after urethral causes have been assessed. Particularly in patients with long-standing obstruction or evidence of bladder wall thickening on imaging or cystoscopy, these patients may develop issues with compliance, urgency, and reflux (Fig. 13.1d). In a study of "LUTS failure" in which LUTS persisted following urethroplasty, pelvic floor dysfunction accounted for one in five cases of failure [37]. Lastly, recurrent urinary tract infections (UTIs) should be evaluated with both a RUG and cystoscope to assess for stricture and sacculation/diverticulum, but also any foreign objects such as hair or calcification.

Surgical Management

Given that most presenting symptoms requiring surgical correction in this patient population are related to urethral complications, our discussion of surgical options will focus on urethroplasty. Generally, urethral strictures in these cases occur in the penile neo-urethra (see Fig. 13.2). These are more common following preputial flaps or grafts and in more proximal repairs [36]. Due to the penile location and the complexity of these strictures, they are generally not amenable to endoscopic management such as dilation or urethrotomy. Moreover, there is evidence to suggest that endoscopic management of urethral strictures is associated with the development of ED in this patient population. In a study by Husman (2021), 100 adults with failed hypospadias repair were surveyed regarding their erectile dysfunction, and direct visual internal urethrotomy was strongly associated with ED, regardless of hypospadias severity ($p < 0.0001$) [38]. Similarly, excision and primary anastomosis (EPA) is limited due to the location of most strictures (penile urethra) and the limited elasticity of the neo-urethra.

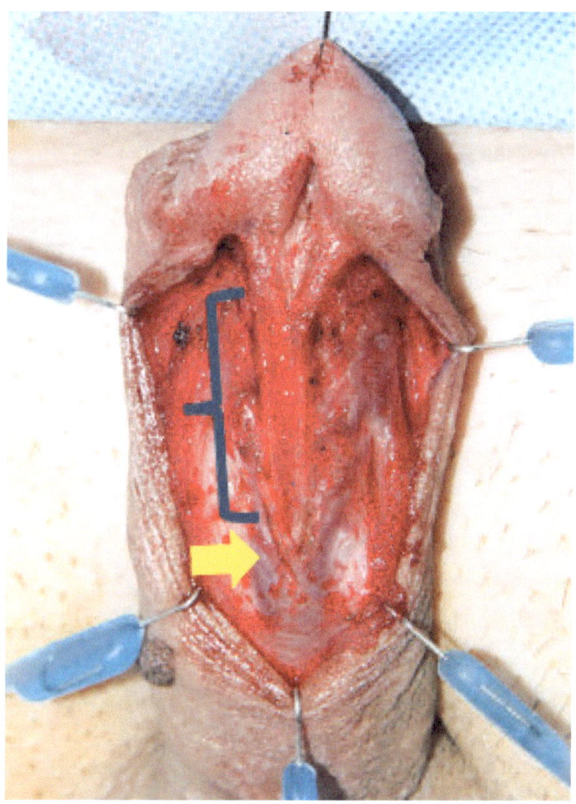

Fig. 13.2 Unrepaired hypospadias with long-segment stricture of the distal penile urethra (*blue bracket*). The corpus spongiosum can be seen terminating and diverging proximal to the segment that is strictured, which is typical of hypospadias (*yellow arrow*)

Vascular Supply

Before any surgical intervention, it is important to note the blood supply to the urethra from the internal pudendal artery, which branches into the dorsal artery and the ventral bulbourethral artery. Circumflex arteries carry blood from the dorsal artery to provide a retrograde blood flow to the urethra. In a recent study by Tsachouridis et al. (2025), the hypospadias urethral plate was found to have fewer subepithelial capillaries and smaller vascular spaces compared to normal urethral tissue [39]. Additionally, prior glansplasty may have excluded retrograde flow through the glans and corpus spongiosum. This may impact wound healing, stricture recurrence, and highlights the need to carefully preserve blood supply and avoid transecting repairs that would eliminate antegrade blood flow via the bulbar arterial supply.

One-Stage

For short (<1–2 cm), nonobliterative strictures, a one-stage dorsal onlay substitution urethroplasty may be appropriate. This is generally preferred compared to the dorsal inlay, given the narrow urethral plate [40]. Briefly, an incision is made through the stricture, extending into healthy tissue. The size of the defect is measured, and a graft is harvested from the buccal mucosa in standard fashion. The graft should be wide enough to stretch the width of the defect and be anchored to the corpora without tension [36]The graft is quilted to a healthy bed of dartos tissue over the corpora using chromic suture. A flap of dartos (if present) may be mobilized and used to cover the suture line before closure. If there is insufficient dartos for a second layer, a tunica vaginalis flap can be used (see Fig. 13.3). Typically, a catheter is left in place for around 3 weeks following a 1-stage repair. Use of prophylactic antibiotics during the postoperative period is variable. Most at least utilize antibiotics around the time of Foley catheter removal, consistent with AUA guidelines for antibiotic prophylaxis [41]. Two-Stage

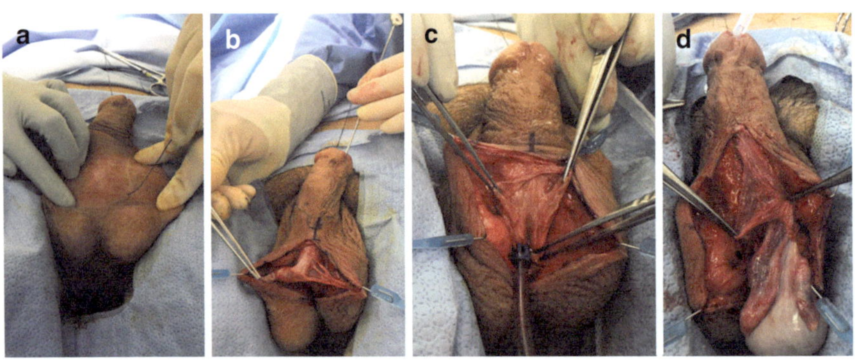

Fig. 13.3 Fistulae are a common presentation in adult life (**a** and **b**). This patient had repair of fistulae (**c**), treatment of associated stricture, and coverage with a tunica vaginalis flap (**d**), as shown

For longer (≥2 cm) and obliterative strictures, a two-stage substitution graft urethroplasty is preferred. This is the most common approach for long-segment and nearly obliterative secondary strictures in adult hypospadias. Five to six months following stage 1, stage 2 tubularization and closure may be performed. Managing obliteration and effacement of the fossa and glans can be particularly difficult. A thorough evaluation of glans size and cleft depth is essential when aiming for a terminal glanular meatus. If the glans is of adequate size and morphology, a two-stage surgical approach is often preferred in these cases. In the first stage, a deep incision is made in the glans to create a width of 2.5–3 cm, ensuring sufficient space for graft placement. An appropriate depth of incision is important for achieving an adequate glans cleft for both functional and aesthetic success. After the incision, a graft—typically buccal mucosa—is applied and allowed to take (Fig. 13.4). Five to six months following stage 1, stage 2 tubularization and closure may be performed. Management of urinary diversion for two-stage repairs is also dependent on surgeon preference. If a glansplasty is performed at the second stage with a goal of a terminal meatus in the glans, many surgeons prefer to fashion a urethral stent out of a piece of catheter and place a suprapubic tube for urinary diversion for 2–3 weeks. A stent (compared to an indwelling Foley) reduces downward pressure on the glans closure to try and prevent "unzipping" of the newly closed glans.

Perineal Urethrostomy

In severe cases, when reconstructive options may be challenging due to the length and degree of the stricture, poor graft availability, penile scarring, patient's candidacy for surgery, an anticipated need for several future endourologic procedures (i.e., recurring kidney stones), or the patient's reluctance to undergo a long course

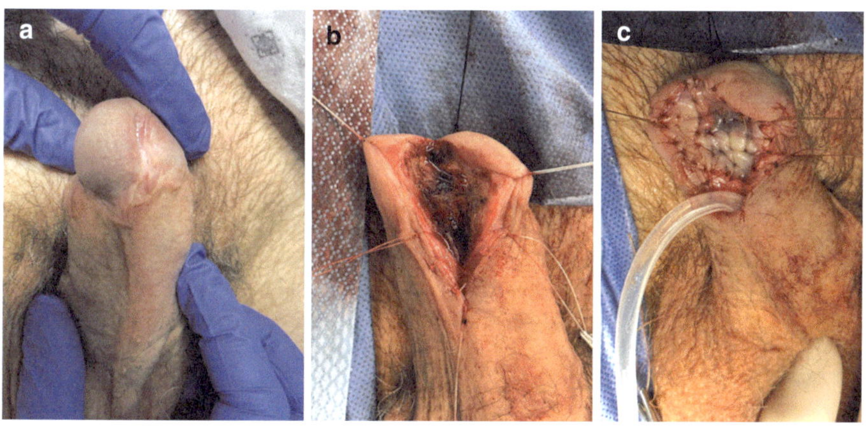

Fig. 13.4 Obliteration and effacement of the fossa and glans can be the most challenging to treat (**a**). For the two-stage approach, the glans is deeply incised to accommodate a width of 2.5–3 cm (**b**) and then grafted (**c**) to close as a second stage, 5–6 months later

for reconstruction, a perineal urethrostomy should be offered. Perineal urethrostomies are a durable treatment option associated with high rates of patient satisfaction among adults with a history of primary hypospadias repair, ranging from 84% to 92% [42–44]. When discussing these options, it is important to establish whether the patient is currently sitting to void and has ever stood to void, as a requirement to sit to void with a perineal urethrostomy can often impair patient acceptance. Many patients who are candidates for perineal urethrostomy have severe forms of hypospadias with a short phallus and have not voided in a standing position for years or decades. In these cases, even if panurethral reconstruction were feasible technically, it is unlikely that the patient would realistically void in a standing position.

Additional reconstructive options, such as the use of nonbuccal grafts, flaps, penile skin revision, and persistent chordee repair, will not be reviewed but are often utilized based on the surgeon's expertise and the specific problem the patient presents with.

Medical Trauma and Psychosocial Outcomes

The literature regarding long-term psychosocial outcomes in adults following hypospadias repair is limited and mixed. One of the earliest studies from Berg, Berg, and Svensson (1982) reported higher rates of anxiety and depression in adults with a history of repair compared to age-matched controls [45]. More contemporary studies have demonstrated mixed results, but some have noted impacts in psychosocial and psychosexual development, including higher rates of depression, anxiety, behavioral/emotional disorders, including attention-deficit hyperactivity disorder [46–49]. The number of lifetime operations for hypospadias has been associated with poorer psychosocial outcomes [50]. Due to a potentially high risk of secondary psychosocial and psychosexual problems, it is appropriate to screen for these conditions in patients presenting and possibly requiring further corrective surgeries as adults. Anecdotally, urologists who work with this patient population are familiar with the high degree of stress and anxiety that these men frequently experience in medical settings. Trauma refers to an event, series of events, or circumstances that an individual perceives as physically or emotionally harmful or life-threatening, leading to long-term negative impacts on their mental, physical, social, emotional, or spiritual well-being [51]. Unfortunately, there is a dearth of literature describing medical trauma and how it shapes patients' future experiences, as well as approaches care providers may take to minimize traumatic triggers. The Substance Abuse and Mental Health Administration (SAMHSA) presents six key principles of a trauma-informed approach: (1) safety, (2) trustworthiness and transparency, (3) peer support, (4) collaboration and mutuality, (5) empowerment, voice, and choice, (6) cultural, historical, and gender issues [51]. We present some suggestions for trauma-informed care based on our experience in Box 13.1.

Box 13.1: Expert Recommendations for Trauma-Informed Care in Patients with Early-Life Genital Surgery

1. Ask the patient about anxiety related to medical visits, procedures, and surgeries. This will not only allow you to practice more informed care but will signal to the patient your consideration of their emotional state and help develop a more trusting relationship. Establishing this dialogue will encourage the patient to raise their concerns more openly.
2. Minimize non-essential personnel in the room for exams and procedures. Do offer a chaperone for the patient for all exams.
3. Ask for verbal consent to proceed with an examination and tell the patient what you are going to do before you do it. While this may seem self-evident, this brief step may be lost in the rhythm of a busy clinic. Patients may anticipate pain and discomfort even from basic physical exams.
4. Give the patient the option of getting dressed before discussing the next steps.
5. Recognize when a patient may not be able to tolerate a procedure or exam and utilize sedation and anesthesia when needed to optimize the patient's comfort and enhance the quality of care. Normalize this experience and offer to reschedule an appointment if needed.
6. Modify your practice to meet patients where they are. From prescribing an anxiolytic for the office-based procedure, coaching the patient in adjunctive procedures (deep breathing, listening to soothing music), to performing cystoscopy in the operating room under monitored anesthesia care, there are several measures one may take to respect the patient's boundaries and psychological needs.

Changing Paradigm

Two separate population-based studies examining rates of hypospadias repair in Australia and Denmark both reported rates of about 60% for surgical management. Virtually all cases managed nonoperatively were milder distal cases [2, 52]. While such studies have not been done in the United States, fewer cases may be managed nonoperatively, given a 1.5-fold overall increase in the rate of hypospadias surgery from 1994 to 2002 [53]. There are cultural differences in the approach to hypospadias, and in the United States, the treatment of distal hypospadias has been more aggressive due to a historical and cultural assertion that cosmetic deviations from normal will negatively impact patients in the future. The evidence for long-term outcomes in adults with unrepaired hypospadias is of variable quality with mixed results. However, a systematic review including eight studies found that men with mild, uncorrected hypospadias had similar functional outcomes and attainment of psychosocial milestones compared to those who underwent surgery in infancy [54]. A prospective study by Dodds et al. (2008) identified 47 men presenting with uncorrected hypospadias, of whom nearly one-third were unaware of their condition, and none wished to undergo surgical correction [55].

In recent years, there has been a growing movement to delay surgical intervention in children with congenital anomalies of the genitalia, including DSD. While most hypospadias cases are unrelated to DSD, these cases may also represent genitalia that appear abnormal but otherwise have no functional deficits. The longstanding philosophy for surgical "correction" in these patients was that ambiguous or abnormal genitalia may cause future distress and isolation. Today, the voices of patients, providers, and caregivers question this precedent, citing concerns for bodily autonomy, psychological trauma, and physical harm [56, 57]. This debate has risen to the level of nongovernmental authorities and legislatures and has been met with varying results [58].

It remains to be seen to what degree this debate will alter patterns of care and care-seeking in the realm of hypospadias. There is some evidence to support early correction in patients with significant associated chordee [59]. For cases where chordee is minimal or none, a minimalist approach to distal hypospadias surgery may be appropriate until which time the patient has the opportunity to participate in decision-making and articulate functional or cosmetic concerns [27]. Increasing acceptance of this approach may mean that more men enter young adulthood with unrepaired hypospadias-associated complaints, which will require different surgical and medical expertise among our adult-reconstructive urologists. Ultimately, management of hypospadias at any stage should be the result of shared decision-making with the well-informed patient/parent and honest disclosure of risks. To understand these risks, hypospadiologists across the lifespan must collect and report their outcomes.

References

1. Baskin L. What is hypospadias? Clin Pediatr (Phila). 2017;56(5):409–18. https://doi.org/10.1177/0009922816684613.
2. Leunbach TL, Berglund A, Ernst A, Hvistendahl GM, Rawashdeh YF, Gravholt CH. Prevalence, incidence, and age at diagnosis of boys with hypospadias: a Nationwide population-based epidemiological study. J Urol. 2024:101097JU0000000000004319. https://doi.org/10.1097/JU.0000000000004319.
3. Yu X, Nassar N, Mastroiacovo P, et al. Hypospadias prevalence and trends in international birth defect surveillance systems, 1980–2010. Eur Urol. 2019;76(4):482–90. https://doi.org/10.1016/J.EURURO.2019.06.027.
4. Christopher J. Long MRZDAC. Hypospadias. In: Partin A, et al., editors. Campbell-Wlash-Wein urology. 12th ed. Elsevier; 2021. p. 905–48.
5. Elawad A, Haroon A, Ahmad J, et al. Megameatus intact prepuce: a systematic review of surgical techniques and long-term outcomes. Pediatr Surg Int. 2024;41(1) https://doi.org/10.1007/S00383-024-05898-4.
6. Hadidi AT. Classification and assessment of hypospadias. In: Hypospadias surgery: an illustrated textbook. 2nd ed; 2022. p. 237–48. https://doi.org/10.1007/978-3-030-94248-9_9.
7. Kolon TF, Herndon CDA, Baker LA, et al. Evaluation and treatment of cryptorchidism: AUA guideline. J Urol. 2014;192(2):337–45. https://doi.org/10.1016/J.JURO.2014.05.005.
8. Halaseh SA, Halaseh S, Ashour M. Hypospadias: a comprehensive review including its embryology, etiology and surgical techniques. Cureus. 2022;14(7) https://doi.org/10.7759/CUREUS.27544.

9. Kass E, Kogan SJ, Manley C, et al. Timing of elective surgery on the genitalia of male children with particular reference to the risks, benefits, and psychological effects of surgery and anesthesia. Pediatrics. 1996;97(4):590–4. https://doi.org/10.1542/PEDS.97.4.590.
10. Perlmutter AE, Morabito R, Tarry WF. Impact of patient age on distal hypospadias repair: a surgical perspective. Urology. 2006;68(3):648–51. https://doi.org/10.1016/J.UROLOGY.2006.03.079.
11. Lucas J, Hightower T, Weiss DA, et al. Time to complication detection after primary pediatric hypospadias repair: a large, single center, retrospective cohort analysis. J Urol. 2020;204(2):338–43. https://doi.org/10.1097/JU.0000000000000762.
12. Pohl HG, Rana S, Sprague BM, Beamer M, Rushton HG. Discrepant rates of hypospadias surgical complications: a comparison of U.S. news & world report and pediatric health information system® data and published literature. J Urol. 2020;203(3):616–22. https://doi.org/10.1097/JU.0000000000000554.
13. Kim JK, Shiff M, Chua ME, et al. Time to event analysis for post-hypospadias repair complications: a single-surgeon experience. World J Urol. 2021;39(10):3913–9. https://doi.org/10.1007/S00345-021-03689-3.
14. Gamidov S, Shatylko T, Gasanov N, et al. Sexual dysfunction in patients with late complications of hypospadias surgery. Andrologia. 2022;54(6) https://doi.org/10.1111/AND.14413.
15. Myers JB, McAninch JW, Erickson BA, Breyer BN. Treatment of adults with complications from previous hypospadias surgery. J Urol. 2012;188(2):459–63. https://doi.org/10.1016/J.JURO.2012.04.007.
16. Snodgrass W, Bush N. Do new complications develop during puberty after childhood hypospadias repair? J Urol. 2022;208(3):696–701. https://doi.org/10.1097/JU.0000000000002738.
17. Lee OT, Durbin-Johnson B, Kurzrock EA. Predictors of secondary surgery after hypospadias repair: a population based analysis of 5,000 patients. J Urol. 2013;190(1):251–6. https://doi.org/10.1016/J.JURO.2013.01.091.
18. Nguyen S, Durbin-Johnson B, Kurzrock EA. Reoperation after hypospadias repair: long-term analysis. J Urol. 2021;205(6):1778–84. https://doi.org/10.1097/JU.0000000000001569.
19. Spinoit AF, Poelaert F, Groen LA, Van Laecke E, Hoebeke P. Hypospadias repair at a tertiary care center: long-term followup is mandatory to determine the real complication rate. J Urol. 2013;189(6):2276–81. https://doi.org/10.1016/J.JURO.2012.12.100.
20. Saltzman AF, Carrasco A, Colvin A, Campbell JB, Vemulakonda VM, Wilcox D. Patients with disorders of sex development and proximal hypospadias are at high risk for reoperation. World J Urol. 2018;36(12):2051–8. https://doi.org/10.1007/S00345-018-2350-3.
21. Long CJ, Chu DI, Tenney RW, et al. Intermediate-term followup of proximal hypospadias repair reveals high complication rate. J Urol. 2017;197(3 Pt 2):852–8. https://doi.org/10.1016/J.JURO.2016.11.054.
22. Weber DM, Landolt MA, Gobet R, Kalisch M, Greeff NK. The penile perception score: an instrument enabling evaluation by surgeons and patient self-assessment after hypospadias repair. J Urol. 2013;189(1):189–93. https://doi.org/10.1016/J.JURO.2012.08.178.
23. Weber DM, Schönbucher VB, Landolt MA, Gobet R. The pediatric penile perception score: an instrument for patient self-assessment and surgeon evaluation after hypospadias repair. J Urol. 2008;180(3):1080–4. https://doi.org/10.1016/J.JURO.2008.05.060.
24. Chertin B, Natsheh A, Ben-Zion I, et al. Objective and subjective sexual outcomes in adult patients after hypospadias repair performed in childhood. J Urol. 2013;190(4 Suppl):1556–60. https://doi.org/10.1016/J.JURO.2012.12.104.
25. Örtqvist L, Fossum M, Andersson M, et al. Long-term followup of men born with hypospadias: urological and cosmetic results. J Urol. 2015;193(3):975–82. https://doi.org/10.1016/J.JURO.2014.09.103.
26. Tack LJW, Springer A, Riedl S, et al. Adolescent and young adult urogenital outcome following childhood hypospadias repair: perfection revisited. J Urol. 2021;206(3):734–44. https://doi.org/10.1097/JU.0000000000001869.

27. Hoy NY, Rourke KF. Better defining the spectrum of adult hypospadias: examining the effect of childhood surgery on adult presentation. Urology. 2017;99:281–6. https://doi.org/10.1016/J.UROLOGY.2016.07.057.
28. Camoglio FS, Bruno C, Zambaldo S, Zampieri N. Hypospadias anatomy: elastosonographic evaluation of the normal and hypospadic penis. J Pediatr Urol. 2016;12(4):199.e1–5. https://doi.org/10.1016/J.JPUROL.2016.02.007.
29. Zhang JJ, Qiao XH, Gao F, et al. A new method of measuring the stiffness of corpus cavernosum penis with ShearWave™ Elastography. Br J Radiol. 2015;88(1048) https://doi.org/10.1259/BJR.20140671.
30. Rynja SP, De Jong TPVM, Bosch JLHR, De Kort LMO. Functional, cosmetic and psychosexual results in adult men who underwent hypospadias correction in childhood. J Pediatr Urol. 2011;7(5):504–15. https://doi.org/10.1016/J.JPUROL.2011.02.008.
31. Yani MS, Eckel SP, Kirages DJ, Rodriguez LV, Corcos DM, Kutch JJ. Impaired ability to relax pelvic floor muscles in men with chronic prostatitis/chronic pelvic pain syndrome. Phys Ther. 2022;102(7) https://doi.org/10.1093/PTJ/PZAC059.
32. Tack LJW, Spinoit AF, Hoebeke P, et al. Endocrine outcome and seminal parameters in young adult men born with hypospadias: a cross-sectional cohort study. EBioMedicine. 2022:81. https://doi.org/10.1016/J.EBIOM.2022.104119.
33. Moriya K, Mitsui T, Tanaka H, Nakamura M, Nonomura K. Long-term outcome of pituitary-gonadal axis and gonadal growth in patients with hypospadias at puberty. J Urol. 2010;184(4 Suppl):1610–4. https://doi.org/10.1016/J.JURO.2010.04.022.
34. Skarin Nordenvall A, Chen Q, Norrby C, et al. Fertility in adult men born with hypospadias: a nationwide register-based cohort study on birthrates, the use of assisted reproductive technologies and infertility. Andrology. 2020;8(2):372–80. https://doi.org/10.1111/ANDR.12723.
35. Morrison CD, Cinà DP, Gonzalez CM, Hofer MD. Surgical approaches and long-term outcomes in adults with complex reoperative hypospadias repair. J Urol. 2018;199(5):1296–301. https://doi.org/10.1016/J.JURO.2017.11.078.
36. Snodgrass WT, Bush NC. Management of urethral strictures after hypospadias repair. Urol Clin North Am. 2017;44(1):105–11. https://doi.org/10.1016/J.UCL.2016.08.014.
37. Chapman DW, Bekkema J, Rourke K. Urinary symptom nonresponse ("LUTS failure") after urethroplasty: incidence and associations. J Urol. 2021;206(4):986–92. https://doi.org/10.1097/JU.0000000000001840.
38. Husmann DA. Erectile dysfunction in patients undergoing multiple attempts at hypospadias repair: etiologies and concerns. J Pediatr Urol. 2021;17(2):166.e1–7. https://doi.org/10.1016/j.jpurol.2020.12.002.
39. Tsachouridis G, Liu X, de Bakker B, Nijman R, de Kort L, de Graaf P. Microscopic and molecular analysis of the urethral plate: a step towards improved hypospadias surgery outcomes. Urology. 2025; https://doi.org/10.1016/J.UROLOGY.2025.01.062.
40. Marshall SD, Raup VT, Brandes SB. Dorsal inlay buccal mucosal graft (Asopa) urethroplasty for anterior urethral stricture. Transl Androl Urol. 2015;4(1):10. https://doi.org/10.3978/J.ISSN.2223-4683.2015.01.05.
41. Lightner D, Wymer K, Sanchez J, Kavoussi L. Best practice statement on urologic procedures and antimicrobial prophylaxis. J Urol. 2020;(203):351. Accessed April 8, 2025. https://www.auanet.org/guidelines-and-quality/quality-and-measurement/quality-improvement/clinical-consensus-statement-and-quality-improvement-issue-brief-(ccs-and-qiib)/urologic-procedures-and-antimicrobial-prophylaxis-(2019)
42. Shinchi M, Horiguch A, Ojima K, et al. Evaluation of the efficacy of perineal urethrostomy for patients with anterior urethral stricture: insights from surgical and patient-reported outcomes. World J Urol. 2021;39(12):4443–8. https://doi.org/10.1007/S00345-021-03795-2.
43. Horiguchi A, Asanuma H, Shinchi M, et al. Efficacy of urethral reconstruction for urethral stricture associated with hypospadias surgery in adults. Int J Urol. 2022;29(12):1470–5. https://doi.org/10.1111/IJU.15015.

44. Joshi EG, VanDyke ME, Langford BT, Franzen BP, Morey AF. Algorithmic midline approach to perineal urethrostomy is associated with long-term success and high patient satisfaction. Urology. 2024;190:133–9. https://doi.org/10.1016/J.UROLOGY.2024.03.016.
45. Berg R, Berg G, Svensson J. Penile malformation and mental health. A controlled psychiatric study of men operated for hypospadias in childhood. Acta Psychiatr Scand. 1982;66(5):398–416. https://doi.org/10.1111/J.1600-0447.1982.TB06721.X.
46. Jin T, Wu W, Shen M, et al. Hypospadias and increased risk for psychiatric symptoms in both childhood and adolescence: a literature review. Front Psych. 2022:13. https://doi.org/10.3389/FPSYT.2022.799335.
47. Gulseth E, Urdal A, Andersen MH, et al. Mental health and health-related quality of life in adolescents surgically treated for hypospadias in childhood. J Pediatr Urol. 2024; https://doi.org/10.1016/J.JPUROL.2024.09.031.
48. Gunawan IPGF, Abbas T, Situmorang GR, et al. Self-reported outcomes in adults with hypospadias: a meta-analysis of patient satisfaction and quality-of-life metrics. J Pediatr Urol. 2025; https://doi.org/10.1016/J.JPUROL.2025.01.004.
49. Örtqvist L, Engberg H, Strandqvist A, et al. Psychiatric symptoms in men with hypospadias—preliminary results of a cross-sectional cohort study. Acta Paediatr. 2019;108(6):1156–62. https://doi.org/10.1111/APA.14658.
50. Tack LJW, Springer A, Riedl S, et al. Psychosexual outcome, sexual function, and long-term satisfaction of adolescent and young adult men after childhood hypospadias repair. J Sex Med. 2020;17(9):1665–75. https://doi.org/10.1016/J.JSXM.2020.04.002.
51. Williams HN, Farley B. Trauma-informed care. Semin Pediatr Neurol. 2024;50:101139. https://doi.org/10.1016/J.SPEN.2024.101139.
52. Schneuer FJ, Holland AJA, Pereira G, Bower C, Nassar N. Prevalence, repairs and complications of hypospadias: an Australian population-based study. Arch Dis Child. 2015;100(11):1038–43. https://doi.org/10.1136/ARCHDISCHILD-2015-308809.
53. Pohl HG, Joyce GF, Wise M, Cilento BG. Cryptorchidism and hypospadias. J Urol. 2007;177(5):1646–51. https://doi.org/10.1016/J.JURO.2007.01.058.
54. Bohane E, Murphy M, Chierigo F, et al. Long term outcomes from uncorrected hypospadias: a scoping review. Actas Urol Esp. 2025;49(1):1–10. https://doi.org/10.1016/J.ACUROE.2024.10.004.
55. Dodds PR, Batter SJ, Shield DE, Serels SR, Garafalo FA, Maloney PK. Adaptation of adults to uncorrected hypospadias. Urology. 2008;71(4):682–5. https://doi.org/10.1016/J.UROLOGY.2007.07.078.
56. Grimstad F, Kremen J, Streed CG, Dalke KB. The health care of adults with differences in sex development or intersex traits is changing: time to prepare clinicians and health systems. LGBT Health. 2021;8(7):439–43. https://doi.org/10.1089/LGBT.2021.0018.
57. Wiesemann C, Ude-Koeller S, Sinnecker GHG, Thyen U. Ethical principles and recommendations for the medical management of differences of sex development (DSD)/intersex in children and adolescents. Eur J Pediatr. 2010;169(6):671–9. https://doi.org/10.1007/S00431-009-1086-X.
58. Mulkey N, Streed CG, Chubak BM. A call to update standard of care for children with differences in sex development. AMA J Ethics. 2021;23(7):E550–6. https://doi.org/10.1001/AMAJETHICS.2021.550.
59. Schlomer B, Breyer B, Copp H, Baskin L, Disandro M. Do adult men with untreated hypospadias have adverse outcomes? A pilot study using a social media advertised survey. J Pediatr Urol. 2014;10(4):672–9. https://doi.org/10.1016/J.JPUROL.2014.01.024.

Varicoceles and Undescended Testicles in the Adolescent and Young Adult Population

14

Samuel R. Donnenfeld, Akanksha Mehta, and Gabreilla J. Avellino

Key Points

1. Varicoceles are a clinical diagnosis based only upon physical examination of a patient in the standing and recumbent position, with and without Valsalva.
2. While there are many approaches to surgical treatment of a varicocele, subinguinal microscopic varicocelectomy has the lowest rates of complications and recurrence.
3. Intervening on testicles with ipsilateral hypotrophy and a varicocele has been shown to improve semen parameters, paternity, as well as serum testosterone.
4. For undescended, entrapped, or ascended testicles in the adult population, orchiectomy is the preferred approach; however, orchiopexy remains a viable alternative.
5. Surgical or procedural treatment of a varicocele for infertility should be considered in patients with abnormal semen analyses, but not for azoospermic patients.

Introduction

Varicoceles have been diagnosed and treated since antiquity. First described in *De Medici* by the Philosopher Celsus in the first century CE, varicocele management has remained nuanced. Many varicoceles are observed for years by pediatric urologists without repair before transitioning to an adult clinician. The workup, natural history, indications for treatment, fertility considerations, complications, and

S. R. Donnenfeld (✉) · G. J. Avellino
Brown University Division of Urology, Providence, RI, USA

A. Mehta
Emory University Department of Urology, Atlanta, GA, USA
e-mail: akansha.mehta@emory.edu

H.-Y. Wu et al. (eds.), *Pediatric Urology for the Adult Urologist*,
https://doi.org/10.1007/978-3-032-10306-2_14

relevant management approaches of a varicocele in a pediatric patient transitioning to an adult provider will be reviewed here. The index patient reviewed will be a late adolescent to early adult male with a known varicocele, mild associated pain, and interest in future fertility without immediate plans to conceive. The chapter will conclude with a brief description of the management of an undescended testicle in the postpubertal patient.

Natural History

Varicoceles are defined by the abnormal dilation and tortuosity of the internal spermatic veins of the pampiniform plexus of the scrotum. They are more commonly left-sided as testicular venous drainage is different between sides. The right gonadal vein drains into the inferior vena cava (IVC), and the left gonadal vein drains into the left renal vein. There is increased venous pressure in the left renal vein as compared to the IVC, which can lead to increased pressure and venous congestion in the left gonadal vein. This can subsequently lead to venous valvular incompetence on the ipsilateral side of the pampiniform plexus, creating a varicocele. While the true adult prevalence is not clear and data are primarily based on fertility studies, varicoceles occur in approximately 10–15% of the pediatric population [1]. Varicoceles tend to be diagnosed after 10 years of age as testicular blood flow increases [2]. Higher varicocele prevalence is also observed in first-degree relatives, such as brothers of patients diagnosed with varicoceles [3]. Across all age groups, only 2–10% of patients with varicoceles present with pain as the main symptom prompting evaluation, as the majority are asymptomatic [4].

Workup

Few guidelines from the American Urological Association (AUA) exist on the management and diagnostic workup of varicoceles. Varicoceles are a clinical diagnosis based upon physical examination. The current grading scale, penned by Dubin and Amelar in 1970, remains the foremost grading scale for varicoceles. This defines varicoceles as small (grade 1), medium (grade 2), and large (grade 3) by physical exam [5]. Due to the widespread availability of ultrasound, there also exists another category of Grade 0 or "subclinical varicocele," which can only be seen on ultrasound of the scrotum but not felt or seen on physical exam, and has no clinical significance.

The grading of a varicocele on physical examination requires visual examination of the scrotum and palpation of the spermatic cords to feel for the dilatation of veins if not visible. The initial examination is performed with the patient in the standing position. Small varicoceles are only palpable in the standing position with the accompanied Valsalva. Moderate varicoceles can be palpated without Valsalva in the standing position. Large varicoceles are visible in the scrotum without palpation and do not reduce when lying down.

Laterality is important as there may be consideration of retroperitoneal pathology underlying cases of an isolated right varicocele. While small case series have shown isolated right-sided varicoceles to be the presenting symptom of adrenal or renal pathology, the largest study of cancer risk and varicocele laterality reported no difference in cancer diagnosis based on laterality of varicocele [6, 7]. Abdominal imaging is more often performed following the diagnosis of a right varicocele compared to the left, without a significantly increased rate of cancer detection [8]. The AUA does not recommend routine abdominal imaging for isolated small or moderate right-sided varicoceles, but does advise further workup in isolated large right-sided varicoceles at the discretion of the clinician. In general, imaging is not needed to diagnose a varicocele, as it is a diagnosis based on physical exam. Scrotal ultrasound, thermography, radionuclide scanning, and spermatic venography should also not be used for the detection of subclinical varicocele in a patient without a palpable varicocele, as they provide little to no clinical significance [9].

When counseling patients and their families, it is important to discuss fertility, as the pediatric or young adult patient may not be actively trying to conceive or family planning, such as in our index patient. While fixing clinically significant varicoceles can improve semen analysis parameters in adults, the presence of a varicocele in childhood may not be a reliable indicator of future fertility. One study published in 2007 by Diamond et al. found no difference in any semen analysis parameters between any grade of varicocele in adolescent patients [10]. Mori et al., however, determined that sperm concentrations were lower in patients with grade 2 or 3 varicoceles than without a varicocele or with a grade 1 on presentation. The population with a grade 1 or no varicocele had an average total motile sperm concentration of 134.1 million, while grades 2 and 3 had 72.7 and 30.3 million, respectively [11]. No long-term follow-up information pertaining to fertility was available for this patient cohort.

All patients transitioning to an adult provider with varicoceles should be offered a baseline semen analysis and can be monitored every 1–2 years at the discretion of the urologist, along with shared decision-making with the patient [12]. Other objective measurements, including sizing of testicles and asymmetry from the contralateral side, should be recorded per AUA guidelines. Varicocele repair may be considered if there are abnormal semen analyses or testicular sizes. Patients should be counseled that data does exist to show that varicoceles over time can contribute to progressively worsening semen analysis measurements and are a known cause of secondary infertility [13, 14].

Testicular Asymmetry

Testicular sizing is an important data point to trend in the workup of pediatric patients with a varicocele transitioning to an adult provider. A pediatric patient or a young adult may present with testicular hypotrophy. There is debate over the most accurate way to measure a testicle. Ideally, a practitioner is consistent with trending this data point, no matter what method is utilized. While there is no established size discrepancy between testicles prompting urologists to intervene, a 20% size discrepancy is often quoted as being significant [10, 15]. European Association of Urology (EAU) guidelines state in adolescents surgery may be offered for varicoceles associated with a persistent small testis using a size difference of greater than 2 ml or 20% with the caveat that measurements should be confirmed on two subsequent visits performed six months apart.

It has been shown that testicles do not grow symmetrically, and therefore, sequential measurements at two points in time are important to determine the presence or absence of testicular atrophy in children [16]. In a 2018 study of 539 adolescent boys ages 11–16 to assess the presence of normal testicular volumes without varicoceles or other pathology, a very large discrepancy was noted in Tanner 3 boys with testicular volumes ranging from 2 to 23 ml. This wide range in the nonvaricocele population has prompted many pediatric urologists to wait on offering varicocelectomy until Tanner 4 or 5 stages, at which point they are more likely to begin seeing an adult provider [17]. Catch-up growth after varicocele repair may be up to 70% in patients in their early 20 s after surgical varicocelectomy [18].

Methods to size testicles include the orchidometer, physical exam via palpation, or ultrasound examination. The percent asymmetry between the sizes can then be calculated. Measurements are fraught with variability. A significant difference ($p < 0.001$) with an interobserver error of 16% was found in estimating testicular size in 23 young men in a study published in 2000 using a Prader orchidometer. The difference in the estimate tended to be greater with increasing testicular size [19]. The two accepted formulas can be found below and often yield different numerical values.

$$\%\text{asymmetry} = \left[\left(\text{vol right}\left(\text{cc}\right) - \text{vol left}\left(\text{cc}\right)\right) / \text{vol right}\left(\text{cc}\right)\right] \times 100$$

$$\%\text{asymmetry} = \left[\left(\text{vol right} - \text{vol left}\right) / \left(\text{vol right} + \text{vol left}\right)\right] \times 100$$

Infertility Indications

Patients presenting with both infertility (defined as 12 months without conception despite regular intercourse with a female partner under 35 years old) and findings of a varicocele are not addressed in this chapter. Still, fertility status should always be clarified. This chapter focuses on patients found to have a varicocele and not currently trying to conceive, but potentially interested in future biological children. The American Society for Reproductive Medicine (ASRM) practice committee, along with the AUA, advises that treatment of a varicocele should be considered in men attempting to conceive who have palpable varicocele(s), infertility, and abnormal semen parameters, except for azoospermic men [20]. The AUA also advises that varicocelectomy should not be considered for azoospermic males as it provides little to no therapeutic value.

Intervening on testicles with ipsilateral hypotrophy and a varicocele has been shown to improve semen parameters, paternity, as well as serum testosterone. In a nonrandomized prospective study of 110 Tanner V boys with at least a 2 ml or 20% difference in testicular size with ipsilateral varicocele in the smaller testicle, semen parameters improved with surgical intervention, but more importantly, so did paternity on 5-year follow-up. Forty-four percent (31/70 boys) of the boys at the 5-year follow-up period who chose to undergo varicocele repair were married, with a paternity rate of 80% (25/31). Amongst those who chose to observe their varicocele at the same 5-year follow-up, 58% (22/40 boys) were married, with a paternity rate of 36% (8/22). Mean years to conception after marriage were 1.5 years for the operative group and 3.5 years for the nonoperative group. While not all were actively trying to conceive, a certain limitation of the study, the two groups present age-matched cohorts and similar populations. At 5-year follow-up for those who had varicocelectomy, serum testosterone also increased from 240 ng/dl to 808 ng/dl (236.66%), while amongst the observation group, there was an increase from 230 ng/dl to 280 ng/dl only (21.74%). The observation group average remained below the 300 ng/dl cutoff for normal serum testosterone recognized by the AUA in adults [21].

Our index patient is not trying to conceive, and thus, counseling regarding a potentially prophylactic surgery is nuanced but can be of importance to the patient or their families. When discussing infertility and varicoceles amongst young adult males, there are several studies which exist to help counsel about future fertility in the setting of a varicocele. Cayan et al. in 2017 studied a nonrandomized cohort of 408 boys in a single center with palpable varicoceles followed for 16 years. Of this group, a larger proportion who underwent microsurgical varicocelectomy were fertile (77.3% vs. 48.4%) with shorter times to conception (11 vs. 17 months) [22]. Clinicians must balance the operative morbidity of an outpatient procedure when counseling patients about varicocelectomy, especially in patients who are not actively attempting to conceive. It is not clear who benefits from prophylactic repair of their varicocele, as men diagnosed with a varicocele in childhood can still conceive without undergoing varicocele repair. In one small study of 13 men with normal baseline semen analysis values and varicoceles, semen parameters were shown to progressively decline over time [23]. Other studies, however, show no such decline, indicating a need for further research in this area. Currently, there is no definitive benefit to early vs. delayed operative intervention on varicoceles when couples are attempting to conceive if they experience infertility [4].

Pain

Scrotal or testicular pain is a common ailment seen by urologists. The presence of a varicocele does not necessarily mean it is the cause of a patient's pain. The grade of varicocele, the nature and duration of pain, body mass index, prior conservative management, and the type of surgical method used are predictors for the success of varicocelectomy when treating pain. Testicular pain associated with a varicocele is typically a dull aching pain that worsens with long periods of standing, exercise, or activity. When elucidating the cause of the pain, it is paramount to discuss aggravating and alleviating factors with an emphasis on urinary habits, bowel movements, associated symptoms, and sexual and physical activities.

It is important to reiterate that the diagnosis of a varicocele remains a physical exam finding, and imaging plays no role in diagnosis. Other conditions causing testicular pain include, but are not limited to, space-occupying tumors, epididymo-orchitis, spermatoceles, and hydroceles. Iatrogenic injury following vasectomy or hernia repair may trigger postprocedural testicular pain. Referred pain from a variety of causes, such as a ureteral stone and the presence of an inguinal hernia, should also be considered in the differential diagnosis of orchialgia or scrotal pain. Importantly, the presence of a varicocele does not automatically rule out these other causes of scrotal pain.

Conservative management remains a cornerstone of treatment for symptomatic varicoceles. A period of observation allows for other subclinical causes of pain to resolve themselves, such as minor trauma or strained groin muscles. Nonoperative treatments, including scrotal elevation, topical or oral nonsteroidal anti-inflammatory agents, and rest from exertional activities, can help alleviate pain associated with varicoceles. Insufficient evidence and few studies exist at this time for the long-term efficacy of acupuncture and acupressure for the treatment of pain associated with a varicocele; however, it remains a low-risk intervention for interested patients. Typically, a period of nonsurgical management should be recommended before operative intervention when the indication is for pain alone and not infertility or size discrepancy. Once conservative options are exhausted, embolization and operative intervention can be safe and effective forms of managing pain associated with varicoceles and will be discussed below.

Conservative management of painful varicoceles causes complete resolution of symptoms in only 4.2–15.2% of cases [24]. The goal of conservative management through the use of warm baths, rest, nonsteroidal anti-inflammatory drugs (NSAIDs), and supportive underwear is to eliminate the need for surgery and not necessarily for complete resolution of symptoms. NSAIDs should be prescribed with appropriate precautions. Still, this can spare the patient from the risks of embolization or surgery. Data varies widely on the amount of pain relieved by nonoperative measures. Pain resolution or mitigation, however, is typically higher when more invasive measures are taken. Kim et al. in 2012 found that of 81 patients who underwent microsurgical varicocelectomy, 58 patients (71.6%) experienced a complete resolution of pain postoperatively, and 16 patients (19.7%) experienced partial resolution. Seven patients (8.6%) experienced no change [25]. Rates of pain relief following embolization are similar. In a 2015 study of 96 varicoceles managed with embolization, 71 patients (74%) had reduced pain, and 28 (30%) had complete resolution of pain; a larger proportion, 23 patients (24%), had no change in symptoms.

Operative Intervention and Embolization

Different operative approaches exist for the treatment of varicoceles, namely, conventional open varicocelectomy (the Palomo technique), laparoscopic varicocelectomy, inguinal, and subinguinal microsurgical varicocelectomy. Other techniques, such as robotic-assisted varicocelectomy and the subinguinal nonmagnified approach, are rarely performed. Another option is percutaneous embolization of scrotal varices, typically performed by interventional radiology. Operative procedures are performed under spinal or general anesthesia, while embolization can be done with moderate sedation.

Conventional open varicocelectomy is done through several different types of abdominal incisions to expose the spermatic vessels at various levels. Typically, the incision is medial and inferior to the ipsilateral anterior superior iliac spine and extends medially. The internal spermatic vessels proximal to the internal inguinal ring are thereby exposed and ligated in the retroperitoneum. Complications, occurring at a rate of 5–30%, include hydroceles, inadvertent arterial ligation, testicular atrophy, injury to the vas deferens, epididymo-orchitis, hematoma, and wound infection. The recurrence or persistence rate, at 10–45%, is also significantly higher than other treatment approaches [26].

In the United States, though several operative methods are utilized, varicocelectomy is dominated by the inguinal nonmicroscopic approach. In an insurance claims review published in 2021, a total of 261,785 subjects were diagnosed with varicocele from 2007 to 2014. Of these, 19,800 (7.6%) underwent varicocelectomy. Inguinal, abdominal, laparoscopic, microsurgery, and embolization surgery were performed in 66%, 19%, 10%, 3%, and 2%, respectively, as initial treatment [27]. Rates vary, however, across the globe. In Germany, for instance, laparoscopic ligation accounts for the majority of cases at 45% [28]. AUA guidelines do not comment on the most appropriate operative technique for varicocelectomy; however, subinguinal microscopic varicocelectomy has been shown to be the safest and most effective approach and will be discussed later in the chapter.

Laparoscopic varicocelectomy is a commonly performed procedure. Typically a transperitoneal procedure, it has also been described with a retroperitoneoscopic approach. Ligation with this approach occurs at or above the level of the internal inguinal ring. Special attention must be taken to avoid injury to the vas deferens, which can be incorporated into the ligation if not identified and spared. The persistence or recurrence rate for laparoscopic varicocelectomy is between 6% and15% [29]. Operative complications occur in 8–12% of the laparoscopic cases, including genitofemoral nerve injury with paresthesias, inadvertent testicular arterial ligation, peritonitis, and intestinal injury. Hydroceles secondary to lymphatic congestion after accidental ligation of the lymphatic vessels can be as high as 40% [30]. While lymphatic sparing laparoscopic varicocelectomy using 10–20× magnification was originally described in 1999, it is technically more difficult and has had little adoption with the advent of the subinguinal microscopic varicocelectomy. Hydrocele rates are significantly lessened with the laparoscopic lymphatic sparing approach when compared to the nonlymphatic sparing laparoscopic approach, but do not limit potential complications of an intraperitoneal procedure [31].

Subinguinal microscopic varicocelectomy remains the gold standard in the treatment of scrotal varices with the lowest pain, recurrence, and complication rates. Performed through a subinguinal incision, this approach allows exposure of the spermatic cord without splitting abdominal musculature or fascia, resulting in less postoperative pain. Injury to the vas deferens and vasal artery is low, reported in 1% of cases [32]. Recurrence rates for the microsurgical subinguinal approach are noted in the literature to be between 0.9% and 2.5% [33], significantly lower than other approaches. A meta-analysis in 2015 showed that hydrocele rates following surgery are also lowest in the subinguinal approach [34]. These factors, when taken together, have led to the increasing adoption of the microsurgical technique in recent years.

Finally, sclerotherapy or embolization remains an option via percutaneous access by Interventional Radiology, typically performed under conscious sedation. In one prospective study of 697 patients, postoperative complications developed in 35 patients (5%), and failure to collapse the varicocele occurred in 63 (9%). Failure rates were similar for different grades and sides, but notably, operator experience played a large role in mitigating recurrence of varicoceles, indicating a steep learning curve for interventional radiologists [35].

There are multiple methods of embolization that can be used by interventional radiologists. While femoral and subclavian vein access are options, the procedure is typically done by accessing the right internal jugular vein, as this provides the easiest access to both the left and right gonadal veins. Options for embolization include mechanical agents (plugs, metallic coils), sclerosants, liquid embolic agents, as well as combinations of the three. There is similar efficacy between the agents utilized [36]. Risks of embolization include postprocedure back pain and hydrocele, which is reported in up to 10% of patients. More serious but rare complications include coil migration to the heart and pulmonary vessels, vessel perforation, and off-target embolization, which can result in testicular infarction [37]. Radiological embolization is typically chosen for recurrent or persistent varicoceles after surgical varicocelectomy, as it avoids the need for repeat surgery.

Conclusions

Diagnosis, counseling, and management of varicoceles requires a multifaceted approach by both pediatric and adult urologists. In patients with clinically relevant varicoceles, physical exam remains the hallmark of diagnosis. Indications for treatment include progressive declines in semen analysis parameters, subfertility, testicular hypotrophy, testicular size discrepancy, cosmetic appearance of visibly engorged veins, or pain. When counseling patients, it is important to consider the morbidities associated with treatment versus a trial of conservative management. Consideration for referral to a microscopic or infertility-trained urologist when transitioning a patient from a pediatric urologist for continued care is important when considering operative intervention or surveillance.

The Undescended Testicle

The undescended testicle is a common condition encountered by pediatric urologists, with an incidence rate of 3% [38]. While most undescended testicles will spontaneously descend by 3 months of age, a persistent undescended testicle increases the risks of testicular malignancy, torsion, and ipsilateral inguinal hernia [38]. Any patient with a history of undescended testicles transitioning care from a pediatric to adult provider should be examined to identify the location, consistency, size, and mobility of one or both testicles.

The AUA recommends that an orchiopexy for a persistent or cryptorchid testicle be performed by 18 months of age [39]. Retractile testicles, which can be maneuvered and then remain in the scrotum during physical exam, are not considered undescended and do not require surgical intervention. For the pediatric patient transitioning to the adult provider, it is important to monitor for an ascending or entrapped testicle, i.e., a testicle that had been at the level of the scrotum but has climbed into or above the inguinal canal. While ascending testicles occur spontaneously, entrapment occurs after another inguinal surgery, such as inguinal hernia repairs. Hernia repair closure can include the spermatic cord, dragging the testicle upward.

In postpubertal patients with undescended testicles for any reason, orchiectomy versus orchiopexy remains an option, with orchiectomy being the preferred management per AUA guidelines. AUA guidelines state that a biopsy can be performed on these testicles at the time of surgery to help determine the correct course of surgical action if a normal contralateral testicle is present; however, the utility of testicular biopsy is not proven. Furthermore, providers should counsel all patients about the underlying risks of infertility and cancer should the testicles be left in place. An undescended testicle in the postpubertal male has a four- to sixfoldincreased cancer risk. If an undescended testicle cannot be monitored for malignancy due to location on physical examination, or if it becomes painful, orchiectomy vs. orchiopexy remains a viable option. While orchiopexy before puberty diminishes cancer risk from a four- to sixfold increase to two- to three times more likely than controls, the rate remains higher than average, and regular self-examination is strongly recommended [40]. Patients with unilateral cryptorchidism typically do not have significantly diminished fertility or hormonal derangements [41]. This is distinct from bilaterally undescended testicles, which have a roughly six times greater risk of experiencing infertility, and 50% of such patients have been shown to have decreased sperm concentrations [42]. An epidemiological study published in 2005 found amongst all patients diagnosed with bilaterally cryptorchid testicles, fertility was found to be 65% compared to 89.7% amongst the unilaterally cryptorchid patients, and 93.2% of men in the control group [43].

In conclusion, while orchiopexy remains an option in the young adult and adolescent population, orchiectomy remains the preferred approach when the contralateral testis is normal. It is important to recognize and differentiate the undescended testicle from other similar diagnoses, such as ascended, entrapped, or retractile testicles. Counseling remains very important with risks of higher malignancy potential not just in the cryptorchid testis but also in the contralateral descended testicle following orchiectomy [44]. As long as a unilaterally undescended testicle does not ascend postpuberty or become entrapped by another procedure, fertility and hormonal parameters should be significantly less impacted than in bilateral undescended testicle cases.

References

1. Akbay E, Cayan S, Doruk E, et al. The prevalence of varicocele and varicocele-related testicular atrophy in Turkish children and adolescents. BJU Int. 2000;86:490–3.
2. Paduch DA, Skoog SJ. Diagnosis, evaluation and treatment of adolescent varicocele. Sci World J. 2004;4(suppl. 1):263–78.
3. De Los Reyes T, Locke J, Afshar K. Varicoceles in the pediatric population: diagnosis, treatment, and outcomes. Can Urol Assoc J. 2017;11(1–2 Suppl 1):S34–9. https://doi.org/10.5489/cuaj.4340.
4. Paick S, Choi WS. Varicocele and testicular pain: a review. World J Mens Health. 2019;37(1):4–11.
5. Diagnosis of clinical and subclinical varicocele: how has it evolved?. ResearchGate. https://www.researchgate.net/figure/Dubin-and-Amelar-varicocele-grading-system_tbl1_284195735.
6. Spittel JA Jr, Deweerd JH, Shick RM. Acute varicocele: a vascular clue to renal tumor. Proc Staff Meet Mayo Clin. 1959;34:134.
7. Cheungpasitporn W, Horne JM, Howarth CB. Adrenocortical carcinoma presenting as varicocele and renal vein thrombosis: a case report. J Med Case Rep. 2011;5:337.
8. Elmer DeWitt M, Greene DJ, Gill B, et al. Isolated right varicocele and incidence of associated cancer. Urology. 2018;117:82.
9. Practice Committee of the American Society for Reproductive Medicine; Society for Male Reproduction and Urology. Report on varicocele and infertility: a committee opinion. Fertil Steril. 2014;102(6):1556–60.
10. Diamond DA, et al. Relationship of varicocele grade and testicular hypotrophy to semen parameters in adolescents. J Urol. 2007;178:1584–8. https://doi.org/10.1016/j.juro.2007.03.169.
11. Mori MM. Does varicocele grade determine extent of alteration to spermatogenesis in adolescents? Fertil Steril. 2008;90:1769–73.
12. Arow JP, Sharlip ID, Belker AM, Lipshultz LI, Sigman M, Thomas AJ, Schlegel PN, Howards SS, Nehra A, Damewood MD, Overstreet JW, Sadovsky R. Best practice policies for male infertility. J Urol. 2002:2138–44. https://doi.org/10.1097/00005392-200205000-00052.
13. Witt MA, Lipshultz LI. Varicocele: a progressive or static lesion? Urology. 1993;42(5):541–3. https://doi.org/10.1016/0090-4295(93)90268-F.
14. Gorelick JI, Goldstein M. Loss of fertility in men with varicocele. Fertil Steril. 1993;59(3):613–6.
15. Franco A, Proietti F, Palombi V, et al. Varicocele: to treat or not to treat? J Clin Med. 2023;12(12):4062. https://doi.org/10.3390/jcm12124062.
16. Minhas S, et al. European association of urology guidelines on male sexual and reproductive health: 2025 update on male infertility. Eur Urol. 2025;87(5):601–16.
17. Vaganée D, Daems F, Aerts W, Dewaide R, van den Keybus T, De Baets K, De Wachter S, De Win G. Testicular asymmetry in healthy adolescent boys. BJU Int. 2018;122(4):654–66. https://doi.org/10.1111/bju.14174. Epub 2018 Mar 23

18. DeCastro GJ, et al. Adolescent varicocelectomy—is the potential for catch-up growth related to age and/or tanner stage? J Urol. 2009;181(1):322–7. https://doi.org/10.1016/j.juro.2008.09.037.
19. Carlsen E, et al. Int J Androl. 2000;23(4):248–53. https://doi.org/10.1046/j.1365-2605.2000.00240.x.
20. Brannigan RE, Hermanson L, Kaczmarek J, et al. Updates to male infertility: AUA/ASRM guideline (2024). J Urol. 2024;
21. Patil N, Javali T. Varicocelectomy in adolescents—does it safeguard future fertility? A single centre experience. J Pediatr Urol. 2022;18(1):5.e1.
22. Çayan S, et al. Paternity rates and time to conception in adolescents with varicocele undergoing microsurgical varicocele repair vs observation only: a single institution experience with 408 patients. J Urol. 2017;198(1):195–201. https://doi.org/10.1016/j.juro.2017.01.066.
23. Chehval MJ, Purcell MH. Deterioration of semen parameters over time in men with untreated varicocele: evidence of progressive testicular damage. Fertil Steril. 1992;57(1):174–7. https://doi.org/10.1016/s0015-0282(16)54796-7.
24. Jarow JP, Coburn M, Sigman M. Incidence of varicoceles in men with primary and secondary infertility. Urology. 1996;47:73.
25. Kim S-O, Jung H, Park K. Outcomes of microsurgical subinguinal varicocelectomy for painful varicoceles. J Androl. 2012;33(5):872–5.
26. Szabo R, Kessler R. Hydrocele following internal spermatic vein ligation: a retrospective study and review of the literature. J Urol. 1984;132:924–5.
27. Park HK, et al. Practice pattern of redo varicocelectomy for recurrent varicocele according to type of initial treatment. World J Mens Health. 2021;
28. Aksoy C, et al. Trends for surgical treatment of testicular varicocele: a German whole-population analysis of inpatient procedures from 2006 to 2021. Eur Urol Open Sci. 2025;75:29.
29. Abdulmaaboud MR, et al. Treatment of varicocele: a comparative study of conventional open surgery, percutaneous retrograde sclerotherapy, and laparoscopy. Urology. 1998;52:294–300.
30. Hassan JM, et al. Hydrocele formation following laparoscopic varicocelectomy. J Urol. 2006;175:1076–9.
31. Kocvara R, Dvorácek J, Sedlácek J, Díte Z, Novák K. Lymphatic sparing laparoscopic varicocelectomy: a microsurgical repair. J Urol. 2005;173(5):1751–4. https://doi.org/10.1097/01.ju.0000154357.72837.43.
32. Chan PT, Wright EJ, Goldstein M. Incidence and postoperative outcomes of accidental ligation of the testicular artery during microsurgical varicocelectomy. J Urol. 2005;173:482–4.
33. Shiraishi K, Oka S, Ito H, Matsuyama H. Comparison of the results and complications of retroperitoneal, microsurgical subinguinal, and high inguinal approaches in the treatment of varicoceles. J Androl. 2012;33:1387–93.
34. Wang J, et al. Inguinal and subinguinal micro-varicocelectomy, the optimal surgical management of varicocele: a meta-analysis. Asian J Androl. 2015;17:74.
35. Galfano A, Novara G, et al. Surgical outcomes after modified antegrade scrotal sclerotherapy: a prospective analysis of 700 consecutive patients with idiopathic varicocele. J Urol. 2008;179(5):1933–7. https://doi.org/10.1016/j.juro.2008.01.042.
36. Favard N, et al. Comparison of three different embolic materials for varicocele embolization: retrospective study of tolerance, radiation and recurrence rate. Quant Imaging Med Surg. 2015;5:806.
37. Neves da Silva HV, et al. Varicoceles: overview of treatment from a radiologic and surgical perspective. Semin Interv Radiol. 2022;39:490.
38. Leslie SW, Sajjad H, Villanueva CA. Cryptorchidism. In: StatPearls, updated 5 May 2024. StatPearls Publishing; 2025. https://www.ncbi.nlm.nih.gov/books/NBK470270/.

39. Kolon TF, Herndon CDA, Baker LA, Baskin LS, Baxter CG, Cheng EY, et al. Evaluation and treatment of cryptorchidism: AUA guideline. J Urol [Internet]. 2014 [cited 2025 Jun 5];192(2):337–45. Available from: https://doi.org/10.1016/j.juro.2014.05.005.
40. Wood HM, Elder JS. Cryptorchidism and testicular cancer: separating fact from fiction. J Urol. 2009;181:452.
41. Rusnack SL, et al. Testis histopathology in boys with cryptorchidism correlates with future fertility potential. J Urol. 2003;169:659.
42. Fawzy F, Hussein A, Eid MM, et al. Cryptorchidism and fertility. Clin Med Insights Reprod Health. 2015;9:39–43. https://doi.org/10.4137/CMRH.S25056.
43. Lee PA. Fertility after cryptorchidism: epidemiology and other outcome studies. Urology. 2005;66(2):427–31.
44. Akre O, Pettersson A, Richiardi L. Risk of contralateral testicular cancer among men with unilaterally undescended testis: a meta-analysis. Int J Cancer. 2009;124:687.

Sexual and Fertility Education

15

Jacob Hartman-Kenzler and William T. Berg

Introduction

Fertility and sexual development are subjects that many patients and clinicians struggle to discuss for several cultural, social, and medical reasons. These complex discussions are made much more nuanced when introducing parent/child dynamics into the conversation. This chapter will serve as an overview of common fertility and sexual developmental concerns for patients from the neonatal stage through adolescence, as well as indications for corrective surgery and reproductive tissue collection and preservation.

As a society and as clinicians, there are commonly accepted definitions regarding sexual development and nomenclature. These definitions do not always align with one another, and understanding of what is "normal" vs. "abnormal" and what should or need to be treated can be difficult to communicate to patients. In this chapter, we include many definitions and labels for gender and sex, which are commonly held in the medical community. However, we recognize that these definitions are constantly changing and being updated to encompass an evolution of societal norms. Furthermore, they may not align with an individual patient's experience. To this end, we attempt to provide a broad understanding of sexual and fertility education in the pediatric population.

J. Hartman-Kenzler · W. T. Berg (✉)
Renaissance School of Medicine at Stony Brook University, Stony Brook, NY, USA
e-mail: jacob.hartman-kenzler@stonybrookmedicine.edu

H.-Y. Wu et al. (eds.), *Pediatric Urology for the Adult Urologist*,
https://doi.org/10.1007/978-3-032-10306-2_15

Developmental Milestones in Sexual and Reproductive Health

There are many ways to divide sexual development in children and adolescents; however, for this chapter, we will focus on anatomical sexual development. Along with anatomic development is the development of gender identity and sexual orientation, which can be influenced by multiple factors, including assigned gender and sex, cultural upbringing, socioeconomic status, and general regional social factors. This figures heavily in discussions surrounding fertility and fertility.

Sexual development is a complex process based on hormonal changes, which typically occurs in the teen years and is associated with puberty. These hormonal changes are mediated by the hypothalamic-pituitary-gonadal (HPG) axis. The first changes are triggered by a pulsatile release of gonadotropin-releasing hormone (GnRH), which leads to the release of luteinizing hormone (LH) and follicle-stimulating hormone (FSH). LH acts on the ovaries (Theca cells) and testicles (Leydig cells) to stimulate the release of estrogens and androgens, as well as to initiate gametogenesis. FSH stimulates the ovarian follicle to produce estrogen and Sertoli cells to support the production of sperm. Subsequently, the rise in estrogen and testosterone facilitates further external anatomic development of breasts and adult male genitalia. The adrenal glands also contribute to the formation of secondary sex characteristics, especially the development of pubic and axillary hair (pubarche). This may coincide with HPG axis maturation; however, pubarche itself is not the best indicator of pubertal development.

When evaluating a new patient for stage of sexual development, a common tool is the Tanner staging system, which is determined by progression of pubic hair growth, breast development (female) (Fig. 15.1a), and testicular size (male) (Fig. 15.1b). It is important to note that the Tanner staging system is quite simplified, and there may be significant variation based on sex, race, ethnicity, environmental factors, and hormone sensitivity.

Normal onset of puberty for females in the United States is 8–13 years old, with white females averaging 10 years and black females averaging 8.9 years old. Thelarche is the development of breast buds and represents entry to Tanner stage 2. Breast tissue grows through pubarche (development of pubic and axillary hair) about 1–1.5 years later. Menarche, the onset of menses, begins at approximately 12.5 years old, about 2.5 years after thelarche. The onset of puberty in males ranges from 9 to 14 years of age and begins with the secondary sexual characteristic of gonadarche (increasing testicular volume). Testicular volume greater than or equal to 4 mL (or long axis greater than or equal to 2.5 cm) indicates Tanner stage 2. Development during Tanner Stage 3 involves increased height velocity. Spermarche is sperm development, and typically occurs during Tanner Stage 4 [2].

While sexual development is highly variable, there are a few commonly accepted norms to keep in mind when evaluating patients. Precocious puberty is defined as puberty occurring before 8 years of age in girls and 9 in boys. Delayed puberty is commonly self-resolving; however, hormonal imbalances such as hypogonadism must be ruled out. Before pursuing any hormone or genetic profile analysis, it is recommended to consult with a pediatric endocrinologist to coordinate care.

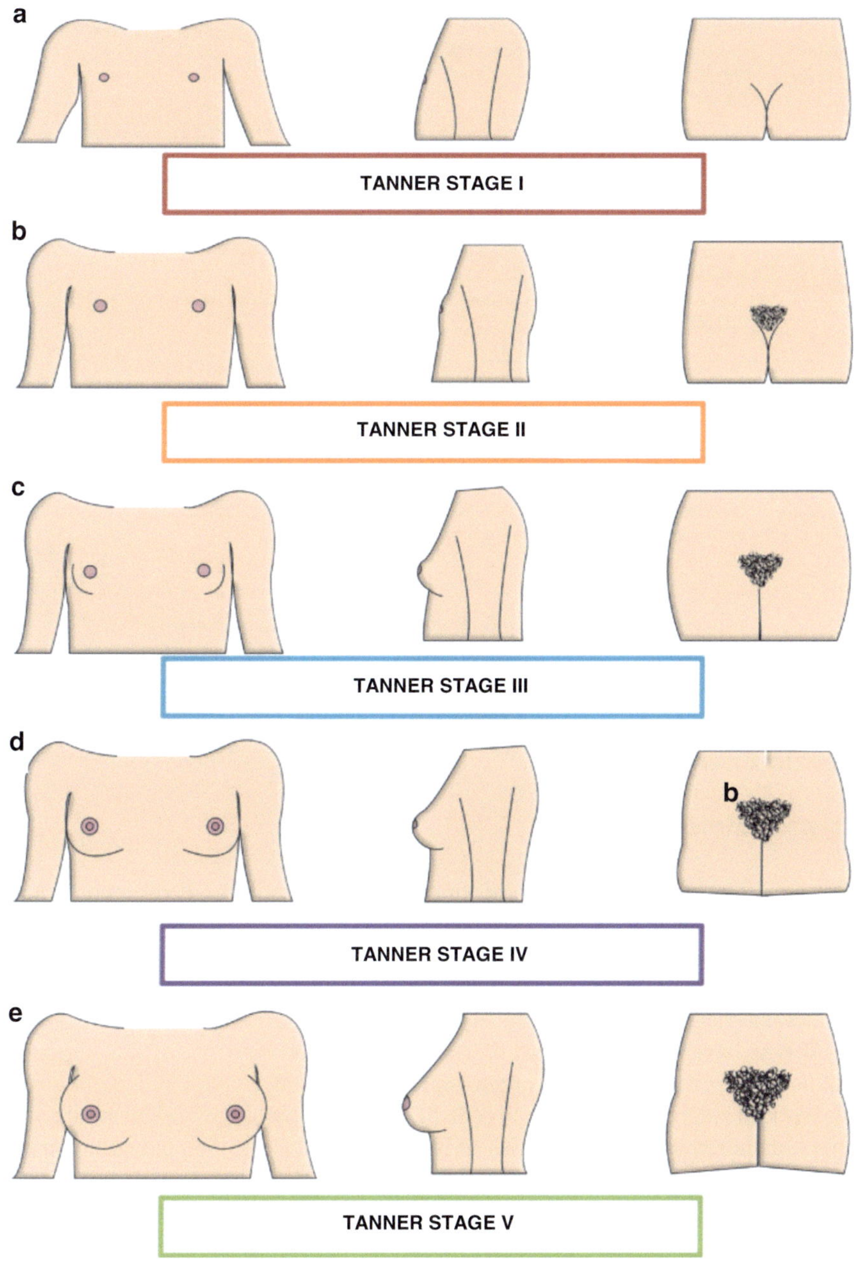

Fig. 15.1 (**a**) Tanner staging tables, female. (https://media.springernature.com/lw685/springer-static/image/chp%3A10.1007%2F978-3-030-49984-6_3/MediaObjects/493040_1_En_3_Fig1_HTML.png). (**b**) Tanner staging tables, male. [1]. (https://media.springernature.com/lw685/springer-static/image/chp%3A10.1007%2F978-3-030-94248-9_12/MediaObjects/510035_2_En_12_Fig7_HTML.jpg)

Stage 1 G1	Preadolescent: testes, scrotum, and penis are about the same size in proportion as in early childhood, Testicular volume < 4 ml or long axis < 2.5 cm
Stage 2 G2	Enlargement of scrotum and of testes. The skin of the scrotum thickens without enlargement of penis, testicular volume 4 ml-8 ml (or 2.5 to 3.3 cm long), 1st pubertal sign in males
Stage 3 G3	Penile enlargement starts. Further growth of testes and scrotum, testicular volume 9 ml-12 ml (or 3.4 to 4.0 cm long)
Stage 4 G4	Increased size of penis, with growth of glans. There is further enlargement of testes and scrotum, testicular volume 15-20 ml (or 4.1 to 4.5 cm long)
Stage 5 G5	Genitalia are adult in size and shape, testicular volume > 20 ml (or > 4.5 cm long)

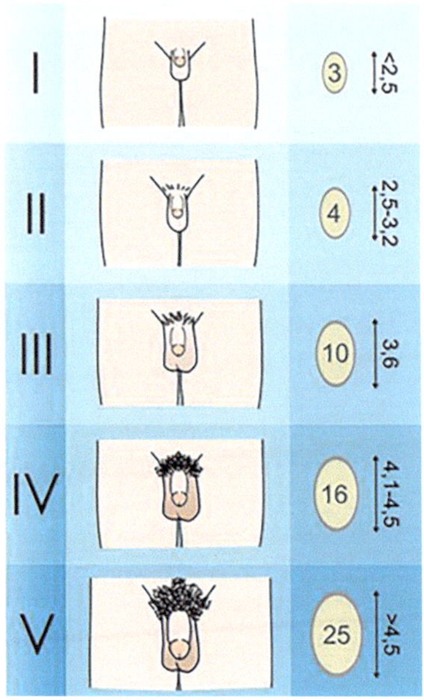

Fig. 15.1 (continued)

Pediatric Urologic Conditions Affecting Sexual and Fertility Development and Health

Cryptorchidism

Testes may be undescended at birth or become acquired; this is different from a retractile testis, which can be manipulated into the scrotum manually and remain there transiently with cremasteric muscle fatigue. Acquired undescended testes may be idiopathic (prior retractile testis), but may also be iatrogenic if there is a history of inguinal hernia repair causing entrapment. Unilateral cryptorchidism is very unlikely to have a negative effect on fertility, and there is no evidence to support a lasting effect on fertility after orchiopexy [3]. Bilateral cryptorchidism, however, has reduced paternity rates of up to 65% [4]. In boys with successful bilateral orchiopexy, there remains a 20–25% risk of infertility. The connection between cryptorchidism and cancer is also significant when counseling patients regarding this condition. This is beyond the scope of this chapter.

Testicular Torsion

Testicular torsion is a twisting of the spermatic cord resulting in the absence of oxygenated blood flow to the testicle. Torsion occurs most commonly in either the neonatal period or during puberty. While fertility is often preserved with one functional testicle, the contralateral testicle is also at risk of torsion in the future. While some studies have demonstrated decreased sperm counts and motility after testicular torsion, longer-term studies have failed to demonstrate a significant impact on overall fertility [5].

Varicocele

A varicocele is an aberrant dilation of the pampiniform venous plexus of the testicle. The fertility implications of varicocele are discussed in Chap. 14.

Hypospadias

Hypospadias is discussed more in depth in Chap. 13; however, we will give a short overview for the purposes of fertility and sexual development discussion.

Fertility is primarily affected by the degree of hypospadias, with a more proximal urethral opening having a more negative effect on fertility. Distal and supracoronal hypospadias may have minimal effect on future fertility; however, the relationship between paternity and the degree of hypospadias is difficult to correlate. Large population-based studies have been performed showing at least some level of negative effect regardless of the degree of hypospadias, although these studies are hindered by a lack of standardization for hypospadias classification. Large-scale studies have shown that men with hypospadias tend to have lower birth rates and are more likely to rely on assisted reproductive technologies. While men who underwent distal hypospadias repairs generally exhibit normal semen quality, those with proximal repairs often have lower sperm concentration and motility. Furthermore, the prevalence of ejaculatory disorders in men with proximal hypospadias remains unknown and likely depends on individual postoperative complications [6].

Sexual dysfunction in individuals with hypospadias is most often linked to the degree of chordee and the specific surgical repair methods used. Although studies have shown that men who underwent hypospadias repair tend to have shorter penile length compared to those without the condition, self-reported surveys indicate no significant differences in sexual satisfaction or libido [7].

Cloacal Malformations

Cloacal malformations include a wide range of presentations, and most often are diagnosed first by identifying an imperforate anus or urinary tract/rectal fistulas. It is important to note that they may be associated with several of the other congenital conditions discussed, including vaginal septae and uterine/vaginal duplication. They may also be associated with long-term bladder dysfunction and spinal cord anomalies. Regarding fertility, concerns surround the internal Müllerian structure duplication in girls, which can lead to hydrocolpos. The obstruction and collection can be secondary to the congenital condition itself or an iatrogenic stricture from prior surgery. This may be associated with pain, obstructive uropathy, infection, and infertility. Typical treatment for hydrocolpos is a drainage procedure.

Exstrophy

This is discussed in Chap. 18.

Transgender Considerations

Standards of care are ever-changing for pediatric transgender patients and are often subject to extensive political and societal pressures. It is the current recommendation to offer fertility preservation to any patient undergoing any gender affirming therapy that may have an impact on future fertility, such as gonadectomy [8]. These conversations should be approached with open consideration to a patient's preference as to their gender assigned at birth, biological sex, and overall fertility desires. These conversations are complex, and the discussion should be framed in the context of preservation for a future decision as an adult.

Fertility Preservation in Pediatric Urology

Fertility preservation may be pursued in pediatric populations whenever an individual's fertility may be put at risk. Fertility risks include congenital etiologies discussed in this chapter, as well as iatrogenic causes, typically related to cancer treatments (discussed in a separate chapter). Principles of counseling apply similarly in both scenarios, as do options for fertility preservation techniques. For prepubertal patients, testicular tissue preservation is an option; however, this is currently experimental and should only be offered in a clinical trial or research setting. Prepubertal oocyte freezing is more established and should be considered when possible. Below is a brief overview of options for fertility preservation in postpubescent minors.

Sperm Cryopreservation

Sperm cryopreservation may be pursued under several circumstances, most commonly before treatment for testicular cancer or exposure to systemic therapies for other cancers. Other possible reasons include hormone or surgical therapies for gender affirming care. Postpubertal males who are capable of ejaculation may provide sperm for storage, which is the simplest way of preserving future fertility. Discussions surrounding this cryopreservation are nuanced and depend heavily on the age and understanding of the patient and parents. It is important to have separate discussions with the patient outside of parental supervision when applicable. If the patient cannot ejaculate or is too young, sperm extraction via testicular sperm extraction can be done with their assent and parental consent. Prepubertal testicular tissue cryopreservation is currently considered experimental but may be an option in the future outside of research settings.

Oocyte Cryopreservation

For fertility preservation in females, the primary option is to undergo ovarian stimulation and oocyte retrieval with subsequent cryopreservation. Oocyte cryopreservation has made recent strides in efficacy. With modern cryopreservation techniques, there is a high rate of oocyte survival after thaw. Mature oocyte cryopreservation in postpubertal females is ideal. Ovarian tissue banking is now recognized as a valid and established method of fertility preservation in prepubertal girls and is no longer classified as experimental. It is currently the only option available for preserving fertility in prepubertal girls, as they are not candidates for ovarian stimulation. Cortical ovarian tissue is cryopreserved after obtaining the tissue via surgical extraction. When fertility is desired, the cryopreserved tissue is then orthotopically transplanted. There have been over 100 reported live births following orthotopic transplantation of previously cryopreserved and thawed ovarian tissue [9].

Teaching Sexual and Reproductive Health

Armed with knowledge and data, the importance of effective communication is not to be downplayed. A key part of addressing sexual and reproductive health in the pediatric population is developing strategies on how to interact and discuss fertility and sexuality with children, adolescents, teenagers, and their parents and guardians in an appropriate way. Tailoring a discussion must consider a child's developmental stage, as well as an understanding of parents' and guardians' ethical and cultural background. Clinicians play a critical role in creating a safe, inclusive, and informative environment.

In young children, the focus of any conversation should be on correct anatomical terms, body autonomy, and discussions around privacy and consent. As children approach and enter puberty, topics should include expected physical changes, relationships, gender identity, and sexual orientation. A conversation around menstruation, erections, and emotional changes should be had while normalizing curiosity and providing fact-based answers. A nonjudgmental approach is paramount. While discussions regarding gender identity are currently popular within the media, rates of gender dysphoria are low. Ensuring that a clinician provides a welcoming atmosphere and opportunities for open dialogue can help foster trust and understanding. The use of open-ended questions can help assess a child's knowledge, values, and concerns. Adolescents and teenagers benefit from confidential and private discussions about sexual behavior, contraception, sexually transmitted infection prevention, and development of healthy relationships [10].

Discussions about sexuality and fertility can be challenging for adolescents, regardless of specific age or gender. They may be uncomfortable raising these topics without direct prompting. The use of health checklists and screening questionnaires can facilitate discussion of sexuality and fertility and other potentially sensitive topics. It is important not to miss the opportunity to have these conversations. When done properly, effective discussions of sexuality can change the way adolescents view and approach sexual discussions with their health care provider. Physicians must be proactive in addressing sexuality issues with adolescents and cannot assume that adolescents will initiate discussions [11]. These discussions can, and should, be incorporated into regular yearly well-child visits with the pediatrician. Initiation of the discussion should not add significant time to the visit. If complex issues arise, we recommend a separate visit be scheduled so that more time is available so as not to rush the conversation. If the discussion ranges outside the scope of practice of general pediatrics or delves into an area unknown to the practitioner, referral can be made to a specialist in sexual medicine. Fellowship-trained sexual medicine practitioners have advanced training and are sometimes more comfortable discussing topics. Rarely, a referral to a therapist is needed, unless there are concerns regarding significant conflicts of sexual identity or paraphilias. If such a referral is needed, the consultant should be experienced with adolescents or sexual therapy.

Parents and guardians play a pivotal role in shaping a child's worldview, and sexuality and reproduction are directly influenced by this. Clinicians should start by validating parental concerns and providing reassurance that early and accurate education is the best support for safe behaviors. Furthermore, anticipatory guidance around normalization of sexual development and encouraging open communication at home provides a safe and supportive environment for the child and adolescent. Early on, before adolescence, clinicians should clarify the importance of confidential practices that create an environment of trust while respecting legal and ethical boundaries [12]. Cultural and ethical considerations should be focused on respecting family values and religious beliefs while ensuring that all youth, including those with disabilities, receive nonjudgmental and inclusive care. The phrase, culturally responsive care, is very relevant in this setting. The clinician should recognize the influence of external/environmental factors that influence personal beliefs and adapt their communication style accordingly. This includes addressing misconceptions and possible resistance to evidence-based information. One must recognize the wide variability in beliefs around sexuality, fertility, gender roles, and the appropriate timing of sexual education. Avoid assumptions and ask families about their values and preferences. Sometimes this conversation may include navigating conflicts between the adolescents' viewpoints and/or rights and parental authority.

Providers are encouraged to self-reflect on their own attitudes and biases, use clear language, and offer opportunities for youth to speak privately, especially regarding issues of abuse, consent, or identity. Having these conversations early and often normalizes the discussion and helps to reduce stigma to support healthy sexual development. Clinicians can frame the discussion around hypothetical scenarios or use indirect language. If uncertainty about an answer arises, being honest about one's limits and providing transparency can help to build trust. Additionally, when communicating complex topics, visual aids and printed resources have been found to help increase comprehension.

Teaching Sexual and Reproductive Health in Special Populations: Exstrophy-Epispadias Complex, Spina Bifida, and Hypospadias

Spina Bifida

Patients with spina bifida have varying anatomic and functional limitations affecting sexual function in adulthood. As patients age, it is important to have candid and informed conversations when counseling to establish reasonable expectations. While sexual satisfaction is lowered in this patient population, sexual desire is less impacted. Over half of adults with spina bifida are sexually active [13]. Unfortunately, research in this area is generally limited by small group size, heterogeneity, and poorly validated questionnaires.

Primary issues with sexual function concern the ability to achieve orgasm and genital sensation [14]. In general, men with intact sacral reflexes or lower spinal lesions will have better overall function. Between 56% and 96% of men will be able to achieve an erection, although this may not be sufficient for penetrative intercourse [15]. Between 20% and 67% will achieve orgasm, while 50–88% will ejaculate, although it often either lacks velocity, is retrograde, or insensate [15]. Treatment with phosphodiesterase-5 inhibitors (PDE5i) is generally safe in sexually active patients of any age. Doses of all strengths are well tolerated with few and often nonsignificant side effects. Alternatives to medication include the use of vibratory devices to induce reflexive erections. Medical-grade devices exist, but are usually not covered by insurance and can be cost-prohibitive. Nonmedical grade devices are easily available and may perform equally as well. High-frequency devices should be recommended as these appear to function better [16].

Research is less available in women; however, they may experience decreased arousal, difficulty achieving orgasm, and dyspareunia secondary to poor vaginal lubrication. Beyond direct effects on sexual function, patients may have a range of physical limitations that may need to be addressed. Some patients may also suffer from bladder and bowel incontinence, which is a bothersome side effect of spina bifida on sexual function and intercourse. Artificial lubrication can be very helpful in improving sexual satisfaction. Vaginal estrogen can also be beneficial if atrophy is present. Positioning during sexual activity can also be a challenge. Open and honest discussions can be constructive.

As in the broader population, spina bifida patients will have different degrees of sexual desire and expectations depending on the type of intercourse they wish to pursue. While these conversations may be awkward or uncomfortable at the beginning, it is important to establish what level of sexual function a patient is seeking.

Counseling can then be tailored to a patient's specific sensory and anatomical limitations. Patients should be counseled on the availability of sexual positioning aids, such as wedges, pillows, and ramps.

Bladder Exstrophy-Epispadias Complex

Bladder exstrophy and epispadias are some of the most complex conditions treated by pediatric urologists and often require multiple procedures from the postnatal period to young adulthood to improve urinary and sexual function. This can lead to psychological distress later in life when patients may wish to pursue sexual activity with a partner. While there is some evidence that there is little difference in sexual satisfaction between these patients and age-matched controls, research in this area is limited by small sample size, single institutions, and older patient data that may not reflect the most current surgical practices [17]. Beyond sexual function, there is a paucity of data on fertility for this patient population.

In men, bladder exstrophy can be accompanied by many penile and lower urinary tract malformations, including epispadias, dorsal chordee, urethral pathologies, and iatrogenic complications. While erectile function is relatively well preserved, many adult men may be unhappy with the cosmetic appearance of their genitals, which may contribute to sexual dissatisfaction. There is also limited data on ejaculatory function, although many of these patients are able to achieve erections sufficient for penetrative intercourse and masturbation [17, 18]. Mental health counseling and therapy may be useful in this population, as male patients may suffer from concerns regarding penile size and appearance. Postpubertal or adult reconstruction can sometimes be helpful, but there are few procedures available to provide changes in penile girth or length. If chordee is recognized as limiting sexual satisfaction or causing painful intercourse, this can be evaluated in the office through intracavernous injection and induced erection for surgical planning. Penile plication should take into account possible further shortening, and grafting may be necessary to achieve an acceptable penile length. Patients should be educated on the possibilities of decreased sensation or erectile dysfunction postoperatively.

Women with bladder exstrophy suffer from numerous anatomical variations that may impair sexual function. These variations involve both internal and external structures. At birth, there may be defects in the lower anterior abdominal wall, genital tubercles, and pubic rami. The internal genitalia may be anteriorly displaced, with the vagina having a more horizontal axis and the cervix entering the vagina close to the introitus. The pubic bones are separated (diastasis) and the pelvic muscles diverge anteriorly, providing less support to the pelvic floor, which leads to a predisposition to pelvic organ prolapse. Before surgical repair, the clitoris is bifid, the labia majora are anteriorly positioned without superior fusion, and the vaginal introitus is narrow [19]. These anomalies and the subsequent surgical correction can lead to significant differences in the appearance and function of sexual organs in adulthood. This has been shown to have a severe psychological impact. The most common issues include narrow vaginal introitus and pelvic organ prolapse. Many patients will seek surgical correction in adulthood to facilitate penetrative intercourse [19]. Similar to men, dialectical behavior therapy (DBT) may be beneficial. DBT is a type of cognitive behavior therapy that helps people understand how their thoughts impact their emotions and behaviors. The word "dialectical" refers to holding onto opposing ideas within your mind at the same time. It involves accepting reality and one's behaviors while learning to change one's unhelpful behaviors and thoughts. Patients should also be counseled on the importance of lubrication. Vaginal dilators may be employed to assist with providing for pain-free penetrative intercourse.

The degree of sexual satisfaction and impairment is heavily dictated by the severity of presentation and outcomes of surgical interventions. For both male and female patients, the most difficult aspect of sexuality appears to be the psychosocial effects of aberrant external anatomy; however, there may also be impaired sensation and function in more severe cases. Furthermore, patients can be educated on strategies to disclose their condition to their partners. Referral to a sexual therapist can also guide patients on nonpenetrative sexual intimacy.

Hypospadias

While hypospadias-related concerns are addressed earlier in this chapter, this section will elaborate on how to counsel and educate patients specifically. Discussions regarding sexual function must start early to normalize and explain possible anatomical differences from peers. Patients should be encouraged to ask questions about their bodies and express curiosity. It is paramount that patients be educated on why surgery was needed and how their condition by impact future issues of ejaculation and erections. There may be concerns regarding perceived small size, evidence of scars/scarring, and residual chordee. Again, most men report adequate erections, and most men are satisfied with their appearance. Again, emphasis on early disclosure can be helpful with acceptance. Concerns may arise in men who were not informed regarding their condition. In a meta-analysis, 88% of patients reported normal erectile function, and 84% of patients are satisfied with their sexual function overall [20]. As with general counseling for all sexual function, parents and guardians can be included in early age discussions, but should transition to confidential counseling as the child matures. Patients should be followed into adulthood and have regular assessments of sexual function, activity, confidence, and relationships. Off-label use of PDE5i is safe in teenage patients who may suffer from mild erectile dysfunction or to build confidence in situations of performance anxiety. Healthcare practitioners may collaborate with psychologists, therapists, or sexual health counselors to provide support, especially during transitional stages such as puberty or entry into romantic relationships. Promoting a positive, affirming approach to genital diversity is crucial for improving psychosexual well-being.

Differences of Sexual Development

Recommendations for sexual education in patients with DSD are very similar to the considerations listed in the sections above. Emphasis is on correct, neutral anatomical terms (e.g., "penis," "vulva," "scrotum," etc.), including discussion of their variation, and should avoid labeling genitals as "boy parts" or "girl parts." Counseling should encompass that bodies can be different and that these differences are normal. Clinicians may reinforce that there are many ways to be male, female, or something in between. If surgeries were performed, information should include age-appropriate discussion of how these might impact sensation, function, and future sexual experiences. A multi-disciplinary approach, including endocrinologists, psychologists, and surgeons, is beneficial.

Conclusion

Understanding and addressing fertility and sexual development in pediatric patients requires not only clinical knowledge but also sensitivity to cultural and social norms. Effective communication with both patients and their families is essential, particularly when navigating evolving definitions of sex, gender, and normal developmental variation. As this chapter highlights, management of this topic is wide-ranging and includes understanding surgical treatments as well as a broad understanding of sexual development and fertility preservation. The emphasis should be on providing individualized treatment plans, meeting the patient and parent or guardian where they are at, while remaining flexible and informed as societal customs shift and as language around sexuality and fertility evolves. Ultimately, a patient-centered, developmentally appropriate, and inclusive approach fosters trust and promotes better health outcomes for children and adolescents.

Key Points

- Sexual education in pediatric and adolescent patients should incorporate clear, age-appropriate explanations about development, sexual maturity, and include normalization of variation in genital appearance.
- Self-perception of genital appearance and body image significantly influences sexual satisfaction and psychosexual development. Education and counseling should occur early and often
- Sexual education must be part of a broader continuum of care that includes routine, structured follow-up from adolescence into adulthood. Many sexual and fertility concerns may not be apparent until adulthood.
- Special considerations may be needed for patients with congenital genitourinary malformations, but most patients are able to achieve satisfactory sexual and fertility function

References

1. Al-Salem AH. Precocious puberty. In: Pediatric gynecology. Cham: Springer; 2020. https://doi.org/10.1007/978-3-030-49984-6_3.
2. Fawzy M, Hadidi AT. Hormones and growth of the genital tubercle. In: Hadidi AT, editor. Hypospadias surgery: an illustrated textbook. Cham: Springer International Publishing; 2022. p. 285–98.
3. Miller KD, Coughlin MT, Lee PA. Fertility after unilateral cryptorchidism. Paternity, time to conception, pretreatment testicular location and size, hormone and sperm parameters. Horm Res. 2001;55(5):249–53. https://doi.org/10.1159/000050005.
4. Lee PA, Coughlin MT. Fertility after bilateral cryptorchidism. Evaluation by paternity, hormone, and semen data. Horm Res. 2001;55(1):28–32. https://doi.org/10.1159/000049960.
5. Zhang X, Zhang J, Cai Z, Wang X, Lu W, Li H. Effect of unilateral testicular torsion at different ages on male fertility. J Int Med Res. 2020;48(4):300060520918792. https://doi.org/10.1177/0300060520918792.
6. Skarin Nordenvall A, Chen Q, Norrby C, Lundholm C, Frisen L, Nordenstrom A, et al. Fertility in adult men born with hypospadias: a nationwide register-based cohort study on birthrates, the use of assisted reproductive technologies and infertility. Andrology. 2020;8(2):372–80. https://doi.org/10.1111/andr.12723.
7. Chertin B, Koulikov D, Fridmans A, Farkas A. Dorsal tunica albuginea plication to correct congenital and acquired penile curvature: a long-term follow-up. BJU Int. 2004;93(3):379–81. https://doi.org/10.1111/j.1464-410x.2003.04621.x.
8. Ethics Committee of the American Society for Reproductive, M. Access to fertility services by transgender persons: an ethics committee opinion. Fertil Steril. 2015;104(5):1111–5. https://doi.org/10.1016/j.fertnstert.2015.08.021.
9. Practice Committee of the American Society for Reproductive Medicine. Electronic address, a. a. o. Fertility preservation in patients undergoing gonadotoxic therapy or gonadectomy: a committee opinion. Fertil Steril. 2019;112(6):1022–33. https://doi.org/10.1016/j.fertnstert.2019.09.013.
10. Hammarstrom S, Bernhardsson S, Nilsen P, Elisson J, Frostholm E, Lindroth M. Ask me, listen to me, treat me well and I shall tell: a qualitative study of Swedish youths' experiences of systematic assessment of sexual health and risk-taking (SEXIT). Sex Reprod Health Matters. 2022;30(1):2146032. https://doi.org/10.1080/26410397.2022.2146032.
11. Sieving RE, McRee AL, Mehus C, Gewirtz O'Brien JR, Wang S, Brar P, et al. Sexual and reproductive health discussions during preventive visits. Pediatrics. 2021;148(2). https://doi.org/10.1542/peds.2020-049411.
12. Song X, Klein JD, Yan H, Catallozzi M, Wang X, Heitel J, et al. Parent and adolescent attitudes towards preventive care and confidentiality. J Adolesc Health. 2019;64(2):235–41. https://doi.org/10.1016/j.jadohealth.2018.08.015.
13. Cardenas DD, Topolski TD, White CJ, McLaughlin JF, Walker WO. Sexual functioning in adolescents and young adults with spina bifida. Arch Phys Med Rehabil. 2008;89(1):31–5. https://doi.org/10.1016/j.apmr.2007.08.124.
14. Hughes TL, Simmons KL, Tejwani R, Barton KD, Wiener JS, Todd Purves J, Routh JC. Sexual function and dysfunction in individuals with spina bifida: a systematic review. Urology. 2021;156:308–19. https://doi.org/10.1016/j.urology.2021.03.042.
15. Streur CS, Corona L, Smith JE, Lin M, Wiener JS, Wittmann DA. Sexual function of men and women with spina bifida: a scoping literature review. Sex Med Rev. 2021;9(2):244–66. https://doi.org/10.1016/j.sxmr.2020.09.001.
16. Sonksen J, Biering-Sorensen F, Kristensen JK. Ejaculation induced by penile vibratory stimulation in men with spinal cord injuries. The importance of the vibratory amplitude. Paraplegia. 1994;32(10):651–60. https://doi.org/10.1038/sc.1994.105.

17. Suominen JS, Santtila P, Taskinen S. Sexual function in patients operated on for bladder exstrophy and epispadias. J Urol. 2015;194(1):195–9. https://doi.org/10.1016/j.juro.2015.01.098.
18. Park W, Zwink N, Rosch WH, Schmiedeke E, Stein R, Schmidt D, et al. Sexual function in adult patients with classic bladder exstrophy: a multicenter study. J Pediatr Urol. 2015;11(3):125 e121-126. https://doi.org/10.1016/j.jpurol.2015.02.001.
19. Deans R, Liao LM, Wood D, Woodhouse C, Creighton SM. Sexual function and health-related quality of life in women with classic bladder exstrophy. BJU Int. 2015;115(4):633–8. https://doi.org/10.1111/bju.12811.
20. Effendi R, Situmorang GR, Wahyudi I, Rodjani A, Raharja PAR, Abbas TO. Adult sexual function following hypospadias repair in childhood: a systematic review and meta-analysis of long-term patient outcomes. Urology. 2025; https://doi.org/10.1016/j.urology.2025.05.015.

Vesicoureteral Reflux

16

Dan Wood

The purpose of this chapter is to give the reader insight into the diagnosis, management, outcomes, and some of the controversies around vesicoureteral reflux (VUR).

Vesicoureteral reflux is defined as the retrograde flow of urine from the bladder into the ureters and upper tracts. It is conventionally classified as either primary or secondary. Primary VUR represents a congenital, anatomical fault in the one-way valve-like mechanism at the vesicoureteral junction, whereas secondary VUR results from mechanical failure of the valve-like mechanism, usually as a result of a sustained and pathological increase in vesical pressure, which may result from bladder outflow obstruction, as seen in posterior urethral valves most commonly, or with neurogenic bladder/outlet.

Primary VUR has an incidence of 1–2% in young children, with 30–50% of first-degree relatives also being affected. Embryonically, the development of the vesicoureteral junction appears to rely on the origin of the ureteric bud from the mesonephric duct. If the ureteral bud originates caudally off the mesonephric duct, the ureteric orifice will be placed cranially and laterally on the bladder floor, and the one-way valve-like mechanism will fail. If this is severe and the interaction with the metanephros (developing kidney) is also affected, then the kidney may also be dysplastic. Whilst researchers have attempted to define a genetic basis for VUR, the exact pathway remains unclear. Inheritance appears to behave in an autosomal dominant fashion with partial penetrance [1].

The important questions that arise in relation to VUR are:

1. Is the return of urine from the bladder into the ureter/kidney in itself harmful?
2. What are the investigations for VUR?
3. When is it appropriate to treat VUR?

D. Wood (✉)
University of Colorado School of Medicine, Aurora, CO, USA
e-mail: dan.wood@childrenscolorado.org

H.-Y. Wu et al. (eds.), *Pediatric Urology for the Adult Urologist*,
https://doi.org/10.1007/978-3-032-10306-2_16

4. What are the treatment options for VUR?
5. What are the outcomes for both treated and untreated VUR?

The reason for highlighting these questions at the start of the chapter is to try and point the reader toward the fact that there remains some controversy about what should be done for patients suffering from VUR.

For secondary VUR, the treatment of the underlying cause is where management should begin; thereafter, some of the treatments and principles applied in the rest of this chapter may apply. The treatment pathways for these are best examined in the context of the primary condition and its management.

Is the Return of Urine from the Bladder into the Ureter/Kidney in Itself Harmful?

At baseline, the answer to this question appears to be no. If urine is sterile and the bladder is functioning at physiological pressures, evidence suggests that reflux alone does not result in scarring nor has a harmful effect on renal growth. VUR is the most common of all the congenital anomalies of the kidneys and urinary tract (CAKUT). Whilst it remains difficult to demonstrate direct harm to the kidneys from pure VUR, it is certainly an important association, and, therefore, needs to be understood in these terms.

In children with end-stage renal failure, VUR nephropathy is implicated in 20% of cases and increases long-term risk in other less severe grades of chronic kidney disease.

Reflux is graded from I to V (see Fig. 16.1).

Urologists with a focus on adult practice will be familiar with a condition for which the morbidity of treatment may outweigh the potential harm from the condition.

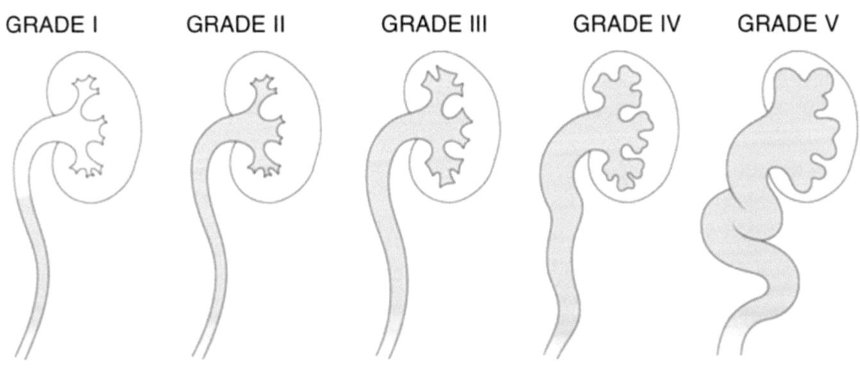

Fig. 16.1 Illustrations of the grades of vesicoureteral reflux. (Source: https://epomedicine.com/medical-students/vesicoureteric-reflux-vur-grading-mnemonic)

Table 16.1 Spontaneous resolution rate and successful outcome in the treatment of VUR (data from Tejwani and Routh in Thomas and Wilcox) [1]

	% Spontaneous resolution (1st year)	% Spontaneous resolution (by 5th year)	Open reimplantation % success	Endoscopic injection % success
Grade I	39	92	99	89
Grade II	28	81	99	83
Grade III	10	42	98	71
Grade IV	6	16	99	59
Grade V	–	–	81	62
Average (all grades)	17	53	97	72

Table 16.1 shows the rate of spontaneous resolution, by grade and outcomes of treatment.

VUR is most commonly diagnosed following presentation with symptomatic UTIs. Traditional teaching was that up to 30% of children with UTIs would be found to have VUR upon investigation, this may be an overestimation when UTIs are further classified into those focused solely on the lower urinary tract versus those affecting the upper tract. The association between VUR and bladder and bowel dysfunction has been clearly established. Pain is an unusual feature of VUR, and if described, consideration should be given to a secondary diagnosis such as pelviureteric junction (PUJ) obstruction. Children may occasionally present with hypertension/renal insufficiency with a minimal history of UTI—the nephropathy, in these cases, may have a congenital element or potentially be associated with unrecognized childhood pyelonephritis.

Given the significant increase in close family members, siblings, and offspring of affected family members should be told that they need investigation if they develop UTIs. The clinical and cost effectiveness of routine screening of family members has never been conclusively demonstrated, although it may persist in some guidelines.

What Are the Investigations for VUR?

The clinical consequences in the form of UTI and reflux nephropathy have been outlined.

For a child who presents with UTI, alongside a general medical evaluation, assessment of voiding patterns and urinalysis and stooling patterns, renal ultrasound (US) is a reasonable starting point for investigation, if required. It is limited as a screening tool as lower grades of reflux (not resulting in renal dilatation) may be missed. Studious examination for a postvoid residual or bladder wall thickening may provide additional clues. The addition of US contrast injected into the bladder (via a catheter) adds an invasive element to the investigation, but may show reflux. Annual US in those diagnosed with VUR is recommended in their follow-up.

Radionuclide testing with technetium-99 m dimercaptosuccinic acid (DMSA) is used to look for renal scarring (DMSA) or, potentially, with the use of an indirect cystogram, to detect reflux [2].

Voiding cystourethrography (VCUG) remains the definitive investigation for VUR. Whilst it remains invasive, it offers the advantages of being reproducible and easy to interpret. The test is performed by placing a bladder catheter and filling the bladder with radiopaque contrast. X-rays are taken in both the filling and voiding stages to look for VUR. If bladder function is a concern, pressure monitoring can be added to perform video urodynamics. It is by VCUG that the grading system above can be specified for a patient.

For children with febrile UTIs, it is largely agreed that VCUG and DMSA are indicated and appropriate. If an initial US showed dilatation or the urine culture grew out an atypical organism, e.g., Pseudomonas or Proteus, these would be additional features that would trigger invasive testing. The more challenging group is children with UTIs and a normal US, in whom, if low-grade VUR were found, may benefit from endoscopic treatment. There is logic in performing an initial US and DMSA in this group and only progressing to VCUG if renal scarring is demonstrated. The principle being that without renal scarring, the probability of significant VUR is very low. The historic approach has been to progress from US to VCUG and progress to a DMSA based on the findings. Both approaches and their proponents and parents/patients need to be given relevant and up-to-date information so they can make sensible decisions for their situation.

Younger children (below the age of 4) are suggested to be at greater risk of renal scarring and hence might trigger a more aggressive investigative approach. Studies examining adult nephrectomy specimens show girls to be at greater risk of pyelonephritic scarring, whereas males more commonly show evidence of congenital nephropathy. Other factors that can influence the disease, including affected parent, sibling, race, ethnicity, comorbidities, and geography, may affect the decisions around investigation and treatment. For older patients, data are lacking either in those who had untreated reflux diagnosed in childhood or those found later in life, but it seems reasonable to apply similar principles, no matter the age, except for infants [1].

What Are the Treatment Options for VUR?

Treatment aims to reduce/remove the occurrence of significant UTIs and prevent renal scarring/nephropathy. The above factors, alongside clinical history, frequency/severity of UTIs, and renal function, will be the triggers to both investigate and subsequently treat. In older teenage and adult patients, it may be helpful to elicit whether infections have been lifelong (in which case VUR may well be a factor) or a more recent phenomenon, which may point more to lifestyle factors, including sexual activity, as being implicated. These features are not mutually exclusive, but may guide the clinician and patient on where to begin treatment.

Treatment options include:

1. Medical management, including comprehensive management of bladder and bowel dysfunction, with the addition of daily antibiotic prophylaxis where indicated.
2. Endoscopic injection to correct VUR.
3. Ureteric reimplantation using either open, laparoscopic, or robotic techniques.

Bladder Bowel Dysfunction

It remains a fundamental urological principle that ineffective or inefficient voiding, manifest by incomplete or infrequent emptying, creates an increased risk of UTI. Increased bladder pressures may exacerbate primary VUR and cause secondary VUR. Constipation is recognized as being an integral and exacerbating/causal factor in these children and probably older patients.

If these factors are not treated and resolved, any further treatment, either medical or surgical, runs the risk of being compromised [2].

Antibiotic Prophylaxis

This has been a key component of medical management since the 1970s. The aim is to reduce the risk of UTI by preventing bacterial accumulation. In turn, this reduces the risk of renal scarring in a patient affected by reflux. The strongest rationale exists in those who are under investigation or newly diagnosed, closely followed but those with lower grades of reflux (I, II, and III), most likely to resolve without the need for surgical intervention. Randomized trial data suggest a threefold reduction in risk of febrile UTI for patients with grade III or IV reflux; however, a significant reduction in the development of scarring has not been convincingly demonstrated (perhaps because most scarring has happened before VUR is diagnosed). The data from published trials suggest that for boys over the age of one, there is little value in antibiotic prophylaxis, but girls seem much more likely to derive benefit. In boys with high-grade VUR, the risk of developing further UTIs is significantly reduced by performing a circumcision [3]. However, as we become more aware of the need for antibiotic stewardship and the potential for resistant infections, greater caution around prolonged antibiotic prophylaxis may be warranted [1, 4–7].

Endoscopic Injection

There have been a range of products marketed for this purpose. The most widely applied technique is performed using a cystoscopy (rigid or flexible), through which a needle for injection is inserted under the open ureteric orifice, or further in if the ureteral orifice (UO) admits the scope. The bulking agent is injected to create a mound, which alters the shape of the UO to a crescent shape. Once the gel has been given a few seconds to solidify, the needle is withdrawn. Success based on this technique is shown in Table 16.1. Recently, authors have suggested that a hydrodistension implantation technique (HIT) or double hydrodistension technique may improve outcomes further. Although overall success is high, around 20% have needed a second injection. The measure of success has been the relative downgrading of VUR or the absence of VUR on a VCUG. Data to support this with clinical outcomes or a reduced risk of renal scarring remains lacking. In addition, there does not appear to be a compromise to the success of ureteral reimplantation in those who have failed endoscopic corrections and require repair of VUR.

The most important complications would be continued VUR, with UTIs and worsening nephropathy or obstruction following the injection, said to occur in 5% and usually to be temporary.

It is worthy of note that in adult patients with a history of VUR and endoscopic injection, the injection site (at the ureteric orifice) is commonly reported as being a VUJ stone on later life imaging.

Ureteric Reimplantation

This can be performed using the following:

- The Leadbetter-Politano technique detaches the ureter from the bladder after initial intravesical mobilization and creates a neocystostomy with an extended submucosal tunnel. This can be useful with dilated ureters, as it is possible to taper the distal portion.
- For less dilated ureters, the cross-trigonal (Cohen) technique extends the submucosal course of the ureter by mobilizing it across the trigone. It has a very high published success rate of approximately 97%. It is important not to separate a duplex system, as that will probably result in devascularization of one or both distal ureters.
- The extravesical technique or Lich-Gregoir can also be used for tapering but has an increased association with postoperative urinary retention, if performed bilaterally.

Minimally invasive techniques are developing and growing in popularity. Data from early adopters is beginning to suggest comparable outcomes, at this stage, which comes with a learning curve to develop the skills. As current trainees emerge, and the use of the robot is more ubiquitous, it seems likely that open techniques may be reserved for those with a history of multiple prior surgeries of some form of anatomical or physiological compromise that excludes the use of a robot [1].

What Are the Outcomes for Both Treated and Untreated VUR?

The majority of children with primary VUR either resolve or are successfully treated in childhood; it follows that adult urologists see and manage it relatively infrequently. Patients who are asymptomatic or whose reflux resolves, we are unlikely to see long-term data, as they will not be followed up with. The same is probably true for those who have treatment (either endoscopic or open) and whose problems resolve, as they will likely be seen for a short period in pediatric practice and may never reappear. However, it is recognized that the association with renal scarring and UTI may predispose them to hypertension, chronic kidney disease, and end-stage renal disease. Adults may present with VUR; whether this is de novo or something that had been asymptomatic and undetected through childhood is impossible to determine [8]. It is tempting to assume this is the cause of the patients' UTIs, and it may be that the same treatment principles are worthy to apply in the adult as in the child. Ensuring bladder and bowel function are optimized, including fluid intake, hygiene, and sexual history, may all be avenues for improvement ahead of intervention. The use of antibiotic prophylaxis is rare in adults, for fear of creating resistance. UTI prevention with adjuncts such as cranberry supplements, D-mannose, topical estrogen, or methenamine may be helpful [9]. Occasionally, a short course of daily prophylaxis (3 months) may act as a reset.

Published data make it difficult to give precise indicators of who is at risk and, therefore, needs follow-up in adulthood. Renal scarring and renal dysplasia are important, but the associations with UTI, severity of VUR, age, and prior correction (or not) are much harder to determine. Those with secondary VUR, e.g., spina bifida or posterior urethral valves, appear to be at greater risk. Patients with scarring or the presence of chronic kidney disease should be educated and monitored for hypertension (and proteinuria), as it has been shown to develop earlier in 20–40% and at an earlier age (between 15 and 30 years). Angiotensin-converting enzyme (ACE) inhibitors have been shown to be effective in slowing renal deterioration in patients with reflux nephropathy. [8]

Data have shown that for those who present with compromised renal function, VUR is the leading cause of ESRD (at around 25%). This group clearly need follow-up in expert hands [10–12].

Pregnancy in women with a prior history of VUR is worthy of consideration. They may be at increased risk of UTI, especially if they have suffered UTI before their initial treatment, have renal scarring, or an abnormal split renal function differential. If they have no renal scars, then their risk of preeclampsia or gestational hypertension appears to be similar to that of an unaffected population. For those who have undergone VUR correction, rates of preeclampsia may be as high as 38% (eclampsia in 10%) with a spontaneous abortion risk of 9–27%, which increases if they have an elevated creatinine or preexisting hypertension. It is also known that pregnancy will accelerate renal deterioration with a background of chronic renal disease. Patients should also be counselled that their offspring are at increased risk of VUR and may be worth screening [8]. For these reasons, patients with a background of VUR and associated risks should be carefully managed by a high-risk obstetrician, nephrologist, and urologist with regular monitoring of maternal and fetal well-being, including renal function, ultrasounds to look for worsening hydronephrosis.

Summary

- Patients with mild VUR have a high chance of spontaneous resolution and may not need any treatment.
- The presence of UTIs and renal scarring is a strong indication for treatment.
- Adult patients with renal scarring should be screened for hypertension and proteinuria.
- Women with a history of intervention for VUR, chronic kidney disease, or renal scarring need careful counselling and management before and during pregnancy.

References

1. Rohit Tejwani JR. Vesicoureteric reflux. In: David Thomas DW, editor. Essentials of pediatric urology. Oxford: Taylor & Francis; 2022.
2. Peters CA, Skoog SJ, Arant BS Jr, Copp HL, Elder JS, Hudson RG, Khoury AE, Lorenzo AJ, Pohl HG, Shapiro E, Snodgrass WT. Management and screening of primary vesicoureteral reflux in children 2017. American Urological Association Guidelines.
3. Singh-Grewal D, Macdessi J, Craig J. Circumcision for the prevention of urinary tract infection in boys: a systematic review of randomised trials and observational studies. Arch Dis Child. 2005;90(8):853–8.
4. Craig JC, et al. Antibiotic prophylaxis and recurrent urinary tract infection in children. N Engl J Med. 2009;361(18):1748–59.
5. Holmdahl G, et al. The Swedish reflux trial in children: II. Vesicoureteral reflux outcome. J Urol. 2010;184(1):280–5.
6. Investigators RT, et al. Antimicrobial prophylaxis for children with vesicoureteral reflux. N Engl J Med. 2014;370(25):2367–76.
7. Wang HH, et al. Efficacy of antibiotic prophylaxis in children with vesicoureteral reflux: systematic review and meta-analysis. J Urol. 2015;193(3):963–9.
8. Friedman AA, Hanna MK. Vesicoureteric reflux and the adult. In: Hadley DW, Wood M, editors. Transition and lifelong care in congenital urology. Cham: Springer International; 2015.
9. Nelson Z, et al. Guidelines for the prevention, diagnosis, and management of urinary tract infections in pediatrics and adults: a WikiGuidelines Group consensus statement. JAMA Netw Open. 2024;7(11):e2444495.
10. Ardissino G, et al. Long-term outcome of vesicoureteral reflux associated chronic renal failure in children. Data from the ItalKid Project. J Urol. 2004;172(1):305–10.
11. Berquist TH, et al. Vesicoureteral reflux in adults. Am J Roentgenol Radium Therapy, Nucl Med. 1975;125(2):314–21.
12. Lackgren G, et al. Management of vesicoureteral reflux: what have we learned over the last 20 years? Front Pediatr. 2021;9:650326.

Urinary Incontinence

17

Julia Drexelius and Meredith C. Wasserman

In the adult population, nonneurogenic urinary incontinence is typically divided into major categories of urgency urinary incontinence (UUI), as part of overactive bladder syndrome (OAB), and stress urinary incontinence (SUI). UUI (previously known as urge urinary incontinence) is the result of involuntary detrusor contractions due to factors such as age-related changes in bladder signaling, bladder irritants (medications, dietary triggers, etc.), or underlying bladder pathology (urinary tract infection, bladder stones or tumors, radiation cystitis, etc.). Conversely, SUI is due to weakening of the urethral closure, resulting in loss of urine with increased intra-abdominal pressure. This can be due to urethral hypermobility or intrinsic sphincter deficiency (ISD). Urethral hypermobility is the result of weakened pelvic floor muscles and/or the supportive structures around the urethra. Risk factors include childbearing, chronic cough, obesity, and pelvic floor dysfunction, to name a few. Conversely, ISD is due to loss of urethral sphincter function leading to a lower resting urethral sphincter pressure, regardless of position or activity, often seen in patients who have had prior pelvic surgery, iatrogenic sphincter damage, and occasionally in neurogenic conditions. Although not considered a major category of urinary incontinence in the general adult population, nocturnal enuresis is another etiology to be considered, specifically in the transitional urology population, and will also be addressed in this chapter. For this chapter, OAB and UUI will be used interchangeably.

J. Drexelius (✉) · M. C. Wasserman
Department of Urology, The Warren Alpert Medical School of Brown University, Providence, RI, USA
e-mail: jdrexelius@brownhealth.org

H.-Y. Wu et al. (eds.), *Pediatric Urology for the Adult Urologist*,
https://doi.org/10.1007/978-3-032-10306-2_17

Urgency Urinary Incontinence

There are many treatment options in the management of UUI, so it is important to take individual patient preferences and circumstances into account, especially in the transition of care from pediatric to adult urology. Although patients should have undergone workup by their pediatric urologist at the time of presentation to the adult urologist at transition of care, a thorough reevaluation, including urinalysis, is recommended. It is essential to understand the prior care received, including workup, interventions, and counseling. It is also important to recognize the changes associated with adolescence and young adulthood, as well as the potential for the development of new comorbidities as patients age. This prepares the urologist to provide well-rounded care that includes the patient in decisions surrounding their care and treatment options.

The treatment approach to OAB has previously followed a stepwise approach from least to most invasive therapies; however, updated guidelines advise the use of shared decision-making to guide the choice of therapy based on individual factors and patient values [1, 2]. Thus, it is no longer required to trial medication before minimally invasive therapies. Conservative management of OAB includes incontinence management strategies, behavioral therapies, and optimization of comorbidities. Pelvic floor physical therapy (PFPT) is one option that has been shown to be effective in the management of adult OAB, and should be revisited at the transition of care [3]. A randomized controlled trial evaluating the efficacy of PFPT in the pediatric population showed that it was equivalent to standard urotherapy, and for those pediatric patients who would benefit from PFPT, it may be difficult to find a facility that offers treatment for their age group [4]. Thus, urologists should discuss the utility of PFPT with these patients at the transition of care to determine if it is a fitting option for the patient. In patients with persistent OAB despite conservative management, the next steps often include the use of pharmacologic therapy and minimally invasive therapies.

Pharmacotherapy

In the transition of pediatric to adult urologic care, patients with an overactive bladder may be established on medication at the time of presentation. If the patient is satisfied with their current regimen, it is not necessary to discontinue or modify treatment simply because they are transitioning care. A stoppage trial can be considered in patients who wish to wean off medications, but there is no evidence specific to the discontinuation of OAB medications at the transition of care that allows for recommendation for or against this option. Regardless, a thorough evaluation of the efficacy and side effects of the current therapy is essential, as well as a review of prior therapies.

Anticholinergics

Anticholinergic medications are often used in the treatment of OAB. Oxybutynin is a commonly used antimuscarinic medication that is Food and Drug Administration (FDA)-approved for the treatment of OAB in children and adults. One important consideration when prescribing oxybutynin is its side effect profile. Due to its anticholinergic properties, common side effects include constipation, dry eyes, dry mouth, flushing, and blurred vision [5–7]. There has also been increasing concern for the central nervous system (CNS)-related adverse events with oxybutynin use, including hallucinations, agitation, sedation, confusion, amnesia, and nightmares. Oxybutynin has also been associated with cognitive decline, especially in older patients [8, 9]. These data are often extrapolated to the other anticholinergic medications used to treat OAB. The exception to this is trospium, which is an antimuscarinic with less ability to cross the blood-brain barrier and thus is thought to have fewer CNS-related adverse events. Other antimuscarinic agents that have been approved for overactive bladder in adults include solifenacin, tolterodine, darifenacin, and propiverine [10]. Overall, oxybutynin and other antimuscarinic medications are a reasonable choice for the treatment of OAB, but their side effect profile must be carefully considered. Studies have shown a poor long-term adherence rate associated with anticholinergic therapy, likely due to unmet expectations or intolerable side effects [11, 12].

Beta-3 Adrenergic Agonists

Beta-3 agonists are another class of medications frequently used in the treatment of OAB that are sometimes preferred for their more favorable side effect profile. Mirabegron is among the most common beta-3 adrenergic agonists prescribed for OAB in adults, as it was the first FDA-approved option. The efficacy of anticholinergics and beta-3 agonists appears to be similar in the treatment of OAB in adults; however, the more favorable side effect profile associated with beta-3 agonists, particularly the lack of associated cognitive issues, makes them a preferred choice among many urologists. Still, beta-3 agonists do carry their own risks, with some of the most common adverse events including hypertension, nasopharyngitis, and urinary tract infections [13–15]. Although it is not FDA-approved for the treatment of nonneurogenic OAB in children, mirabegron may be less likely to be self-discontinued by patients, resulting in better therapeutic outcomes [16]. One consideration in prescribing beta-3 agonists is cost; however, a generic version of mirabegron is now available and becoming more accessible through insurance companies [17].

When using pharmacotherapy for the treatment of OAB in children, it is important to closely monitor adverse events and medication adherence. In the transition of care from pediatric to adult urologic care, it is reasonable to adjust or change medication classes based on individual patient factors to limit side effects while maintaining efficacy of treatment. Medical management of OAB can have poor long-term compliance due to adverse effects or unachieved patient expectations; thus, minimally invasive therapies should not be excluded for this population [12].

Minimally Invasive Therapies (MIT)

Minimally invasive therapies are a great option for many patients with OAB and may be preferred over more conservative treatment options depending on various patient factors. The 2024 American Urological Association (AUA) guidelines on the treatment of idiopathic OAB advise the use of shared decision-making to guide the choice of therapy based on individual factors and patient values, regardless of level of invasiveness [3]. Instead, therapy should be guided by the individual patient's needs, desires, and side effect tolerance. It is not required to trial patients on medication before considering minimally invasive therapies. If the patient has a good response to a minimally invasive treatment, their medication for OAB can be discontinued; however, if symptoms recur, medication should be restarted [3]. Of note, although the guidelines do not require failure of pharmacotherapy before use of MIT, many insurance companies do still require a pharmacotherapy trial before approval of MIT; thus, a thorough history is a critical portion of workup in this population.

Sacral Neuromodulation

Sacral neuromodulation (SNM) is FDA-approved for the treatment of urgency incontinence, frequency, and nonobstructive urinary retention in adults. SNM has been shown to be safe and efficacious in the treatment of OAB in adults [18–21]. The development of rechargeable and magnetic resonance imaging (MRI)-compatible systems has been foundational for the increasing application of SNM. The advances in technology over the years have resulted in a variety of devices of different sizes, battery life, and MRI-compatibility that are currently in use.

There are many factors to consider for patients interested in SNM, particularly in transitional urology. Patients may undergo changes in weight during young adulthood that can affect device positioning or have cosmetic preferences regarding battery size. One question that may arise for female patients considering SNM is its effect on pregnancy. In a literature review, there were no significant negative effects of SNM on fetus, mother, or device reported [22]. However, it is recommended that the device remain deactivated during pregnancy as there are no randomized controlled trials assessing safety.

For patients who present with an existing implantable device with changes in urinary symptoms, one should proceed with a history including changes in lifestyle, medications, behaviors, etc. Additionally, the urologist must perform a thorough evaluation of the device to ensure appropriate impedances are present and the battery is still functional. A pelvic x-ray should be done to rule out migration of the lead if stimulation and sensations have changed or impedances are out of range. In patients where a lead fragment is retained during implant removal or replacement, the urologist must determine if the patient is safe to undergo an MRI, if necessary. In Medtronic devices with SureScan technology, lead fragments must meet certain conditions to be eligible for MRI: [1] total length of metallic content ≤6 cm, [2] distance to other metallic components ≥2 cm, [3] lead fragment location is sacral, and [4] lead fragment is MRI-eligible [23].

Botulinum Toxin Injections

Botulinum toxin injections (BTX) have been FDA-approved for the treatment of overactive bladder since 2013. BTX has been shown to be a safe and effective therapy for patients with urgency urinary incontinence, with the most common adverse events being UTI and urinary retention requiring catheterization [20]. The recommended starting dosage of BTX for nonneurogenic OAB is 100 units [24]. The standard injection technique is 20 injections of 0.5 mL each (100u BTX diluted in 10 mL). There are increasing studies on varying injection templates, such as ten injections of 1 mL or five injections of 2 mL, that have shown similar efficacy when given throughout the posterior bladder wall, sparing the trigone [25].

The urologist performing BTX injections must regularly inquire about patients' use of BTX for other indications to ensure they remain within the recommended dosage limits of 400 units within a 3-month period, especially in the young adult population, when patients may begin using BTX for cosmetic purposes [26].

Tibial Nerve Stimulation

Tibial nerve stimulation is safe and effective in treating OAB. Percutaneous tibial nerve stimulation (PTNS) has been found to improve frequency, nocturia, urgency, and urgency incontinence episodes [27]. PTNS requires weekly office visits for 12 weeks, followed by monthly visits for maintenance, making it a difficult option for some patients. Transcutaneous tibial nerve stimulation (TTNS) uses a surface electrode rather than a needle to stimulate the tibial nerve and has also shown effectiveness in treating OAB symptoms. TTNS is lower cost and less invasive than PTNS and may be preferred by some patients [28]. There are now two FDA-approved implantable tibial nerve devices with more in clinical trials. The early data available suggest these devices offer equivocal, if not superior, efficacy compared to PTNS; however, long-term studies are not available [29].

Nocturnal Enuresis

Enuresis is attributed to the combination of abnormalities in nocturnal urine production, bladder storage capacity, and the ability to arouse from sleep. The abnormal increase in urine volume with concurrent decrease in urine osmolality during the night is attributed to nocturnal vasopressin deficiency [30–32]. Although an annual spontaneous remission rate of 15% is cited for enuresis, not all patients grow out of the condition. Interestingly, more frequent episodes of enuresis have been associated with decreased chances of becoming dry without treatment [31, 33]. In the workup and treatment of enuresis, it is important to keep other conditions in mind, including constipation, sleep apnea, diabetes, and urinary tract infections. In the young adult population, one must also consider the introduction of alcohol or other drugs and their effects on nocturnal enuresis.

Initial treatment for enuresis involves behavioral modifications and alarm therapy. If this fails, patients may trial desmopressin. Efficacy is seen within one to two weeks, though the drug does have a low rate of cure and is often continued for several years [31]. When the decision is made to discontinue desmopressin, a taper of the drug is recommended to decrease the risk of relapse [34]. The most serious adverse effect of desmopressin is hyponatremia, which, when severe, can cause more serious complications. The hyponatremia due to desmopressin is dilutional in nature, so it is more commonly observed following excess fluid intake or with illnesses that predispose to fluid and electrolyte balance (i.e., fever, vomiting, and diarrhea) [35]. Patients must be counseled appropriately on these risks and strategies to mitigate them, including fluid restriction and pausing treatment during certain acute illnesses.

While nocturnal enuresis is seen more commonly in pediatric patients, a few cases can persist into adolescence and early adulthood. There is scarce literature on the management of these patients, but one review of the literature suggests a stepwise approach for patients with enuresis at the transition from pediatric to adult care. A multidisciplinary care team, as well as a transition coordinator, can be helpful in these cases. The transition process should be initiated early to ensure adequate communication between the provider, patient, and their family, including patient-specific characteristics and comorbidities, as well as expectations for continued management [36].

Stress Urinary Incontinence

Many patients with childhood-onset stress urinary incontinence may continue to experience symptoms into adulthood or have recurrence of symptoms once beyond the care of the pediatric urologist. Adult urologists play a critical role in the long-term follow-up of these patients. Understanding their history and prior interventions is essential to providing appropriate management and ensuring continuity of care.

There are many etiologies of stress urinary incontinence in patients transitioning from pediatric urology that may fall into the categories of congenital, developmental, or iatrogenic. Some patients may have stress incontinence because of intrinsic sphincter deficiency due to underlying neurologic dysfunction or prior surgical alteration of the bladder outlet. Conversely, SUI may develop because of pelvic floor dysfunction or other nonneurogenic etiologies. A comprehensive approach is necessary to capture all prior care. A detailed history with review of prior pediatric treatments, including conservative management strategies and/or surgical interventions, should be obtained. A thorough physical examination is completed, paying particular attention to pelvic floor dysfunction and identifying surgical scars, if present, and confirming the presence of SUI with a full bladder cough stress test. In patients who have undergone prior therapies, have a mixed symptom presentation, or do not exhibit SUI on exam, pressure-flow studies may be utilized to evaluate detrusor function, rule out any negative effects of prior therapies such as obstruction, and evaluate sphincter competence. Workup can also include imaging to evaluate for mesh or bulking implants; these modalities may include ultrasound, MRI, or CT.

Treatment counseling includes the options of observation, pelvic floor muscle therapy, continence vaginal inserts, and surgical procedures, including bulking agents, urethral suspensions, and sling procedures with or without synthetic mesh. The ultimate choice for intervention will depend on patient risk factors and their own goals for treatment in a shared decision-making process.

In young women, surgical counseling must address future or current plans for pregnancy and childbirth. Pregnancy and mode of delivery may affect the efficacy of previous anti-incontinence procedures. The direct effects of pregnancy and delivery on urethral bulking agents have not been well-studied. However, the less durable nature of urethral bulking agents as compared to other anti-incontinence procedures suggests that pregnancy may impact their efficacy. Given the relatively low-risk nature of the procedure and that it does not preclude future sling placement, it is a reasonable first step for an anti-incontinence procedure in patients planning future childbearing. There is now more literature on the effects of pregnancy and childbirth on synthetic midurethral slings (MUSs) and autologous fascial slings. One recent meta-analysis concluded that there was a 22% risk of SUI recurrence with childbirth in women who previously underwent midurethral sling and a 5% reintervention rate, with no difference in the mode of delivery [37]. The current AUA/Society of Urodynamics, Female Pelvic Medicine & Urogenital Reconstruction (SUFU) guidelines on surgical treatment of stress urinary incontinence recommend, in most cases, delaying any surgical treatment until after childbearing is complete [38].

One additional consideration is the presence of mixed urinary incontinence (MUI) in patients, specifically when nonurge predominant. The Effects of Surgical Treatment Enhanced with Exercise for Mixed Urinary Incontinence (ESTEEM) trial demonstrated that 85% of women with stress predominant or equal bother MUI who underwent insertion of midurethral sling had a significant improvement in UUI in addition to SUI [39]. Although not proven through a randomized controlled trial, this theory has been extrapolated to urethral bulking as a primary modality in MUI patients as well. Thus, in patients with nonurge predominant MUI, one is not required to treat the UUI before addressing SUI.

Summary

1. Initial workup of any urinary incontinence in the transitional urology patient includes a detailed history with specific focus on prior therapies, a thorough physical exam, urinalysis, and postvoid residual; consider uroflowmetry or imaging based on symptoms or prior diagnoses.
2. Shared decision-making is prioritized over stepwise therapy in managing urgency urinary incontinence; patients should pursue treatments based on preference rather than mandatory progression.
3. When deciding on pharmacotherapy for urgency incontinence, medication choice will likely be most influenced by insurance plan, making close follow-up

of adverse outcomes and adherence important. Similarly, minimally invasive therapies may be influenced by insurance coverage but should also include consideration of long-term needs (i.e., imaging) and repeat access to care.

4. Nocturnal enuresis is multifactorial, and etiologies may change with maturity; ensure a thorough evaluation of lifestyle factors and changes in medical history.
5. Stress urinary incontinence (SUI) management is individualized, and surgical intervention is typically deferred until after childbearing.

References

1. Thom M, Campigotto M, Vemulakonda V, Coplen D, Austin PF. Management of lower urinary tract dysfunction: a stepwise approach. J Pediatr Urol. 2012;8(1):20–4. https://doi.org/10.1016/j.jpurol.2011.01.004.
2. Cameron AP, Chung DE, Dielubanza EJ, et al. The AUA/SUFU guideline on the diagnosis and treatment of idiopathic overactive bladder. J Urol. 2024;212(1):11–20. https://doi.org/10.1097/ju.0000000000003985.
3. Cho ST, Kim KH. Pelvic floor muscle exercise and training for coping with urinary incontinence. J Exerc Rehabil. 2021;17(6):379–87. https://doi.org/10.12965/jer.2142666.333.
4. van Gool JD, de Jong TP, Winkler-Seinstra P, Tamminen-Möbius T, Lax H, Hirche H, Nijman RJ, Hjälmås K, Jodal U, Bachmann H, Hoebeke P, Walle JV, Misselwitz J, John U, Bael A, European Bladder Dysfunction Study (EU BMH1-CT94-1006). Multi-center randomized controlled trial of cognitive treatment, placebo, oxybutynin, bladder training, and pelvic floor training in children with functional urinary incontinence. Neurourol Urodyn. 2014;33(5):482–7. https://doi.org/10.1002/nau.22446. Epub 2013 Jun 15. PMID: 23775924.
5. Van Arendonk KJ, Austin JC, Boyt MA, Cooper CS. Frequency of wetting is predictive of response to anticholinergic treatment in children with overactive bladder. Urology. 2006;67(5):1049–53; discussion 1053-4. https://doi.org/10.1016/j.urology.2005.11.060.
6. Van Arendonk KJ, Knudson MJ, Austin JC, Cooper CS. Improved efficacy of extended release oxybutynin in children with persistent daytime urinary incontinence converted from regular oxybutynin. Urology. 2006;68(4):862–5. https://doi.org/10.1016/j.urology.2006.04.034.
7. Ramsay S, Bolduc S. Overactive bladder in children. Can Urol Assoc J. 2017;11(1–2Suppl1):S74–s79. https://doi.org/10.5489/cuaj.4337.
8. Gish P, Mosholder AD, Truffa M, Johann-Liang R. Spectrum of central anticholinergic adverse effects associated with oxybutynin: comparison of pediatric and adult cases. J Pediatr. 2009;155(3):432–4. https://doi.org/10.1016/j.jpeds.2009.01.074.
9. Kay GG, Abou-Donia MB, Messer WS Jr, Murphy DG, Tsao JW, Ouslander JG. Antimuscarinic drugs for overactive bladder and their potential effects on cognitive function in older patients. J Am Geriatr Soc. 2005;53(12):2195–201. https://doi.org/10.1111/j.1532-5415.2005.00537.x.
10. Ramsay S, Lapointe É, Bolduc S. Comprehensive overview of the available pharmacotherapy for the treatment of non-neurogenic overactive bladder in children. Expert Opin Pharmacother. 2022;23(8):991–1002. https://doi.org/10.1080/14656566.2022.2072212.
11. Veenboer PW, Bosch JL. Long-term adherence to antimuscarinic therapy in everyday practice: a systematic review. J Urol. 2014;191(4):1003–8. https://doi.org/10.1016/j.juro.2013.10.046.
12. Benner JS, Nichol MB, Rovner ES, et al. Patient-reported reasons for discontinuing overactive bladder medication. BJU Int. 2010;105(9):1276–82. https://doi.org/10.1111/j.1464-410X.2009.09036.x.
13. Kim JK, De Jesus MJ, Lee MJ, et al. β3-Adrenoceptor Agonist for the Treatment of Bladder Dysfunction in Children: A Systematic Review and Meta-Analysis. J Urol. 2022;207(3):524–33. https://doi.org/10.1097/ju.0000000000002361.

14. Nitti VW, Khullar V, van Kerrebroeck P, et al. Mirabegron for the treatment of overactive bladder: a prespecified pooled efficacy analysis and pooled safety analysis of three randomised, double-blind, placebo-controlled, phase III studies. Int J Clin Pract. 2013;67(7):619–32. https://doi.org/10.1111/ijcp.12194.
15. Kelleher C, Hakimi Z, Zur R, et al. Efficacy and tolerability of mirabegron compared with antimuscarinic monotherapy or combination therapies for overactive bladder: a systematic review and network meta-analysis. Eur Urol. 2018;74(3):324–33. https://doi.org/10.1016/j.eururo.2018.03.020.
16. Song YS, Lee HY, Park JJ, Kim JH. Persistence and adherence of anticholinergics and beta-3 agonist for the treatment of overactive bladder: systematic review and meta-analysis, and network meta-analysis. J Urol. 2021;205(6):1595–604. https://doi.org/10.1097/ju.0000000000001440.
17. Shapiro K, Dusetzina SB, Brucker BM, Escobar CM. Analyzing access and costs of oral medications for overactive bladder: uncovering disparities. Urology. 2024;183:57–62. https://doi.org/10.1016/j.urology.2023.09.020.
18. Lo CW, Wu MY, Yang SS, Jaw FS, Chang SJ. Comparing the efficacy of OnabotulinumtoxinA, Sacral Neuromodulation, and peripheral tibial nerve stimulation as third line treatment for the management of overactive bladder symptoms in adults: systematic review and network meta-analysis. Toxins (Basel). 2020;12(2):128. https://doi.org/10.3390/toxins12020128.
19. Yang G, Xu Y, Qu G, Zhang Y. Refractory overactive bladder patients who chose sacral neuromodulation therapy after failed OnabotulinumtoxinA treatment: a systematic review and meta-analysis. *PLoS One*. 2020;15(3):e0230355. https://doi.org/10.1371/journal.pone.0230355.
20. Amundsen CL, Komesu YM, Chermansky C, et al. Two-year outcomes of Sacral Neuromodulation versus OnabotulinumtoxinA for refractory urgency urinary incontinence: a randomized trial. Eur Urol. 2018;74(1):66–73. https://doi.org/10.1016/j.eururo.2018.02.011.
21. Siegel S, Noblett K, Mangel J, et al. Five-year followup results of a prospective, multicenter study of patients with overactive bladder treated with sacral neuromodulation. J Urol. 2018;199(1):229–36. https://doi.org/10.1016/j.juro.2017.07.010.
22. Salehi-Pourmehr H, Atayi M, Mahdavi N, Aletaha R, Kashtkar M, Sharifimoghadam S, Hassanzadeh R, Hajebrahimi S. Is sacral neuromodulation effective and safe in pregnancy? A systematic review. Neurourol Urodyn. 2023;42(6):1329–43. https://doi.org/10.1002/nau.25224. Epub 2023 Jun 8. PMID: 37288591.
23. Medtronic MRI Guidelines for InterStim™ systems, M980291A032 Rev A.
24. Nitti VW, Dmochowski R, Herschorn S, et al. OnabotulinumtoxinA for the treatment of patients with overactive bladder and urinary incontinence: results of a phase 3, randomized, placebo controlled trial. J Urol. 2013;189(6):2186–93. https://doi.org/10.1016/j.juro.2012.12.022.
25. DiCarlo-Meacham AM, Dengler KL, Welch EK, et al. Reduced versus standard intradetrusor OnabotulinumtoxinA injections for treatment of overactive bladder. Neurourol Urodyn. 2023;42(1):366–74. https://doi.org/10.1002/nau.25107.
26. Chiu SY, Patel B, Burns MR, et al. High-dose botulinum toxin therapy: safety, benefit, and endurance of efficacy. Tremor Other Hyperkinet Mov (N Y). 2020:10. https://doi.org/10.7916/tohm.v0.749.
27. Peters KM, Carrico DJ, Perez-Marrero RA, et al. Randomized trial of percutaneous tibial nerve stimulation versus Sham efficacy in the treatment of overactive bladder syndrome: results from the SUmiT trial. J Urol. 2010;183(4):1438–43. https://doi.org/10.1016/j.juro.2009.12.036.
28. Manríquez V, Guzmán R, Naser M, et al. Transcutaneous posterior tibial nerve stimulation versus extended release oxybutynin in overactive bladder patients. A prospective randomized trial. Eur J Obstet Gynecol Reprod Biol. 2016;196:6–10. https://doi.org/10.1016/j.ejogrb.2015.09.020.
29. Vollstedt A, Gilleran J. Update on Implantable PTNS devices. Curr Urol Rep. 2020;21(7):28. https://doi.org/10.1007/s11934-020-00980-5.
30. Nevéus T. Pathogenesis of enuresis: towards a new understanding. Int J Urol. 2017;24(3):174–82. https://doi.org/10.1111/iju.13310.

31. Nevéus T, Fonseca E, Franco I, et al. Management and treatment of nocturnal enuresis-an updated standardization document from the International Children's Continence Society. J Pediatr Urol. 2020;16(1):10–9. https://doi.org/10.1016/j.jpurol.2019.12.020.
32. Rittig S, Knudsen UB, Nørgaard JP, Pedersen EB, Djurhuus JC. Abnormal diurnal rhythm of plasma vasopressin and urinary output in patients with enuresis. Am J Physiol. 1989;256(4 Pt 2):F664–71. https://doi.org/10.1152/ajprenal.1989.256.4.F664.
33. Hirasing RA, van Leerdam FJ, Bolk-Bennink L, Janknegt RA. Enuresis nocturna in adults. Scand J Urol Nephrol. 1997;31(6):533–6. https://doi.org/10.3109/00365599709030657.
34. Chua ME, Silangcruz JM, Chang SJ, et al. Desmopressin withdrawal strategy for pediatric enuresis: a meta-analysis. Pediatrics. 2016;138(1):e20160495. https://doi.org/10.1542/peds.2016-0495.
35. Lucchini B, Simonetti GD, Ceschi A, Lava SA, Faré PB, Bianchetti MG. Severe signs of hyponatremia secondary to desmopressin treatment for enuresis: a systematic review. J Pediatr Urol. 2013;9(6 Pt B):1049–53. https://doi.org/10.1016/j.jpurol.2013.02.012.
36. Karamaria S, Mauel R, Van den Ende M, et al. Transition in enuresis patients: Identifying the gaps and opportunities for the future. Neurourol Urodyn. 2024;43(5):1118–26. https://doi.org/10.1002/nau.25460.
37. Ruffolo AF, Lallemant M, Garabedian C, Deseure A, Kerbage Y, Rubod C, Cosson M. The impact of pregnancy and childbirth on stress urinary incontinence in women previously submitted to mid-urethral sling: a systematic review and metanalysis. Neurourol Urodyn. 2024;43(7):1631–46. https://doi.org/10.1002/nau.25485. Epub 2024 May 10. PMID: 38725418.
38. Kobashi KC, Albo ME, Dmochowski RR, Ginsberg DA, Goldman HB, Gomelsky A, Kraus SR, Sandhu JS, Shepler T, Treadwell JR, Vasavada S, Lemack GE. Surgical treatment of female stress urinary incontinence: AUA/SUFU guideline. J Urol. 2017;198(4):875–83. https://doi.org/10.1016/j.juro.2017.06.061. Epub 2017 Jun 15. PMID: 28625508.
39. Sung VW, Borello-France D, Newman DK, Richter HE, Lukacz ES, Moalli P, Weidner AC, Smith AL, Dunivan G, Ridgeway B, Nguyen JN, Mazloomdoost D, Carper B, Gantz MG, NICHD Pelvic Floor Disorders Network. Effect of behavioral and pelvic floor muscle therapy combined with surgery vs surgery alone on incontinence symptoms among women with mixed urinary incontinence: the ESTEEM randomized clinical trial. JAMA. 2019;322(11):1066–76. https://doi.org/10.1001/jama.2019.12467. PMID: 31529007; PMCID: PMC6749544.

Neurogenic Bladder and Exstrophy 18

Konrad M. Szymanski and Rosalia Misseri

Key Points

- Management: life-long surgical and multidisciplinary
- Key Issues: urinary issues (including continence), renal function, sexual/reproductive function, and psychosocial health must be monitored across the lifespan
- Women: preconception counseling, obstetric referral to a tertiary center, monitor for prolapse and sexual dysfunction
- Men: erectile and ejaculatory function and infertility

Bladder Exstrophy-Epispadias Complex

Bladder exstrophy-epispadias complex (BEEC) is a rare congenital urologic anomaly characterized by defects in the abdominal wall, bladder, genitalia, pelvic bones, and musculature. It occurs in approximately 1 in 50,000 live births, displaying a male-to-female ratio of 2:1 in the United States [1]. While bladder and abdominal wall abnormalities are immediately apparent at birth, associated genital, pelvic, and musculoskeletal anomalies present significant lifelong challenges. Cloacal exstrophy (CE), a rarer and more severe variant, involves incomplete separation of the cloaca into urinary and gastrointestinal tracts, resulting in additional complex abnormalities such as omphaloceles, rudimentary hindgut, imperforate anus, and distinct separation of phallic structures. Renal function can be severely compromised in CE due to associated spinal and renal anomalies. Lifelong management of urinary, sexual, reproductive, and general health is essential for optimal patient outcomes [2, 3].

K. M. Szymanski · R. Misseri (✉)
Riley Children's Health, Indiana, USA

Indiana University School of Medicine, Indiana, USA
e-mail: rmisseri@iu.edu

H.-Y. Wu et al. (eds.), *Pediatric Urology for the Adult Urologist*,
https://doi.org/10.1007/978-3-032-10306-2_18

Bladder and Kidney Health

Renal function can be compromised due to anatomical anomalies, urinary tract infections, vesicoureteral reflux, and obstruction related to reconstructive procedures [4]. Associated spinal anomalies and morphologic abnormalities of the kidneys may more significantly affect the function of people with CE. Long-term renal monitoring and proactive management strategies, including antibiotic prophylaxis, reflux management, and surgical intervention when necessary, help maintain renal function and prevent progressive renal impairment [5, 6].

People with bladder exstrophy (BE) typically require multiple surgical interventions after closure of the exstrophied bladder over their lifetime, including bladder neck procedures, augmentation cystoplasty, and, in some cases, urinary diversion [7–10]. Clean intermittent catheterization (CIC) is frequently necessary, especially in those with augmented bladders or after bladder neck closure. Long-term outcomes indicate that a majority of adults with exstrophy will require CIC, and only a minority will void volitionally per urethra without catheterization or diversion [7–11].

Regular assessment of renal health, continence, and bladder function is very important and optimally should be performed annually. Renal function should be monitored lifelong with annual assessment of basic metabolic panel including serum creatinine (or estimated glomerular filtration rate [eGFR]), cystatin C and vitamin B12 (in bladder augmentation), urinalysis for proteinuria, and blood pressure measurement, as chronic kidney disease and upper tract abnormalities are more common than in the general population; 8% of adults live with chronic kidney disease stage 3 or higher and up to 5% of patients experience end-stage kidney disease by 30 years old [4]. Periodic imaging with renal and bladder ultrasounds should be used to evaluate for hydronephrosis, gross scarring, or calculi. Urodynamic evaluation is particularly important when there are changes in continence, upper tract changes, or recurrent urinary tract infections (UTIs) [7, 9–13]. For patients with augmented or reconstructed bladders, additional monitoring for metabolic disturbances (e.g., annual basic metabolic panel) and periodic assessment of bladder emptying (e.g., postvoid residuals) is warranted, as recommended by the American Urological Association [1–3].

Sexual and Reproductive Function

Sexual and reproductive function is significantly impacted in individuals with BEEC.

Females

Anatomical deviations include distal vaginal stenosis, anterior displacement of the vagina, a bifid clitoris, and divergence of the labia and mons pubis due to pubic diastasis. Additionally, the cervix is positioned closer to the introitus. These anatomical alterations and prior reconstructive surgeries can result in sexual dysfunction, infertility, body image issues, reduced self-esteem, and relationship difficulties. Vaginal stenosis, present in up to half of reconstructed females, further complicates sexual activity and reproductive potential. The prevalence of uterine prolapse is significantly higher than in the general population and often requires surgical intervention at earlier ages [14, 15].

Reproductive outcomes indicate that many women with BEEC achieve satisfactory sexual function and successful pregnancies; however, these pregnancies are often associated with higher risks. There is a notable increase in the incidence of spontaneous abortions (15–35%), stillbirth (7%), and uterine prolapse (up to 60%) during pregnancy. Consequently, pregnancies in this population require specialized obstetric care and careful preconception counseling, addressing genetic risks and potential pregnancy-related complications. Due to these risks, cesarean delivery supervised by experienced urologists is recommended, particularly for women with previous bladder augmentation, catheterizable channels, or bladder neck reconstructions. At our institution, these cesarean sections are typically scheduled at >37 weeks of gestation. The preferred incision is midline, as it is commonly present in women with prior reconstructive surgery. This is particularly helpful when the bladder is augmented, as it may facilitate takedown of adhesions between the bladder and the uterus. In cases where the patient has only a continent catheterizable channel and a prior Pfannenstiel incision, a repeat Pfannenstiel approach may be considered [16]. Temporary urinary incontinence during and after pregnancy further underscores the importance of specialized multidisciplinary care for this patient population [17–19].

Males

Men with BE may experience erectile dysfunction and ejaculatory issues due to altered anatomy, surgical scarring, and psychological factors. Anatomic anomalies such as epispadias and previous reconstructive surgeries may affect penile sensation and function, potentially impairing sexual satisfaction and performance.

Fertility can be compromised by issues such as abnormal ejaculation, impaired semen quality, or obstruction due to scarring from surgical reconstruction. Men may also experience significant psychosocial distress related to genital appearance, sexual performance anxiety, and concerns about masculinity. Appropriate evaluation, including semen analysis, fertility counseling, sexual health interventions, and psychological support, is a critical component of management [3, 19, 20].

Orthopedic Considerations

Orthopedic considerations in individuals with BEEC include significant musculoskeletal abnormalities such as pubic diastasis, acetabular dysplasia, and abnormal pelvic morphology. These structural deviations predispose patients to potential musculoskeletal pain and mobility issues across their lifespan. While data on long-term musculoskeletal outcomes remain sparse, clinicians should maintain a high index of suspicion for orthopedic complications and actively pursue orthopedic evaluations as necessary. Interdisciplinary management involving orthopedic specialists is crucial in addressing these complex musculoskeletal challenges [21–25].

Lifelong and Adult Urologic Management

Comprehensive management of adults with BEEC necessitates collaboration among specialists in reconstructive urology, orthopedics, reproductive medicine, plastic surgery, and psychology. Ideally, care should be provided within multidisciplinary centers that specialize in transitional urology, which facilitates the shift from pediatric to adult care. Given the complexity of the malformation, a thorough history of reconstructive procedures is very beneficial. Effective transition programs ensure continuity of care, improving long-term outcomes and enhancing quality of life for patients. When specialized multidisciplinary centers are unavailable, it is critical for healthcare providers to recognize their limitations and refer patients to appropriate specialized centers as needed [3, 20, 25].

In conclusion, BEEC presents lifelong challenges that necessitate a holistic, multidisciplinary approach to care. Continued attention to urinary, reproductive, orthopedic, and psychosocial needs is imperative for optimal patient outcomes. Comprehensive care models and specialized transition programs significantly enhance health outcomes and quality of life in this unique patient population.

Spina Bifida

Spina bifida (SB) is the most common congenital spinal cord anomaly, impacting 3.4/10,000 births each year (https://www.cdc.gov/spina-bifida/data/index.html). It often results in chronic health problems that require specialized care, including problems with mobility, hydrocephalus, as well as urinary and bowel incontinence [26], that are best coordinated within a multidisciplinary team composed of a urologist with interest and expertise in management of this population, a neurosurgeon familiar with SB pathology to monitor for shunt malfunctions and symptoms of spinal cord retethering, as well as, ideally, a primary care provider, a physical medicine and rehabilitation specialist, a nephrologist, a gastroenterologist, social worker, and an occupational therapist. Annual tests include blood pressure measurement, renal/bladder ultrasound (RBUS), kidneys, ureters, and bladder X-ray (KUB film), and a basic metabolic panel, including creatinine, cystatin C, and vitamin B12 (in patients with bladder augmentation).

While such a clinic offers valuable expertise and resources, access is at times limited by geography and availability. For this reason, local care by an adult urologist is greatly appreciated and, at times, necessary. Goals of urological care for adults with SB focus on recognizing and preventing complications, such as emergency room visits, illnesses, surgeries, and mortality, as well as addressing patient-centered care goals, which may include incontinence, sexual function, and fertility concerns.

Bladder Emptying

Most people with SB are unable to safely empty their bladders through volitional voiding, even with the Valsalva or a Credé maneuver. To prevent urinary incontinence, upper tract deterioration, and urinary tract infections, up to 80% of adults with SB rely on clean intermittent catheterization (CIC) [26]. Although the practice is sometimes abandoned in adulthood, the need for it does not typically change with age unless the patient undergoes an incontinent diversion.

Urinary Tract Infections

While SB patients are at a high risk of developing urinary tract infections (UTIs), antibiotics should be used judiciously to prevent the development of multidrug resistance. Recurrent UTIs warrant investigation for a nidus of infection through imaging (RBUS, KUB to rule out stones, incomplete emptying, or hydronephrosis), cystoscopy (to rule out foreign bodies, including permanent sutures protruding from previous surgeries), and urodynamics (bladder deterioration and diverticula).

Renal Function

Monitoring of hypertension and renal function is essential to long-term longevity, particularly since adults with SB have a 100 times higher risk of end-stage kidney disease (ESKD) than the general population [27]. How to best capture estimated glomerular filtration rates (eGFR) is controversial, given the limitations of existing formulas in people with SB who have low muscle mass and creatinine alone being a late marker of irreversible renal deterioration [28, 29]. The same formula should be used over time to track changes prospectively. Formulas combining cystatin C and creatinine are more accurate than those relying on creatinine alone: the Chronic Kidney Disease in Children Under 25 (CKiD U25) formula, for younger patients, https://kidney.wiki/gfr-calculator/ [30], and the Chronic Kidney Disease Epidemiology Collaboration (CKD-EPI) formula (https://www.kidney.org/professionals/gfr_calculator) [31].

Upper Tracts

Regular RBUS helps monitor hydronephrosis, as well as kidney and bladder stones, especially when combined with a kidneys, ureters, and bladder (KUB) radiograph. Alternatively, adults with significant obesity and/or scoliosis may best be monitored with a low-dose stone protocol computer tomography of the abdomen and pelvis.

Bladder and Kidney Stones

Adults with SB are at high risk of developing urolithiasis due to a combination of risk factors, including immobility, urinary stasis, mucus production in the presence of bowel, and recurrent urinary tract infections. The risk is elevated without and with bladder augmentation, but 7–16% of patients develop nephrolithiasis 10 years after bladder augmentation [32, 33].

Depending on the stone burden and anatomical considerations, bladder stones can be managed endoscopically, percutaneously, or through a cystotomy. Ureteroscopy and percutaneous treatment of renal stones have higher complication rates than people without SB [34] and can be challenging due to difficulties with positioning, difficulty cannulating previously reimplanted ureters, and small access windows in the setting of scoliosis, limb contractures, and obesity [32, 35]. Referral to a stone specialist is frequently recommended.

Sexual and Reproductive Function

Adults with SB report normal sexual interest and desire compared to the general population, but also significant sexual dysfunction. Most men and women with SB engage in sexual activity [36]. Furthermore, 40% of men reported nongenital erogenous zones as most pleasurable [36, 37], similar to women (unpublished data). Urinary and bowel incontinence during sexual activity is reported by 70% and 45% of adults with SB, respectively; when it occurs, it is virtually always bothersome [38]. Consequently, emptying the bladder and bowel before engaging in sexual activity, a frank discussion between partners, and baseline incontinence management are recommended.

Females

Since women with SB are typically able to conceive and carry a pregnancy to term, they should be counselled about folate supplementation at a higher dose than the general population (4 mg PO daily for 3 months before and after conception) [38, 39], family planning options, and the need for specialized care once pregnant. During pregnancy, special consideration should be given to daily antibiotic UTI prophylaxis; difficulties with catheterizing channels are best managed with indwelling catheters, and symptomatic hydronephrosis, which may require temporary nephrostomy placement [16]. Pregnant women with SB with a history of genitourinary reconstruction should consult with a high-risk obstetrician and an experienced urologist to go over potential complications specific to previous bladder and bowel surgery, to create follow-up and delivery plans. It should be noted that even with a transition urologist assisting in the delivery, risks of intraoperative complications during cesarean delivery, including cystotomies, have been reported at 40% [16].

Males

Between 55% and 75% of men with SB have erectile dysfunction [16, 37, 40, 41]. Phosphodiesterase type 5 inhibitors have been reported to improve erections, intercourse, and satisfaction in 56–80% of men in observational studies and a randomized controlled trial [37, 42], supporting use in interested individuals. While most men with SB can experience orgasm, abnormal ejaculations are typical, including retrograde ejaculations [37, 43].

Bowel Management

Pediatric urologists frequently manage the bowels of people with SB, particularly those administering antegrade enemas through a cecostomy or a catheterizable channel (antegrade continence enema [ACE]). The annual ACE disuse rate is 1% among patients followed at a multidisciplinary clinic [44], but higher in those without this follow-up [45]. Although resources exist to help troubleshoot ACE issues [46], this topic is beyond the scope of this chapter. Briefly, treating ACE catheterization issues is similar to urinary channels (see below), and balloon catheters should be avoided. Individuals unable to or unwilling to manage their bowel with a current bowel regimen may benefit from a colostomy to simplify care, relieve constipation, and fecal incontinence.

Previous Genitourinary Reconstruction Considerations for People with BEEC and SB

Urinary Channels

Urinary continent catheterizable channels (CCC) made from the appendix (appendicovesicostomy) or retubularized ileum (Monti channel) simplify bladder care and increase independence. As the continence mechanism for CCC is a submucosal tunnel, trauma from a balloon catheter can cause irreversible incontinence. When a catheter needs to be anchored, one without a balloon should be taped or sutured in place. Most people with CCCs made in childhood continue to use them for decades, with an annual disuse rate of 1% [46, 47]. Since the single greatest risk factor for disusing a channel is reliance on others for CIC, maintaining self-catheterization is of utmost importance.

Difficult catheterizations are the most common channel complication. Emptying the bladder per urethra, if it has not been reconstructed with a bladder neck procedure, can frequently relieve channel angulation and allow for the passage of a well-lubricated catheter. A curved tip catheter can help navigate tortuosity as well. Endoscopic placement of a catheter over a wire and leaving it in place for 3–7 days after traumatic catheterization can prevent up to 50% of revisions [48].

At 10 years after creation of the CCC, 10% require a stomal revision (typically for stenosis), while 9% of appendicovesicostomies and 16–32% of Monti channels require a subfascial revision (typically due to angulation leading to difficult catheterizations) [49]. Stomal stenosis can be prevented by using a prefabricated stoma stopper or a "home-made" L-stent, a knotted catheter, placed across the stoma and taped in [49, 50].

Bladder Neck Surgery

Patients with a history of bladder neck repairs should not be catheterized per urethra, as this risks urethral incontinence. Artificial urinary sphincter cuffs must be deflated before catheterizations.

Bladder Augmentation

Bladder augmentation, typically with bowel, decreases storage pressures and increases volumes in hostile bladders unresponsive to maximal medical therapy, intending to protect the upper tracts and treat incontinence. Unfortunately, most patients will experience at least one complication from this surgery, including 44% having a surgical complication at 10 years [51]. Surgery for bladder stones is the most common (28% risk), followed by bladder perforation (10%), small bowel obstruction (5%), as well as tumors, both benign (2%) and malignant (<1%).

Mucus produced by the bowel serves as a nidus of infection and stones. Daily bladder irrigations with two or more syringes (≥120 mL) of saline to clear mucus are routinely recommended, but are rarely performed [51, 52]. Patients should be regularly reminded of the technique, its benefits, and needed supplies. Metabolic derangements, including hypokalemic hypochloremic metabolic acidosis and B12 deficiency, occur after bladder augmentation using ileum [53]. When a bladder malignancy, usually transitional cell carcinoma, when detected, it is typically at an advanced stage and carries a poor prognosis [54]. Given its rarity, similar risks comparing people with SB who were and not augmented, expense of screening and lack of evidence it alters the clinical course, routine surveillance in asymptomatic patients is not recommended.

The risk of life-threatening bladder perforation is 10% at 10 years [51]. It most often occurs after a prolonged period of not catheterizing and/or relatively minor trauma. Being an intraperitoneal perforation with chronically colonized urine in the frequent presence of a ventriculoperitoneal shunt, it represents a surgical emergency. Decreased abdominal sensation among people with SB can render the physical exam unreliable. Prompt recognition with a computed tomography (CT) cystogram, rather than a plain cystogram, is more sensitive [55]. Perforations are treated with laparotomy, copious peritoneal irrigation, drainage, and, at times, shunt externalization.

Urinary Diversion

An incontinent diversion may be appropriate for adults who are unable to or unwilling to maintain their previous bladder regimen. This includes individuals with a history of (multiple) bladder perforations, upper tract deterioration, and recalcitrant urinary incontinence, which is bothersome and/or leads to decubitus ulcers.

Overview of Bladder Exstrophy-Epispadias Complex (BEEC)

- *Incidence*: 1 in 50,000 live births; male-to-female ratio is 2:1 (Campbell's).
- *Pathophysiology*: Involves defects in the abdominal wall, bladder, genitalia, and pelvis. CE (cloacal exstrophy) is a more severe variant involving omphalocele, imperforate anus, and split bladder.
- *Management*: Surgical and multidisciplinary; lifelong follow-up needed.
- *Focus*: The chapter emphasizes classic BE due to the rarity of isolated epispadias and CE.
- *Key Issues*: Urinary, sexual/reproductive, and psychosocial health must be monitored across the lifespan.
  References: [1], [2], [3]

Sexual and Reproductive Function

A. *In Women*
  - *Anatomy*:
    - Bifid clitoris, divergent labia/mons due to pubic diastasis.
    - Shortened, anteriorly displaced vagina.
    - Normal proximal vaginal caliber; distal stenosis in ~50%.
    - Uterine duplication in 95% of patients. [16]
  - *Sexual Function*:
    - Painful intercourse, body image concerns, low orgasm rates. [39]
    - FSFI scores often meet dysfunction thresholds; coital incontinence common. [13], [40]

- *Fertility*:
  - Up to 66% achieve successful pregnancies [149, 159].
  - Increased risk of uterine prolapse (up to 60%) [69]; cesarean delivery usually recommended [36].
  - Offspring have ~400-fold increased risk of BE.
- *Recommendations*:
  - Preconception counseling.
  - Obstetric referral to tertiary center.
  - Monitor for prolapse and sexual dysfunction.
  - *References*: [3]–[5], [13], [16], [32], [35], [36], [38], [39], [40], [149], [153], [159]
- *In Men*
- *Evaluation*: *Erectile* and ejaculatory function, semen analysis if fertility desired.
- *Risks*:
  - Infertility, sexual dysfunction, body image issues.

    References: [3], [4], [7]

B. *Multidisciplinary Support*
   - Includes psychosocial, sexual, fertility, and surgical interventions.
   - Mental health support essential to address anxiety, depression, and self-esteem issues.

     References: [2], [3], [4], [9]

Orthopedic Considerations

- *Common Abnormalities*:
  - Pubic diastasis, acetabular dysplasia, spinal curvature.
- *Clinical Implications:*
  - Musculoskeletal pain may occur with age.
  - Limited data on adult outcomes, but orthopedic follow-up may be warranted.

  References: [1], [2], [3], [4], [5]

Lifelong and Adult Urologic Management

- *Challenges*:
  - Complex reconstructions, prior surgeries, and ongoing risk of complications.
  - Continuity of care essential; benefit from specialty centers.
- *Provider Needs*:
  - Familiarity with reconstruction, urinary diversion, and congenital anomalies.
- *Care Models*:
  - Transition programs from pediatric to adult care strongly recommended.
  - General urologists should refer to tertiary centers as needed.

  References: [1], [2], [3]

Key References by Section

General and Pathophysiology

1. Ebert AK et al., *Orphanet J Rare Dis*, 2009.
2. Haddad E et al., *Pediatr Nephrol*, 2024.
3. Wood D et al., *Eur Urol*, 2019.

Sexual and Reproductive Function

1. Rubenwolf P et al., *J Urol*, 2016.
2. Abdellaoui S et al., *BJU Int*, 2025.
3. Weiss DA et al., *J Urol*, 2024.
4. Wiener JS et al., *World J Urol*, 2021.
5. Harris TGW et al., *J Pediatr Urol*, 2022.
6. Diamond DA, *Dial Pediatr Urol*, 1990.
7. Deans R et al., *Am J Obstet Gynecol*, 2012.
8. Woodhouse CR, *BJU Int*, 1999.
9. Stein R et al., *J Urol*, 1999.
10. Woodhouse CRJ et al., *Int Urogynecol J*, 2012.
11. Park et al., *J Pediatr Urol*, 2023.
12. Harris TGW et al., *J Pediatr Urol*, 2022.
13. Harris K et al., *J Urol*, 2021.
14. Park et al., *J Pediatr Urol*, 2023.
15. Deans R et al., *Am J Obstet Gynecol*, 2012.

Orthopedic

1. Mundy A et al., *J Pediatr Orthop*, 2016.
2. Kaar SG et al., *J Pediatr Orthop*, 2002.
3. Kantor R et al., *Clin Orthop Relat Res*, 1997.
4. Suominen JS et al., *J Pediatr Surg*, 2012.

Transition and Adult Management

1. Peycelon M, Misseri R., *World J Urol*, 2021.
2. Venkatramani V et al., *Urology*, 2014.

References

1. Ebert A-K, Reutter H, Ludwig M, Rösch WH. The exstrophy-epispadias complex. Orphanet J Rare Dis. 2009;4(October):23.
2. Haddad E, Hayes LC, Price D, Vallery CG, Somers M, Borer JG. Ensuring our exstrophy-epispadias complex patients and families thrive. Pediatric Nephrol (Berlin, Germany). 2024;39(2):371–82.
3. Wood D, Baird A, Carmignani L, De Win G, Hoebeke P, Holmdahl G, Manzoni G, Nijman RJM, Taylor C, Tekgul S. Lifelong congenital urology: the challenges for patients and surgeons. Eur Urol. 2019;75(6):1001–7.
4. Roth JD, Bowen D, Fuchs ME, Gargollo PC, Gottlich H, Hains DS, Strine AC, Szymanski KM. End-stage and chronic kidney disease in classic bladder exstrophy: a retrospective muti-institutional cohort study. J Pediatr Urol. 2025;21(1):41–6.

5. Ginsberg DA, Boone TB, Cameron AP, Gousse A, Kaufman MR, Keays E, Kennelly MJ, et al. The AUA/SUFU guideline on adult neurogenic lower urinary tract dysfunction: diagnosis and evaluation. J Urol. 2021;206(5):1097–105.
6. Handa N, Bowen DK, Guo J, Chu DI, Kielb SJ. Long-term kidney outcomes in exstrophy-epispadias complex: how patients present as adults. Urology. 2021;154(August):333–7.
7. Abdellaoui S, Cazzorla F, Morel-Journel N, Bidault V, Neuville P, Ruffion A, Mouriquand PDE, Demède D. Long-term urinary outcomes in classic bladder exstrophy: results of an extensive follow-up. BJU Int. 2025;135(6):1018–24.
8. Bolduc S, Capolicchio G, Upadhyay J, Bagli DJ, Khoury AE, McLorie GA. The fate of the upper urinary tract in exstrophy. J Urol. 2002;168(6):2579–82; discussion 2582
9. Maruf M, Manyevitch R, Michaud J, Jayman J, Kasprenski M, Zaman MH, Benz K, et al. Urinary continence outcomes in classic bladder exstrophy: a long-term perspective. J Urol. 2020;203(1):200–5.
10. Szymanski KM, Fuchs M, Mcleod D, Rosoklija I, Strine AC, VanderBrink B, Whittam B, Yerkes E, Gargollo PC, Pediatric Urology Midwest Alliance (PUMA). Probability of bladder augmentation, diversion and clean intermittent catheterization in classic bladder exstrophy: a 36-year, multi-institutional, retrospective cohort study. J Urol. 2019;202(6):1256–62.
11. van Leeuwen MA, Dik P, Klijn AJ, de Kort LMO, de Jong TPVM. Primary repair of bladder exstrophy followed by clean intermittent catheterization: outcome of 15 years' experience. Urology. 2006;67(2):394–8; discussion 398–99
12. Dickson AP. The management of bladder exstrophy: the Manchester experience. J Pediatr Surg. 2014;49(2):244–50.
13. Gargollo PC, Borer JG, Diamond DA, Hendren WH, Rosoklija I, Grant R, Retik AB. Prospective followup in patients after complete primary repair of bladder exstrophy. J Urol. 2008;180(4 Suppl):1665–70; discussion 1670
14. Stein R, Fisch M, Black P, Hohenfellner R. Strategies for reconstruction after unsuccessful or unsatisfactory primary treatment of patients with bladder exstrophy or incontinent epispadias. J Urol. 1999;161(6):1934–41.
15. Woodhouse CR. The gynaecology of exstrophy. BJU Int. 1999;83 Suppl 3(April):34–8.
16. Roth JD, Casey JT, Whittam BM, Szymanski KM, Kaefer M, Rink RC, Schubert FP, Cain MP, Misseri R. Complications and outcomes of pregnancy and cesarean delivery in women with neuropathic bladder and lower urinary tract reconstruction. Urology. 2018;114(April):236–43.
17. Deans R, Banks F, Liao L-M, Wood D, Woodhouse C, Creighton SM. Reproductive outcomes in women with classic bladder Exstrophy: an observational cross-sectional study. Am J Obstet Gynecol. 2012;206(6):496.e1–6.
18. Nakhal RS, Deans R, Creighton SM, Wood D, Woodhouse CRJ. Genital prolapse in adult women with classical bladder exstrophy. Int Urogynecol J. 2012;23(9):1201–5.
19. Rubenwolf P, Thomas C, Thüroff JW, Stein R. Sexual function and fertility of women with classic bladder exstrophy and continent urinary diversion. J Urol. 2016;196(1):140–5.
20. Wiener JS, Huck N, Blais A-S, Rickard M, Lorenzo A, Mccaffrey Di Carlo HN, Mueller MG, Stein R. Challenges in pediatric urologic practice: a lifelong view. World J Urol. 2021;39(4):981–91.
21. Kaar SG, Cooperman DR, Blakemore LC, Thompson GH, Petersilge CA, Elder JS, Heiple KG. Association of bladder exstrophy with congenital pathology of the hip and lumbosacral spine: a long-term follow-up study of 13 patients. J Pediatr Orthop. 2002;22(1):62–6.
22. Kantor R, Salai M, Ganel A. Orthopaedic long term aspects of bladder exstrophy. Clin Orthop Relat Res. 1997;335(February):240–5.
23. Mundy A, Kushare I, Jayanthi VR, Samora WP, Klingele KE. Incidence of hip dysplasia associated with bladder exstrophy. J Pediatr Orthop. 2016;36(8):860–4.
24. Suominen JS, Helenius I, Taskinen S. Long-term orthopedic outcomes in patients with epispadias and bladder exstrophy. J Pediatr Surg. 2012;47(10):1821–4.
25. Venkatramani V, Chandrasingh J, Devasia A, Kekre NS. Exstrophy-epispadias complex presenting in adulthood: a single-center review of presentation, management, and outcomes. Urology. 2014;84(5):1243–7.

26. Szymanski KM, Misseri R, Whittam B, Raposo S-M, King SJ, Kaefer M, Rink RC, Cain MP. QUAlity of life assessment in spina bifida for adults (QUALAS-A): development and international validation of a novel health-related quality of life instrument. Qual Life Res. 2015a;24(10):2355–64.
27. Adams CM, Misseri R, Roth JD, Whittam BM, Guckien ZE, King SJ, Kaefer M, Rink RC, Szymanski KM. Age-based risk of end-stage kidney disease in patients with myelomeningocele. J Pediatr Urol. 2023;19(2):195.e1–7.
28. Chu DI, Balmert LC, Arkin CM, Meyer T, Rosoklija I, Li B, Hodgkins KS, et al. Estimated kidney function in children and young adults with spina bifida: a retrospective cohort study. Neurourol Urodyn. 2019;38(7):1907–14.
29. Szymanski KM, Szymanski AJ, Salama AK, Hains DS, Cain MP, Misseri R. Estimating and tracking renal function in children and adults with spina bifida. J Pediatr Urol. 2020a;16(2):169–77.
30. Pierce CB, Muñoz A, Ng DK, Warady BA, Furth SL, Schwartz GJ. Age- and sex-dependent clinical equations to estimate glomerular filtration rates in children and young adults with chronic kidney disease. Kidney Int. 2021;99(4):948–56.
31. Inker LA, Schmid CH, Tighiouart H, Eckfeldt JH, Feldman HI, Greene T, Kusek JW, et al. Estimating glomerular filtration rate from serum creatinine and cystatin C. N Engl J Med. 2012;367(1):20–9.
32. Salama AK, Misseri R, Hollowell N, Hahney B, Whittam B, Kaefer M, Cain MP, Rink RC, Szymanski KM. Incidence of nephrolithiasis after bladder augmentation in people with spina bifida. J Pediatr Urol. 2021;17(4):521.e1–7.
33. Schlomer BJ, Copp HL. Cumulative incidence of outcomes and urologic procedures after augmentation cystoplasty. J Pediatr Urol. 2014;10(6):1043–50.
34. Wang H-HS, Wiener JS, Ferrandino MN, Lipkin ME, Routh JC. Complications of surgical management of upper tract calculi in spina bifida patients: analysis of nationwide data. J Urol. 2015;193(4):1270–4.
35. Mitchell S, Gurung PMS, Choong S, Morris T, Smith D, Woodhouse C, Philp T. Percutaneous nephrolithotomy and spina bifida: complex major stone surgery? J Endourol. 2018;32(3):205–12.
36. Hensel DJ, Misseri R, Wiener JS, Roth JD, Whittam BM, Cain MP, Szymanski KM. Solo and partnered sexual behavior among an international sample of adults with spina bifida. J Sex Med. 2022;19(12):1766–77.
37. Szymanski KM, Roth JD, Hensel DJ, Wiener JS, Younsi N, Stein R, Whittam B, et al. Sexual activity and function of adult men with spina bifida. J Pediatr Urol. 2023b;19(3):308.e1–9.
38. Roth JD, Hensel DJ, Wiener JS, Younsi N, Stein R, Misseri R, Szymanski KM. Urinary and fecal incontinence during sexual activity is common and bothersome among adults with spina bifida. Urology. 2024;186(April):54–60.
39. Wilson RD, O'Connor DL. Guideline no. 427: folic acid and multivitamin supplementation for prevention of folic acid-sensitive congenital anomalies. J Obstet Gynaecol Can. 2022;44(6):707–19.e1.
40. Gamé X, Moscovici J, Gamé L, Sarramon J-P, Rischmann P, Malavaud B. Evaluation of sexual function in young men with spina bifida and myelomeningocele using the international index of erectile function. Urology. 2006;67(3):566–70.
41. Shiomi T, Hirayama A, Fujimoto K, Hirao Y. Sexuality and seeking medical help for erectile dysfunction in young adults with spina bifida. Int J Urol. 2006;13(10):1323–6.
42. Palmer JS, Kaplan WE, Firlit CF. Erectile dysfunction in patients with spina bifida is a treatable condition. J Urol. 2000;164(3 Pt 2):958–61.
43. Sandler AD, Worley G, Leroy EC, Stanley SD, Kalman S. Sexual function and erection capability among young men with spina bifida. Dev Med Child Neurol. 1996;38(9):823–9.
44. Szymanski KM, Roth JD, Szymanski AJ, King SJ, Whittam B, Kaefer M, Rink RC, Cain MP, Misseri R. People with spina bifida use their MACE on long-term follow-up: a single institutional retrospective cohort study. J Pediatr Urol. 2023a;19(4):405.e1–7.

45. Yardley IE, Pauniaho S-L, Baillie CT, Turnock RR, Coldicutt P, Lamont GL, Kenny SE. After the honeymoon comes divorce: long-term use of the antegrade continence enema procedure. J Pediatr Surg. 2009;44(6):1274–6; discussion 1276–77
46. Roth JD, Bennett WE, Szymanski KM, Whittam BM, Cain MP, Rink RC, King S, Misseri R. Troubleshooting problems with antegrade continent enema flushes: the Indiana University algorithm. J Pediatr Urol. 2021;17(4):446.e1–6.
47. Griffin Y, Meng, Rosalia M, Joshua DR, Benjamin MW, Pankaj D, Shelly K, Kirstan KM, et al. Use and disuse of catheterizable channels as the primary method of emptying the neuropathic bladder: a single institutional cohort study. J Urol. 2025;213(3):361–9.
48. Casey JT, Zhang M, Chan KH, Szymanski KM, Judge B, Whittam B, Kaefer M, Misseri R, Rink RC, Cain MP. Does endoscopy of difficult to catheterize channels spare some patients from formal open revision? J Pediatr Urol. 2016;12(4):248.e1–6.
49. Szymanski KM, Whittam B, Misseri R, Flack CK, Hubert KC, Kaefer M, Rink RC, Cain MP. Long-term outcomes of catheterizable continent urinary channels: what do you use, where you put it, and does it matter? J Pediatr Urol. 2015b;11(4):210.e1–7.
50. Mickelson JJ, Yerkes EB, Meyer T, Kropp BP, Cheng EY. L stent for tomal stenosis in catheterizable channels. J Urol. 2009;182(4 Suppl):1786–91.
51. Szymanski KM, Misseri R, Whittam B, Hollowell N, Hardacker RE, Swenson CR, Kaefer M, Rink RC, Cain MP. Additional surgeries after bladder augmentation in patients with spina bifida in the 21st century. J Urol. 2020b;203(6):1207–13.
52. Peycelon M, Szymanski KM, Monn MF, Salama AK, Risk H, Cain MP, Misseri R. Adherence with bladder irrigation following augmentation. J Pediatr Urol. 2020;16(1):33.e1–8.
53. Hensle TW, Gilbert SM. A review of metabolic consequences and long-term complications of enterocystoplasty in children. Curr Urol Rep. 2007;8(2):157–62.
54. Rove KO, Husmann DA, Wilcox DT, Vricella GJ, Higuchi TT. Systematic review of bladder cancer outcomes in patients with spina bifida. J Pediatr Urol. 2017;13(5):456.e1–9.
55. Karmazyn B, Gurram S, Marine MB, Mathew WR, Cain MP, Rink RC, Eckert GJ, Jennings SG, Kaefer M. Is CT cystography an accurate study in the evaluation of spontaneous perforation of augmented bladder in children and adolescents? J Pediatr Urol. 2015;11(5):267.e1–6.

Chronic Stone Formers from Childhood: Managing Cystinuria and Primary Hyperoxaluria in Adult Urology

19

Jared Goldstein and Gyan Pareek

Introduction

In this chapter, we aim to focus on two of the most complex causes of pediatric stone disease, cystinuria and primary hyperoxaluria, as summarized in Table 19.1. These conditions highlight some of the most difficult aspects of nephrolithiasis management in the most vulnerable of populations, including metabolic and medical management. Practical insights for optimizing care in pediatric patients transitioning to adulthood will be provided to the reader through an algorithmic approach.

Cystinuria

Cystinuria is a genetic disorder that results due to defective amino acid transporters in the nephron. Specifically, the amino acids cystine, ornithine, lysine, and arginine are no longer reabsorbed in the proximal convoluted tubule of the nephron. Although cystinuria is often considered a rare genetic cause of nephrolithiasis and only accounts for 1% of all cases, it is a more common cause of kidney stones in pediatric patients, contributing to 6–8% of stone cases in this group [1]. This condition is reported to be inherited in a genetic autosomal recessive manner, although autosomal dominant inheritance with variable penetrance has also been observed [1]. Most individuals with cystinuria experience kidney stones within the first two decades of

J. Goldstein
Division of Urology, Alpert Medical School, Brown University/Brown University Health, Providence, RI, USA

G. Pareek (✉)
Krishnamurthi Family Professor and Chief of Urology, Alpert Medical School, Brown University/Brown University Health, Providence, RI, USA
e-mail: gyan_pareek@brown.edu

H.-Y. Wu et al. (eds.), *Pediatric Urology for the Adult Urologist*,
https://doi.org/10.1007/978-3-032-10306-2_19

Table 19.1 Comparison of cystinuria and primary hyperoxaluria

Feature	Cystinuria	Primary hyperoxaluria (PH)
Genetics	Autosomal recessive (or sometimes autosomal dominant with variable penetrance) disorder affecting renal tubular transport of amino acids	Autosomal recessive disorder caused by mutations in AGXT, GRHPR, or HOGA1 genes, leading to hepatic overproduction of oxalate
Pathophysiology	Defective reabsorption of cystine, ornithine, lysine, and arginine in the proximal tubule, leading to cystine stone formation	Overproduction of oxalate in the liver results in excessive urinary oxalate excretion, causing calcium oxalate stone formation and nephrocalcinosis
Stone composition	Cystine stones (hexagonal, radiolucent on X-ray, harder than calcium stones)	Calcium oxalate stones (often associated with nephrocalcinosis)
Clinical presentation	Recurrent cystine kidney stones, often starting in childhood or adolescence	Recurrent calcium oxalate stones, progressive nephrocalcinosis, and potential progression to kidney failure
Diagnosis	Urinary cyanide–nitroprusside test, 24-hour urine cystine levels, genetic testing	24-hour urine oxalate levels (>45 mg/day/1.73m^2), plasma oxalate, kidney biopsy (calcium oxalate crystals), and genetic testing
Imaging findings	Cystine stones less radiopaque on X-ray, better visualized on ultrasound or CT	Nephrocalcinosis and calcium oxalate stones, detected on ultrasound or CT
Management	Hydration (≥3 L/day), sodium/protein restriction, urinary alkalinization (pH ≥7.5), thiol-based chelators (e.g., tiopronin and d-penicillamine) for severe cases	Hydration, pyridoxine (for PH1), urinary alkalinization, calcium-based oxalate binders, RNA-based therapy (lumasiran for PH1), dialysis, and liver/kidney transplant for severe cases
Urological intervention	Frequent need for surgical stone removal due to large, recurrent, and resistant stones PCNL preferred for large stones; URS or SWL less effective due to stone hardness Preventive approaches focus on dissolution strategies	Less frequent need for surgical intervention unless obstruction occurs URS or SWL may be used for calcium oxalate stones, but long-term management focuses on reducing oxalate burden rather than stone removal
Prognosis	Lifelong risk of recurrent stones, potential CKD from recurrent obstruction, and surgical interventions	High risk of progressive CKD and ESRD, particularly in PH1, requiring liver/kidney transplantation in severe cases

life, and unfortunately, many will endure repeated stone events throughout their lives. The frequency of these events is common and varies with individual disease severity, and often, the number of events depends on patient compliance with treatment. A study by Pareek et al. revealed that patients who adhered to medical treatment had a higher stone-free rate (73% versus 33%) and required fewer surgical procedures on average (1.0 versus 4.0) compared to non-adherent patients [2]. Similarly, a study by Steeper et al. found that patients had stone events every

12–14 months on average, leading to as many as seven endourologic procedures by middle age [3]. These frequent stone events can severely impact patients' quality of life. In addition, repeated obstructions and surgical interventions increase the risk of scarring in the renal collecting systems and have been associated with higher rates of chronic kidney disease (CKD) and hypertension [4, 5]. Such scarring can complicate future stone treatments, highlighting the need for early detection and management to slow stone formation and protect renal function.

Cystine stone disease presents similar to other forms of urolithiasis with clinical manifestations ranging from ureteral obstruction with or without renal colic to incidental detection of stones within the ureter or renal collecting system on imaging. It is important to note that small cystine stones are less radiopaque and may not be visible on plain film X-ray until they reach a larger size. Due to this characteristic, ultrasound or non-contrast computed tomography (CT) is recommended as the initial imaging modality for evaluating suspected cystine stones during an acute episode [6]. Ultrasound is often preferred for long-term monitoring of these patients given the recurrent nature of the condition and the potential for stone formation. This approach helps to minimize the patient's exposure to ionizing radiation.

Cystine stones are typically treated with a combination of surgical and medical management strategies. A key component of nonsurgical management involves dietary modifications aimed at reducing factors that promote cystine precipitation. Adequate hydration is paramount, with patients generally advised to drink up to 3 l of fluid daily to reduce urinary cystine concentrations to below 250–300 mg/L [6]. Limiting sodium intake is also recommended as reported by Norman et al. [7]. Additionally, reducing animal protein intake is advised due to its decreased methionine content, which is a precursor to the amino acid cystine. Since acidic urine decreases the solubility of cystine, urinary alkalinization is frequently used as an adjunct therapy. Dietary changes alone are often insufficient. Urinary alkalinization is achieved with medications like sodium bicarbonate or potassium citrate, with the goal urinary pH of 7.0 or higher. In patients who are unresponsive to dietary modifications and urinary alkalinization or those with large recurrent cystine stone burdens, the American Urological Association (AUA) guidelines from 2019 recommend cystine-binding thiol drugs, such as tiopronin [8]. This works by forming a mixed disulfide bond with cystine, thereby increasing its solubility and reducing stone formation. The treatment goal when using thiol drugs is to achieve a urinary cystine concentration of less than 250 mg/L, as levels above this threshold increase the risk of stone formation. The availability of thiol drugs outside the United States is limited; thus, alternative chelation therapy with alpha-mercaptopropionyl glycine or d-penicillamine may be used instead [8, 9]. Of note, these medications require interval monitoring of patients' serum chemistries and urine studies due to their potentially significant side effects and risk profiles that may impact patient adherence [6].

It is crucial for patients to strictly adhere to these dietary and medicinal treatments to maximize efficacy, especially in the pediatric population. At our institution, a comprehensive patient education plan is critical for prevention and management. Adherence to an aggressive hydration protocol and alkalinization therapy is recurrently emphasized by our nutritionists through visits every 3 months.

Additionally, for those patients on medical therapy, compliance with pharmaceutical regimens is reviewed and assessed through 24-hour cystine levels at visits. The importance of maintaining cystine levels below 250 mg/l of urine is a standard goal, along with a urine pH of 7.0. Recent improvements in dosing regimens of tiopronin should help with compliance, reducing pill regimens from 9x to 3x a day. As mentioned previously, personalized nutrition support is a critical part of management. Finally, connecting patients and their caregivers with support groups for cystinuria can provide invaluable peer support and offer strategies for coping with the condition.

Cystine stones are largely treated in similar fashion to stones of other compositions in accordance with the AUA guidelines on surgical management of nephrolithiasis. When a patient presents with an uncomplicated (normal renal function, lack of urinary tract infection) and symptomatic ureteral stone ≤10 mm, a 4- to 6-week trial of medical expulsion therapy is an appropriate option if the patient meets observation criteria and is amenable [9, 10]. However, cystinuria patients requiring definitive stone management should be offered timely intervention with complete stone clearance when possible to minimize the potential insult to renal function associated with repeated or persistent ureteral obstruction [9].

Shock wave lithotripsy (SWL) is the least invasive option for definitive stone treatment in adults with renal stone burden ≤20 mm in the upper and/or midpole or ≤10 mm in the lower pole but is associated with a lower stone-free rate (SFR) than ureteroscopy (URS) or percutaneous nephrolithotomy (PCNL) [11, 12]. SWL, in general, may also be less effective with cystine stones due to their hard nature, but the data are not conclusive and SWL has been demonstrated to be effective in select cystinuric patients [13–15]. "Rough" cystine stones, or those exhibiting void regions on CT, have been showed to have increased susceptibility to SWL. These stones, which present with lower Hounsfield units and visible internal heterogeneity, require significantly fewer shock waves for comminution compared to more homogeneous appearing cystine stones. A study by Kim et al. found that stones with CT-visible internal structures needed 650 ± 312 SW/g for total fragmentation, whereas those without such features required 1046 ± 307 SW/g ($P < 0.004$). Furthermore, both average and minimum CT numbers correlated with stone fragility, suggesting that helical CT imaging could serve as a predictive tool for identifying cystine stones more amenable to SWL [13]. It should also be noted that given the propensity for this population to undergo numerous procedural stone interventions, patients are inherently at increased risk of developing complications such as ureteral strictures (e.g., URS stricture rates of 0.3–4.9% have been reported [16]). SWL should be avoided in patients with anatomic or functional obstruction of the collecting system distal to the location of a stone [9].

URS or retrograde intrarenal surgery (RIRS) is an effective and safe treatment option for ureteral and renal stones ≤20 mm with SFR ranging from 59% to 100% in patients with cystine stones across multiple studies [12]. Technologic advances in lasers and ureteroscopes have made treatment of stones >2 cm quite feasible, but patients should be counseled on the potentially increased risk of a staged procedure [17]. As cystine stones commonly occur bilaterally, bilateral URS has been shown as a viable and safe option with a SFR of 84.2% with stone-free rates assessed by CT and similar complication rates to unilateral URS [18]. Distorted renal anatomy such as sclerosed renal pelvis, narrow infundibula, excluded calyces, and altered calyceal anatomy is seen at higher rates after prior surgical stone procedures [19]. This anatomic variation can increase the difficulty and decrease the efficacy of subsequent RIRS [19].

PCNL is widely recommended as the first-line surgical treatment for symptomatic renal stones larger than 20 mm [10]. PCNL has higher stone-free rates (SFRs) compared to URS and SWL for lower pole stones greater than 10 mm, though it may be associated with a higher incidence of morbidity [10]. Despite the elevated complication rate compared to URS or SWL, most of these complications are minor (Clavien–Dindo I–II) while maintaining excellent SFR (up to 95%) [20].

The invasive nature of PCNL inherently causes some degree of trauma to the renal parenchyma at the access site, contributing to concern among clinicians regarding the long-term implications from both an anatomic and functional perspective. Certain prospective studies have suggested that PCNL may negatively impact renal function, especially when multiple access tracts are used or in patients with chronic kidney disease (CKD) [21, 22]. Additional studies have evaluated quantitative technetium-99 m dimercaptosuccinic acid (DMSA) single-photon emission computed tomography (SPECT/CT) in patients after PCNL and found evidence of slight regional renal function loss at the treated kidney site [23]. However, several studies including the study using DMSA SPECT/CT as well as a recent systematic review found no statistically significant decline in global renal function (e.g., glomerular filtration rate or serum creatinine) after PCNL [23–25]. Other studies have even shown improved renal function post-procedure due to relief of renal obstruction [26]. Anatomic complications after PCNL such as infundibular stenosis or ureteral strictures may occur with implications on success of future stone procedures. A recent Cochrane review demonstrated similar rates as compared to RIRS, challenging these findings [27]. Though PCNL appears to be a safe procedure, dedicated studies are needed studying complication rates of patients of these high-risk patients who often undergo multiple endourologic procedures over their lifetime.

Advancements in technology have led to less invasive versions of PCNL, mainly mini-PCNL and ultra-mini-PCNL. These procedures utilize smaller access sheaths and therefore cause less parenchymal trauma. Techniques like these as well as endoscopic combined intrarenal surgery (ECIRS) or combined PCNL with URS have provided alternative approaches that maintain comparable SFR, while potentially reducing complication rates and the need for multiple access tracts [11, 28]. Considering these innovations, and in our institutional experience, PCNL should be considered a second-line option for patients with larger stones (20 mm or more) in the upper or mid poles and stones ranging from 10 to 20 mm in the lower pole in order to minimize morbidity. This is particularly relevant for cystinuric patients who may require multiple interventions over their lifetime. If performing standard (full-size) PCNL due to the above parameters, the ultrasonic and ballistic lithotrite is preferable due to both effectiveness and efficiency in our experience. Concomitant ureteroscopy and/or nephoscopy with laser lithotripsy (ECIRS) is preferable to us for patients with large and complex cystine stones that are unable to be cleared with a single percutaneous access tract. This circumvents the need for multiple percutaneous access tracts, thus reducing morbidity. When performing miniaturized PCNL at our institution, we utilize holmium or thulium laser energy as compared to ultrasonic or pneumatic lithotrite. We find that the 16.5-Fr access sheath in mini PCNL allows for removal of large stone fragments, making laser lithotripsy an effective tool for overall stone clearance in our experience. To our knowledge, no comparative analysis has been done for pneumatic, ballistic, and/or ultrasonic lithotripsy versus laser lithotripsy in cystine stones specifically.

Finally, open or robotic-assisted stone removal remains an effective but more invasive option compared to the aforementioned procedures. These approaches should be reserved for patients with no other viable alternatives (e.g., ureteral strictures, narrow infundibula, or excluded calyces) or those with nonfunctioning kidneys experiencing symptomatic obstruction or recurrent infections.

Primary Hyperoxaluria

Primary hyperoxaluria (PH, types I, II, and III) is a rare autosomal recessive disorder caused by defects in hepatic peroxisomal enzymes, most notably alanine–glyoxylate aminotransferase (AGT), a pyridoxal phosphate-dependent enzyme. This dysfunction leads to the overproduction of oxalate, a metabolic by-product that is excreted through the kidneys. Due to the insolubility of calcium oxalate in the urine, affected individuals are prone to nephrolithiasis and/or nephrocalcinosis [29]. The diagnosis of PH should be considered in patients with recurrent calcium oxalate stones, nephrocalcinosis, a family history of the condition, and/or unexplained progression of CKD. Diagnostic criteria include urinary oxalate levels exceeding 45 mg/day/1.73 m^2 body surface area, significantly elevated plasma oxalate levels, kidney biopsy findings of parenchymal calcium oxalate crystals, and molecular testing of the AGXT, GRHPR, and HOGA1 genes [30]. Genetic testing and counseling should be recommended for affected families at the time of diagnosis. The prevalence of PH is estimated to range from 1 in 50,000 to 1 in 100,000 individuals [31]. Of the three types, PH type I (PH1) is the most severe form, with initial symptoms typically presenting around ages 5–6 [29] with progression to end-stage renal disease (ESRD) occurring at a median age of 24 [32].

The management of PH requires a multidisciplinary approach, incorporating metabolic, nephrological, and occasionally surgical interventions. First-line therapy emphasizes reducing oxalate production and enhancing renal clearance. Key strategies include aggressive hydration, with a recommended daily intake of 3–4 l to dilute urinary oxalate. In pediatric patients unable to achieve the hydration goal orally, gastrostomy tube placement may be considered [33].

Citrate supplementation as an inhibitor of calcium oxalate crystallization has demonstrated efficacy by binding free calcium and increasing urinary pH. Dosing should be individualized, targeting a urinary pH of 6.5–7.5 [30]. Although dietary oxalate intake has only a modest effect on urinary oxalate excretion, studies have reported median intestinal oxalate absorption rates of up to 7% [33], suggesting that limiting dietary oxalate could have some benefit.

Pyridoxine (vitamin B6) is a cornerstone therapy for patients with PH1 as it reduces hepatic oxalate production. Vitamin B6 serves as a co-factor in the hepatic oxalate pathway enhancing the expression, catalytic activity, and peroxisomal import of AGT. The biochemical intervention results in restoring the enzymatic function in PH1. For individuals with specific genotypes, such as Gly170Arg and Phe152Ile, pyridoxine use has been associated with a 20–50% reduction in urinary oxalate levels [30, 32].

Emerging therapies for PH include RNA interference (RNAi) products such as lumasiran and nedosiran. These liver-directed therapies target key enzymes in the oxalate-producing pathway: glycolate oxidase (lumasiran) and lactate dehydrogenase (nedosiran). By inhibiting these enzymes, the therapies aim to shift the metabolic pathway toward producing more soluble by-products that can be renally excreted, thereby reducing oxalate accumulation [30]. Additional studies are needed to understand the long-term efficacy of RNAi.

From a urologic surgical standpoint, the treatment of nephrolithiasis in PH should prioritize complete stone eradication with minimally invasive approaches when able as similarly discussed in the cystinuria section. However, we must take into consideration some disease specific factors. The predominant stone composition in PH is calcium oxalate monohydrate. These stones have been shown to be somewhat resistant to SWL; nonetheless, SWL has been used to successfully treat select patients. Patients with small (mean 8 mm) pelvic and ureteric stones as well as those with PH2 as compared to PH1 have been shown to achieve higher rates of success after SWL [34]. In a retrospective review by Al-Abbadi and Hulton in 2013, those with PH1, upper pole stones, and lower pole stones were shown to have 47%, 66.7%, and 89.9% rates of no improvement after treatment, respectively [34]. Though its rate of overall success is suboptimal, SWL remains an existing minimally invasive option that should be offered to patients who have been informed of the moderate possibility of failure and need for multiple treatments. Ureteral stents may be used alongside SWL to facilitate fragment passage, provide pain relief, and protect against further kidney injury, particularly in cases of obstructive stones, postsurgical swelling, or high-risk patients with compromised renal function. Stents can also be beneficial in managing infected obstructing stones and preventing hydronephrosis in patients awaiting transplantation [34, 35]. The benefit and necessity of ureteral stenting (i.e., after URS) must be weighed with the risk of rapid encrustation, which is higher in this patient population due to higher concentrations of calcium and oxalate within the urine [36].

While these interventions may help mitigate symptoms and slow disease progression, the only definitive treatment for PH is a liver transplant, as oxalate production occurs in the liver. A combined liver–kidney transplant has demonstrated significantly better kidney graft survival rates compared to kidney transplantation alone—76% versus 14% at 5 years, respectively [37]. Continued research and advancements in medical treatment techniques and transplantation remain crucial to improving long-term outcomes for patients with PH.

Conclusion

As pediatric patients transition to adult urology care, it is crucial to consider the unique management and underlying causes of stones in this population. Previous studies have indicated that intensive metabolic testing for pediatric nephrolithiasis offers limited benefits, with no significant reduction in recurrence risk [38]. A multidisciplinary, patient-centered approach is essential to caring for these patients and improving long-term outcomes. Particularly, in those with cystinuria and PH, clinicians should aim to optimize medical and behavioral management while utilizing the most effective and least invasive surgery when necessary, with a goal of maximizing complete stone clearance and minimizing morbidity.

Key Points

- *Cystinuria and primary hyperoxaluria (PH) require distinct management approaches*: Cystinuria treatment focuses on urinary alkalinization and thiol-based therapies, while PH management increasingly involves RNA-based therapies to reduce oxalate production.
- *Early and aggressive intervention is critical*: Patients with PH are at high risk of early end-stage kidney disease, often necessitating dual liver–kidney transplantation, whereas patients with cystinuria benefit from lifelong medical therapy and minimally invasive stone removal techniques when able in order to preserve renal function and minimize morbidity.
- *Surgical intervention strategies*: Maximizing stone clearance while minimizing morbidity in a single surgical procedure should be prioritized in patients with PH or cystinuria as they tend to form recurrent stones and are likely to require many interventions in their lifetime.
- *Long-term monitoring and multidisciplinary care*: Involving nephrologists, urologists, dietitians, and patient support groups play a vital role in optimizing outcomes and enhancing quality of life for affected individuals with these conditions.

References

1. Chillarón J, Font-Llitjós M, Fort J, Zorzano A, Goldfarb DS, Nunes V, Palacín M. Pathophysiology and treatment of cystinuria. Nat Rev Nephrol. 2010;6(7):424–34.
2. Pareek G, Steele TH, Nakada SY. Urological intervention in patients with cystinuria is decreased with medical compliance. J Urol. 2005;174(6):2250–2.
3. Streeper NM, Wertheim ML, Nakada SY, Penniston KL. Cystine stone formers have impaired health-related quality of life compared with noncystine stone formers: a case-referent study piloting the Wisconsin stone quality of life questionnaire among patients with cystine stones. J Endourol. 2017;31(S1):S-48.
4. Prot-Bertoye C, Lebbah S, Daudon M, Tostivint I, Bataille P, Bridoux F, et al. CKD and its risk factors among patients with cystinuria. Clin J Am Soc Nephrol. 2015;10(5):842–51.

5. Döven SS, Delibaş A, Taşkınlar H, Naycı A. O impacto da intervenção cirúrgica sobre a função renal na cistinúria. Braz J Nephrol. 2018;40:256–60.
6. Norman RW, Manette WA. Dietary restriction of sodium as a means of reducing urinary cystine. J Urol. 1990;143(6):1193–5.
7. Thomas K, Wong K, Withington J, Bultitude M, Doherty A. Cystinuria—a urologist's perspective. Nat Rev Urol. 2014;11(5):270–7.
8. Pearle MS, Goldfarb DS, Assimos DG, Curhan G, Denu-Ciocca CJ, Matlaga BR, et al. Medical management of kidney stones: AUA guideline. J Urol. 2014;192(2):316–24.
9. Servais A, Thomas K, Strologo LD, Sayer JA, Bekri S, Bertholet-Thomas A, et al. Cystinuria: clinical practice recommendation. Kidney Int. 2021;99(1):48–58.
10. Assimos D, Krambeck A, Miller NL, Monga M, Murad MH, Nelson CP, et al. Surgical management of stones: American Urological Association/Endourological Society guideline, PART I. J Urol. 2016;196(4):1153–60.
11. Clark CS, Gnanappiragasam S, Thomas K, Bultitude M. Cystinuria: an overview of challenges and surgical management. Front Surg. 2022;9:812226.
12. Ripa F, Pietropaolo A, Geraghty R, Griffin S, Cook P, Somani B. Outcomes of paediatric cystine stone management: results of a systematic review. Curr Urol Rep. 2023;24(8):371–80.
13. Kim SC, Burns EK, Lingeman JE, Paterson RF, McAteer JA, Williams JC. Cystine calculi: correlation of CT-visible structure, CT number, and stone morphology with fragmentation by shock wave lithotripsy. Urol Res. 2007;35:319–24.
14. Vinit N, Khoury A, Lopez P, Heidet L, Botto N, Traxer O, et al. Extracorporeal shockwave lithotripsy for cystine stones in children: an observational, retrospective, single-center analysis. Front Pediatr. 2021;9:763317.
15. Biyani CS, Cartledge JJ. Cystinuria—diagnosis and management. EAU-EBU Update Series. 2006;4(5):175–83.
16. Moretto S, Saita A, Scoffone CM, Talso M, Somani BK, Traxer O, et al. Ureteral stricture rate after endoscopic treatments for urolithiasis and related risk factors: systematic review and meta-analysis. World J Urol. 2024;42(1):234.
17. Karakoyunlu N, Goktug G, Şener NC, Zengin K, Nalbant I, Ozturk U, et al. A comparison of standard PCNL and staged retrograde FURS in pelvis stones over 2 cm in diameter: a prospective randomized study. Urolithiasis. 2015;43:283–7.
18. Ingimarsson JP, Rivera M, Knoedler JJ, Krambeck AE. Same-session bilateral ureteroscopy: safety and outcomes. Urology. 2017;108:29–33.
19. Quiroz Madarriaga Y, Badenes Gallardo A, Llorens de Knecht E, Motta Lang G, Palou Redorta J, Bujons Tur A. Can cystinuria decrease the effectiveness of RIRS with high-power ho: yag laser in children? Outcomes from a tertiary endourology referral center. Urolithiasis. 2022;50(2):229–34.
20. Jones P, Bennett G, Dosis A, Pietropaolo A, Geraghty R, Aboumarzouk O, et al. Safety and efficacy of day-case percutaneous nephrolithotomy: a systematic review from European Society of Uro-technology. Eur Urol Focus. 2019;5(6):1127–34.
21. Yadav R, Agarwal S, Sankhwar S, Goel A, Kumar M, Singh M, et al. A prospective study evaluating impact on renal function following percutaneous nephrolithotomy using Tc99m ethylenedicysteine renal scan: does multiplicity of access tracts play a role? Investig Clin Urol. 2019;60(1):21–8.
22. Hegarty NJ, Desai MM. Percutaneous nephrolithotomy requiring multiple tracts: comparison of morbidity with single-tract procedures. J Endourol. 2006;20(10):753–60.
23. Moskovitz B, Sopov V, Halachmi S, Mullerad M, Barbara Y, Kastin A, et al. 1905: the effect of percutaneous nephrolithotripsy (PCNL) on renal function: assessment with quantitative SPECT of TC 99M-DMSA (QDMSA) renal scintigraphy. J Urol. 2004;171(4S):503.
24. Pérez-Fentes D, Cortés J, Gude F, García C, Ruibal Á, Aguiar P. Does percutaneous nephrolithotomy and its outcomes have an impact on renal function? Quantitative analysis using SPECT-CT DMSA. Urolithiasis. 2014;42:461–7.

25. Dawaba MS, Shokeir AA, Hafez AT, Shoma AM, El-Sherbiny MT, Mokhtar A, et al. Percutaneous nephrolithotomy in children: early and late anatomical and functional results. J Urol. 2004;172(3):1078–81.
26. Reeves T, Pietropaolo A, Gadzhiev N, Seitz C, Somani BK. Role of endourological procedures (PCNL and URS) on renal function: a systematic review. Curr Urol Rep. 2020;21:1–11.
27. Soderberg L, Ergun O, Ding M, Parker R, Borofsky M, Pais V, Dahm P. Percutaneous nephrolithotomy vs retrograde intrarenal surgery for renal stones: a Cochrane review. BJU Int. 2024;133(2):132–40.
28. Hughes T, Tzelves L, Somani BK. Cystine stones: developments in minimally invasive surgery and their impact on morbidity and stone clearance. Res Rep Urol. 2023;15:175–85.
29. Cochat P, Liutkus A, Fargue S, Basmaison O, Ranchin B, Rolland MO. Primary hyperoxaluria type 1: still challenging! Pediatr Nephrol. 2006;21:1075–81.
30. Michael M, Harvey E, Milliner DS, Frishberg Y, Sas DJ, Calle J, et al. Diagnosis and management of primary hyperoxalurias: best practices. Pediatr Nephrol. 2024;39(11):3143–55.
31. Hopp K, Cogal AG, Bergstralh EJ, Seide BM, Olson JB, Meek AM, et al. Phenotype-genotype correlations and estimated carrier frequencies of primary hyperoxaluria. J Am Soc Nephrol. 2015;26(10):2559–70.
32. Shee K, Stoller ML. Perspectives in primary hyperoxaluria—historical, current and future clinical interventions. Nat Rev Urol. 2022;19(3):137–46.
33. Sikora P, Von Unruh GE, Beck B, Feldkötter M, Zajączkowska M, Hesse A, Hoppe B. [13C2] oxalate absorption in children with idiopathic calcium oxalate urolithiasis or primary hyperoxaluria. Kidney Int. 2008;73(10):1181–6.
34. Cochat P, Rumsby G. Primary hyperoxaluria. N Engl J Med. 2013;369(7):649–58.
35. Al-Abadi E, Hulton SA. Extracorporal shock wave lithotripsy in the management of stones in children with oxalosis—still the first choice? Pediatr Nephrol. 2013;28:1085–9.
36. Ureteral stent encrustation: epidemiology, pathophysiology, management and current technology. Erratum. J Urol. 2022;208(1):225. https://doi.org/10.1097/JU.0000000000002737.
37. Harambat J, van Stralen KJ, Espinosa L, Groothoff JW, Hulton SA, Cerkauskiene R, et al. Characteristics and outcomes of children with primary oxalosis requiring renal replacement therapy. Clin J Am Soc Nephrol. 2012;7(3):458–65.
38. Schwarz RD, Dwyer NT. Pediatric kidney stones: long-term outcomes. Urology. 2006;67(4):812–6.

Fertility and Sexual Health in Survivors of Pediatric Urologic Tumors

20

Liza M. Aguiar and Bradley D. DeNardo

Key Points

- Pediatric genitourinary (GU) tumors are managed in multimodal fashion, incorporating chemotherapy, surgery, and radiation, resulting in a lifetime risk for infertility and reproductive toxicity.
- Pelvic radiotherapy and systemic chemotherapy, consisting of high cumulative doses of alkylating agents, such as cyclophosphamide, are treatments considered particularly high risk for infertility.
- Fertility preservation (FP) is an important component of care for children and individuals of reproductive age diagnosed with cancer.
- The effects of treatment can have a profound impact on patients' sexual health and self-esteem.

Introduction

Pediatric urologic tumors, although relatively rare, present unique challenges in their diagnosis and management, often necessitating aggressive treatment approaches that can have lasting implications on patients' fertility and sexual health.

L. M. Aguiar (✉)
Department of Urology, Hasbro Children's Hospital and the Warren Alpert Medical School of Brown University, Providence, RI, USA
e-mail: liza_aguiar@brown.edu

B. D. DeNardo
Division of Pediatric Hematology/Oncology, Hasbro Children's Hospital and the Warren Alpert Medical School of Brown University, Providence, RI, USA
e-mail: bradley_denardo@brown.edu

H.-Y. Wu et al. (eds.), *Pediatric Urology for the Adult Urologist*,
https://doi.org/10.1007/978-3-032-10306-2_20

Advances in the treatment of pediatric urologic tumors through multimodal therapy, including surgery, chemotherapy, and radiotherapy, have significantly improved survival rates. With rising survival rates among children treated for cancer, there is growing focus on the long-term toxicities of these therapies. Among the most critical of these are the late effects on fertility and sexual health, which can profoundly impact survivors' quality of life as they grow into adolescence and adulthood.

This chapter explores how modern treatment approaches to pediatric genitourinary (GU) malignancies impact the reproductive system. Special focus will be given to the long-term toxicity of particular chemotherapeutic agents and how they may impair fertility. By examining current evidence, we aim to clarify how specific therapies influence reproductive outcomes later in life, offering a clearer understanding of the challenges faced by survivors as they mature.

We also will discuss how cancer effects extend beyond physical ailments, influencing psychological well-being and interpersonal relationships. Understanding the interplay between physical side effects and emotional health is essential for supporting young survivors holistically.

Treatment Modalities and Their Impact

The treatment of pediatric urologic tumors encompasses a range of modalities, each posing distinct risks for long-term toxicity and late effects. We will focus our discussion on the late effects associated with surgery, chemotherapy, and radiation therapy for the most common childhood genitourinary (GU) malignancies. Approximately 10% of all pediatric cancers are genitourinary tumors, including Wilms' tumor, rhabdomyosarcoma, and gonadal germ cell tumors [1].

Different chemotherapeutic protocols vary in their effects on long-term fertility, and certain agents are associated with significant reproductive toxicity. The alkylating agents commonly used in rhabdomyosarcoma, such as cyclophosphamide and ifosfamide, have been highlighted in the literature for their potential to induce gonadal damage, leading to reduced fertility rates among survivors. The timing and dosage of chemotherapy also play pivotal roles. Higher doses and prolonged treatment courses are correlated with greater risks of infertility based on cumulative lifetime exposure to particular agents [2].

Radiation therapy, commonly used in most GU rhabdomyosarcoma and higher-stage Wilms' tumor, can have profound effects on reproductive health. The dosage and targeted area of radiation are crucial in determining the extent of damage to reproductive organs. Radiation to the pelvic area poses significant risks of delayed puberty, gonadal dysfunction, and infertility. Although modern radiotherapy techniques minimize exposure to adjacent critical structures, even low doses of photon and proton radiation can adversely affect ovarian function and spermatogenesis, thereby compromising fertility.

Multimodal treatment approaches, combining systemic chemotherapy with radiation and/or surgery, are common for nearly all pediatric GU tumors and lead to more complex interactions regarding fertility outcomes. Patients undergoing combinations of these modalities face compounded risks compared to those treated with singular modalities. The cumulative effects of exposure to various agents and techniques can result in a higher incidence of reproductive health concerns, necessitating a detailed understanding of each patient's unique treatment plan.

Treatment Overview of Common Pediatric Genitourinary Tumors

Wilms' Tumor is the most common pediatric renal tumor with approximately 500–650 new cases per year in the United States. The majority of cases are unilateral with a median age of diagnosis between 3 and 4 years. Only 5–7% of Wilms' tumor is bilateral [3]. Standard management of unilateral Wilms' tumor consists of complete nephrectomy of the involved kidney as well as multiagent chemotherapy depending on the stage and molecular features of the tumor. Vincristine, dactinomycin, and doxorubicin represent the most commonly used agents; cyclophosphamide and etoposide are incorporated for higher-stage disease. Adjuvant radiotherapy is reserved for patients with residual disease confined to the abdomen post-nephrectomy (Children's Oncology Group stage III) and metastatic disease (stage IV). Radiation is administered either to the involved flank or as whole abdominal radiotherapy depending on extent of residual disease.

Rhabdomyosarcoma is the most common pediatric soft tissue sarcoma and can arise anywhere in the body with approximately 350 cases per year in the United States. Over 25% of rhabdomyosarcoma occurs in GU sites, most commonly as the less aggressive embryonal histologic variant in children less than 5 years old [4]. Male GU rhabdomyosarcoma most commonly occurs in the bladder or prostate, or as a paratesticular tumor. Tumors can occur anywhere in the female GU tract, including uterine, cervical, vulvar, and vaginal rhabdomyosarcoma. Modern management consists of systemic chemotherapy combined with local control including surgery, radiation, or a combination of both.

Rhabdomyosarcoma chemotherapy typically consists of the VAC combination: vincristine, dactinomycin, and cyclophosphamide, which frequently includes high cumulative doses of the alkylating agent cyclophosphamide. Local control principles balance the role of surgery and radiation according to the location and resectability of the primary tumor with the goal of preserving form and function of the anatomic site; surgical debulking lacks benefit and is not recommended. Local control considerations for bladder/prostate rhabdomyosarcoma are complex and individualized; radical cystoprostatectomies are not recommended, and definitive radiation is commonly employed following induction chemotherapy.

Paratesticular rhabdomyosarcoma is most commonly managed with upfront radical orchiectomy; most cases occur as the embryonal subtype in patients <10 years old and do not require retroperitoneal lymph node sampling, although modified template retroperitoneal lymph node dissection is recommended for ages >10 years old and for the more aggressive alveolar histologic subtypes. Among female patients with GU rhabdomyosarcoma, radiotherapy including brachytherapy is preferred over attempts at radical resection. Vulvar and vaginal rhabdomyosarcoma typically respond well to chemotherapy, allowing for local control strategies that minimize surgery and radiation. Cervical and uterine rhabdomyosarcoma do not respond as well to chemotherapy, and definitive radiation is typically favored, although hysterectomy that spares the ovaries and distal vagina can be considered.

Surgical treatment involving the reproductive organs can have significant implications for future fertility. In the past, surgery played a central role in managing genitourinary (GU) rhabdomyosarcoma. However, advances in multimodal therapy have shifted the approach. Today, surgery is no longer considered the first-line treatment for most GU rhabdomyosarcoma tumors. Modern surgical guidelines advocate for reserving surgical resection for situations where complete tumor removal is both feasible and can be achieved without compromising critical structures, maintaining both form and function of involved anatomy. Delaying primary tumor excision until chemotherapy has enhanced resectability and is a commonly accepted approach. This evolution in surgical approach reflects a growing emphasis on preserving organ function and minimizing long-term reproductive harm while still achieving effective tumor control.

Fertility Outcomes

Studies have shown that a significant number of childhood cancer survivors can retain fertility despite treatment with chemotherapy and radiation.

An assessment of fertility outcomes has been conducted by the Childhood Cancer Survivor Study (CCSS), which represents the largest analyzed cohort of pediatric cancer survivors. Among 6224 male survivors who were not surgically sterile, compared to their siblings these survivors were approximately half as likely to sire a pregnancy when adjusted for marital status and other variables (HR 0.56; 95% CI 0.49–0.63). Multivariate analysis demonstrated cumulative alkylator dose and testicular radiation >7.5 Gy as independent risk factors for infertility. Similarly, 5149 female survivors had a 0.81 relative risk of ever being pregnant compared to their siblings. Dose-dependent alkylator exposure and ovarian/uterine radiation >5 Gy were identified as independent risk factors (Table 20.1). [5, 6]

Factors Influencing Fertility and Reproductive Outcomes

The likelihood of preserving fertility posttreatment is influenced by several factors:

- *Age at treatment*: Younger patients, particularly prepubertal children, have a higher chance of preserving fertility [7]. This is because they have a larger number of primordial germ cells, which are less susceptible to damage from chemo-

Table 20.1 Reproductive and fertility toxicities associated with pediatric GU tumor therapy

Disease	Intervention	Risk	Toxicity
Wilms' tumor			
	Chemotherapy Alkylating agents: cyclophosphamide (typically used in stages 3 and 4)	Dependent on cumulative dose High if male >4 g/m^2 High if prepubertal female >12 g/m^2 High if postpubertal female >8 g/m^2	Gonadotoxic Premature ovarian insufficiency, diminished ovarian reserve, premature menopause, infertility Oligo/azoospermia, infertility
	Chemotherapy Heavy metal agents: carboplatin (used in diffuse anaplastic Wilms and relapsed disease)	Minimal	Gonadotoxic
	Whole abdominal radiation Only used for abdominal dissemination (preoperative tumor rupture, peritoneal seeding, etc.)	Ovarian High if >15 Gy prepubertal High if >10 Gy postpubertal	Gonadotoxic
		Uterine Intermediate	Uterine insufficiency, low uterine volume, preterm labor, low birth weight infant
	Flank radiation Only used if post-nephrectomy residual disease (lymph node metastases, positive surgical margins, extension into vena cava, etc.)	Minimal	Fetal malposition, preterm labor, low birth weight infant
Rhabdomyosarcoma			
	Chemotherapy Alkylating agents: cyclophosphamide	Dependent on cumulative dose High if male >4 g/m^2 High if prepubertal female >12 g/m^2 High if postpubertal female >8 g/m^2	Gonadotoxic Premature ovarian insufficiency, diminished ovarian reserve, premature menopause, infertility Oligo/azoospermia, infertility
Bladder/prostate rhabdomyosarcoma			
	Cystectomy/prostatectomy Rarely performed for local control	High	Erectile dysfunction
	Radiotherapy	Intermediate	Erectile dysfunction

(continued)

Table 20.1 (continued)

Disease	Intervention	Risk	Toxicity
Paratesticular rhabdomyosarcoma			
	Retroperitoneal lymph node sampling Only indicated if alveolar histology, age > 10 years old, or clinical lymph node involvement	Intermediate	Retrograde ejaculation
	Scrotal radiotherapy Only indicated if alveolar histology or scrotal dissemination	High if >4 Gy	Gonadotoxic
Female GU rhabdomyosarcoma			
	Primary radical surgery Not recommended in modern treatment strategies	High	Sexual dysfunction, infertility, primary hypogonadism,
	Pelvic radiotherapy	Cervical, vaginal, vulvar High	Sexual dysfunction
		Ovarian High if >15 Gy prepubertal High if >10 Gy postpubertal	Gonadotoxic
		Uterine High	Uterine insufficiency, low uterine volume, preterm labor, low birth weight infant

therapy and radiation. However, the developing reproductive organs are still vulnerable to gonadotoxic therapies, and the long-term effects can vary based on the type and intensity of treatment.

- *Type and dose of chemotherapy*: Chemotherapeutic agents, specifically alkylating agents like cyclophosphamide and ifosfamide, as well as heavy metals including cisplatin and carboplatin, are known to be gonadotoxic. These drugs can cause irreversible damage to the ovaries and testes, resulting in acute ovarian failure or premature menopause and azoospermia or oligospermia, respectively. The risk of infertility increases with the cumulative dose of these agents [2].
- *Radiation exposure*: Radiation therapy can adversely affect fertility, particularly when the reproductive organs are within the radiation field. The degree of damage depends on the radiation dose, fractionation schedule, and the specific organs exposed. Testicular radiation and radiotherapy to the ovaries are directly gonadotoxic, resulting in oligo/azoospermia and acute ovarian failure. Delayed puberty may also be encountered. In particular, pelvic radiotherapy >10 Gy in postpubertal females and >15 Gy in prepubertal females is considered high risk for infertility. Doses above 20 Gy to the ovaries are more likely to lead to permanent infertility. Additionally, radiation affecting the uterus can impair uterine development, leading to complications such as reduced uterine volume and vascular

insufficiency, which may affect pregnancy outcomes later in life [8]. The National Wilms' Tumor Study Group demonstrated an increased risk of fetal malposition, premature labor, and low birth weight among pregnancies from female survivors of Wilms' tumor treated with flank radiation [9]. Radiotherapy for bladder/prostate rhabdomyosarcoma can result in erectile dysfunction that may require treatment [10].

- *Surgical considerations*: Oophorectomy, hysterectomy, and surgical resection of cervical and vaginal tumors for the management of female genitourinary tract rhabdomyosarcoma represent significant risk factors for long-term reproductive health. Surgical intervention for bladder/prostate rhabdomyosarcoma may have similar detrimental late effects in males including erectile dysfunction and anejaculation, although cystectomy and prostatectomy are rarely pursued in modern treatment paradigms. Retroperitoneal lymph node dissection and pelvic tumor resections pose similar long-term risks including retrograde ejaculation.

Fertility Preservation Strategies in the Pediatric Patient

Fertility preservation (FP) is an important component of care for children and individuals of reproductive age diagnosed with cancer. It is crucial to address fertility concerns early in the treatment planning process and continue to consider them throughout survivorship [11].

Sperm and Oocyte Cryopreservation

For postpubertal males and females, sperm and egg cryopreservation are standard fertility preservation methods. These procedures involve the collection and freezing of sperm or eggs before cancer treatment. If obtaining an ejaculate is not possible, sperm can be retrieved through epididymal aspiration or testicular biopsy in sexually mature men. It is not uncommon for sperm quality to be poor in cancer patients at the time of diagnosis. However, advances in assisted reproductive technologies, particularly intracytoplasmic sperm injection (ICSI), can result in biological parenthood. These options are not available to prepubertal patients, necessitating the development of alternative strategies like tissue cryopreservation.

Ovarian Tissue Cryopreservation

Ovarian tissue cryopreservation remains an experimental technique. It involves surgically removing and freezing the ovarian cortex, which contains primordial follicles. The tissue can be thawed and reimplanted after cancer treatment to restore fertility [12, 13]. This approach can be considered for prepubertal girls who are not candidates for traditional egg freezing.

Testicular Tissue Cryopreservation

For prepubertal boys, testicular tissue cryopreservation is an emerging option. It is experimental and should only be offered in a clinical trial. This involves the removal and freezing of testicular tissue containing spermatogonial stem cells. Recent research in nonhuman primates has shown promising results in restoring fertility through the transplantation of these stem cells [14].

Ovarian Transposition

Ovarian transposition involves surgically relocating the ovaries outside the radiation field to protect them from damage during pelvic radiation therapy. This procedure aims to preserve ovarian function and fertility, though its success depends on the precise location of the ovaries and the extent of radiation exposure [15, 16].

Psychosocial Effects and Quality of Life

Fertility issues are increasingly being acknowledged as a significant concern for newly diagnosed patients and their families. The inability to achieve parenthood may place significant psychosocial stress on patients and their families, negatively affecting their overall well-being [17].

In addition to the biological implications for fertility, treatment modalities also bring about psychological concerns related to sexual health among pediatric urologic tumor survivors. The physical and emotional changes following aggressive treatment regimens can drastically affect self-esteem, body image, and the ability to engage in intimate relationships. Survivors may experience anxiety surrounding their sexual health, especially if they have received treatment that is known to potentially harm reproductive capacity. This highlights the importance of psychosocial support during and after treatment, addressing the interrelated nature of physical health and mental well-being as children grow into adolescence and adulthood. Counseling can help mitigate the adverse psychological effects, fostering a more holistic approach to survivorship care.

Mental health challenges specific to survivors of pediatric urologic tumors can vary widely. Many face issues such as anxiety, depression, and post-traumatic stress disorder (PTSD) as they cope with the residual effects of their illness and treatments. Research indicates that the emotional burden of cancer can lead to long-lasting mental health consequences. Survivors may grapple with fears related to recurrence, uncertainties regarding future health, and the impact of their illness on their identity. These mental health struggles can interfere with their ability to engage fully in social relationships and life activities, resulting in diminished quality of life [18, 19].

As survivors of pediatric urologic tumors move into adulthood, the implications of their treatment experiences can significantly impact their sexual health and self-esteem. Educating survivors about potential treatment-related outcomes is essential for facilitating informed decisions about family planning and reproductive options. Healthcare providers must take an active role in discussing fertility preservation strategies with families at the onset of treatment. This proactive approach can enhance the quality of life for survivors, empowering them to take charge of their reproductive health as they transition to adulthood.

Conclusion

The exploration of the effects of pediatric urologic tumor treatments on long-term fertility and sexual health reveals a pressing need for action and awareness among healthcare providers. Survivorship care must encompass not only medical interventions but also psychosocial support to address the multifaceted challenges faced by survivors. One key recommendation for healthcare providers is to develop and implement tailored strategies for managing the long-term fertility and sexual health of pediatric urologic tumor survivors. This includes integration of fertility preservation discussions into treatment planning, as well as establishing protocols for regular follow-up that provide resources for managing sexual health.

Patient and family education plays a critical role in fostering awareness and preparedness among young survivors regarding potential reproductive health challenges. By providing comprehensive resources about fertility options and sexual health, healthcare providers can ensure that survivors are informed as they transition into adulthood. This proactive approach not only equips survivors with the knowledge they need but also instills confidence as they navigate their personal journeys toward building families in the future.

References

1. Steliarova-Foucher E, Colombet M, Ries LAG, Moreno F, Dolya A, Bray F, Hesseling P, Shin HY, Stiller CA. IICC-3 contributors. International incidence of childhood cancer, 2001-10: a population-based registry study. Lancet Oncol. 2017;18(6):719–31.
2. Poorvu PD, Frazier AL, Feraco AM, Manley PE, Ginsburg ES, Laufer MR, AS LC, Diller LR, Partridge AH. Cancer treatment-related infertility: a critical review of the evidence. JNCI Cancer Spectr. 2019;3(1):pkz008.
3. Siegel RL, Kratzer TB, Giaquinto AN, Sung H, Jemal A. Cancer statistics, 2025. CA Cancer J Clin. 2025;75(1):10–45.
4. MT ME, Siegel DA, Dai S, Okcu MF, Zobeck M, Venkatramani R, Lupo PJ. Pediatric rhabdomyosarcoma incidence and survival in the United States: an assessment of 5656 cases, 2001–2017. Cancer Med. 2023;12(3):3644–56.
5. Green DM, Kawashima T, Stovall M, Leisenring W, Sklar CA, Mertens AC, Donaldson SS, Byrne J, Robison LL. Fertility of male survivors of childhood cancer: a report from the Childhood Cancer Survivor Study. J Clin Oncol. 2010;28(2):332–9.
6. Green DM, Kawashima T, Stovall M, Leisenring W, Sklar CA, Mertens AC, Donaldson SS, Byrne J, Robison LL. Fertility of female survivors of childhood cancer: a report from the childhood cancer survivor study. J Clin Oncol. 2009;27(16):2677–85.
7. Wallace WH, Anderson RA, Irvine DS. Fertility preservation for young patients with cancer: who is at risk and what can be offered? Lancet Oncol. 2005;6(4):209–18.
8. Green DM, Sklar CA, Boice JD Jr, Mulvihill JJ, Whitton JA, Stovall M, Yasui Y. Ovarian failure and reproductive outcomes after childhood cancer treatment: results from the Childhood Cancer Survivor Study. J Clin Oncol. 2009;27(14):2374–81.
9. Green DM, Lange JM, Peabody EM, Grigorieva NN, Peterson SM, Kalapurakal JA, Breslow NE. Pregnancy outcome after treatment for Wilms tumor: a report from the national Wilms tumor long-term follow-up study. J Clin Oncol. 2010;28(17):2824–30.

10. Frees S, Rubenwolf P, Ziesel C, Faber J, Gutjahr P, Grossmann A, Thüroff JW, Stein R. Erectile function after treatment for rhabdomyosarcoma of prostate and bladder. J Pediatr Urol. 2016;12(6):404.e1–6.
11. Fertility preservation and reproduction in patients facing gonadotoxic therapies: an Ethics Committee opinion. Fertil Steril. 2018;110:380–6.
12. Gellert SE, Pors SE, Kristensen SG, Bay-Bjørn AM, Ernst E, Yding Andersen C. Transplantation of frozen-thawed ovarian tissue: an update on worldwide activity published in peer-reviewed papers and on the Danish cohort. J Assist Reprod Genet. 2018;35(4):561–70.
13. Donnez J, Dolmans MM. Fertility preservation in women. N Engl J Med. 2018;378(4):400–1. https://doi.org/10.1056/NEJMc1715731.
14. Fayomi AP, Peters K, Sukhwani M, Valli-Pulaski H, Shetty G, Meistrich ML, et al. Autologous grafting of cryopreserved prepubertal rhesus testis produces sperm and offspring. Science. 2019;363:1314–9.
15. Irtan S, Orbach D, Helfre S, Sarnacki S. Ovarian transposition in prepubescent and adolescent girls with cancer. Lancet Oncol. 2013;14(13):e601–8.
16. Arian SE, Goodman L, Flyckt RL, Falcone T. Ovarian transposition: a surgical option for fertility preservation. Fertil Steril. 2017;107(4):e15.
17. Nahata L, Caltabellotta NM, Yeager ND, Lehmann V, Whiteside SL, O'Brien SH, et al. Fertility perspectives and priorities among male adolescents and young adults in cancer survivorship. Pediatr Blood Cancer. 2018;65(7):e27019.
18. Kazak AE, Alderfer M, Rourke MT, Simms S, Streisand R, Grossman JR. Posttraumatic stress disorder (PTSD) and posttraumatic stress symptoms (PTSS) in families of adolescent childhood cancer survivors. J Pediatr Psychol. 2004;29(3):211–9.
19. Marusak HA, Iadipaolo AS, Paulisin S, Harper FW, Taub JW, Dulay K, Elrahal F, Peters C, Sala-Hamrick K, Crespo LM, Rabinak CA. Emotion-related brain organization and behavioral responses to socioemotional stimuli in pediatric cancer survivors with posttraumatic stress symptoms. Pediatr Blood Cancer. 2019;66(1):e27470.

Index

H.-Y. Wu et al. (eds.), *Pediatric Urology for the Adult Urologist*, https://doi.org/10.1007/978-3-032-10306-2

D

E